Physiology, Biochemistry, and Pharmacology of Transporters for Organic Cations

Physiology, Biochemistry, and Pharmacology of Transporters for Organic Cations

Editor

Giuliano Ciarimboli

MDPI • Basel • Beijing • Wuhan • Barcelona • Belgrade • Manchester • Tokyo • Cluj • Tianjin

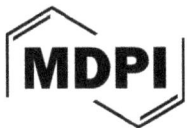

Editor
Giuliano Ciarimboli
University Hospital of Münster
Germany

Editorial Office
MDPI
St. Alban-Anlage 66
4052 Basel, Switzerland

This is a reprint of articles from the Special Issue published online in the open access journal *International Journal of Molecular Sciences* (ISSN 1422-0067) (available at: https://www.mdpi.com/journal/ijms/special_issues/toc).

For citation purposes, cite each article independently as indicated on the article page online and as indicated below:

LastName, A.A.; LastName, B.B.; LastName, C.C. Article Title. *Journal Name* **Year**, *Volume Number*, Page Range.

ISBN 978-3-0365-0562-6 (Hbk)
ISBN 978-3-0365-0563-3 (PDF)

© 2021 by the authors. Articles in this book are Open Access and distributed under the Creative Commons Attribution (CC BY) license, which allows users to download, copy and build upon published articles, as long as the author and publisher are properly credited, which ensures maximum dissemination and a wider impact of our publications.

The book as a whole is distributed by MDPI under the terms and conditions of the Creative Commons license CC BY-NC-ND.

Contents

About the Editor vii

Preface to "Physiology, Biochemistry, and Pharmacology of Transporters for Organic Cations" ix

Giuliano Ciarimboli
Physiology, Biochemistry, and Pharmacology of Transporters for Organic Cations
Reprinted from: *Int. J. Mol. Sci.* 2021, 22, 732, doi:10.3390/ijms22020732 1

Matthias Gorecki, Simon F. Müller, Regina Leidolf and Joachim Geyer
Trospium Chloride Transport by Mouse Drug Carriers of the Slc22 and Slc47 Families
Reprinted from: *Int. J. Mol. Sci.* 2021, 22, 22, doi:10.3390/ijms22010022 5

Melodi A. Bowman, Melissa Vitela, Kyra M. Clarke, Wouter Koek and Lynette C. Daws
Serotonin Transporter and Plasma Membrane Monoamine Transporter Are Necessary for the Antidepressant-Like Effects of Ketamine in Mice
Reprinted from: *Int. J. Mol. Sci.* 2020, 21, 7581, doi:10.3390/ijms21207581 17

Leandro Ceotto Freitas-Lima, Alexandre Budu, Adriano Cleis Arruda, Mauro Sérgio Perilhão, Jonatan Barrera-Chimal, Ronaldo Carvalho Araujo and Gabriel Rufino Estrela
PPAR-α Deletion Attenuates Cisplatin Nephrotoxicity by Modulating Renal Organic Transporters MATE-1 and OCT-2
Reprinted from: *Int. J. Mol. Sci.* 2020, 21, 7416, doi:10.3390/ijms21197416 39

Saskia Floerl, Annett Kuehne and Yohannes Hagos
Functional and Pharmacological Comparison of Human, Mouse, and Rat Organic Cation Transporter 1 toward Drug and Pesticide Interaction
Reprinted from: *Int. J. Mol. Sci.* 2020, 21, 6871, doi:10.3390/ijms21186871 55

Jan Amrhein, Susanne Drynda, Lukas Schlatt, Uwe Karst, Christoph H. Lohmann, Giuliano Ciarimboli and Jessica Bertrand
Tofacitinib and Baricitinib Are Taken up by Different Uptake Mechanisms Determining the Efficacy of Both Drugs in RA
Reprinted from: *Int. J. Mol. Sci.* 2020, 21, 6632, doi:10.3390/ijms21186632 71

Teerasak Wongwan, Varanuj Chatsudthipong and Sunhapas Soodvilai
Farnesoid X Receptor Activation Stimulates Organic Cations Transport in Human Renal Proximal Tubular Cells
Reprinted from: *Int. J. Mol. Sci.* 2020, 21, 6078, doi:10.3390/ijms21176078 85

Marta Kantauskaitė, Anna Hucke, Moritz Reike, Sara Ahmed Eltayeb, Chuyan Xiao, Vivien Barz and Giuliano Ciarimboli
Rapid Regulation of Human Multidrug and Extrusion Transporters hMATE1 and hMATE2K
Reprinted from: *Int. J. Mol. Sci.* 2020, 21, 5157, doi:10.3390/ijms21145157 99

Bayram Edemir
Identification of Prognostic Organic Cation and Anion Transporters in Different Cancer Entities by In Silico Analysis
Reprinted from: *Int. J. Mol. Sci.* 2020, 21, 4491, doi:10.3390/ijms21124491 115

Darcy C. Engelhart, Priti Azad, Suwayda Ali, Jeffry C. Granados, Gabriel G. Haddad and Sanjay K. Nigam
Drosophila SLC22 Orthologs Related to OATs, OCTs, and OCTNs Regulate Development and Responsiveness to Oxidative Stress
Reprinted from: *Int. J. Mol. Sci.* **2020**, *21*, 2002, doi:10.3390/ijms21062002 129

Darcy C. Engelhart, Jeffry C. Granados, Da Shi, Milton H. Saier Jr., Michael E. Baker, Ruben Abagyan and Sanjay K. Nigam
Systems Biology Analysis Reveals Eight SLC22 Transporter Subgroups, Including OATs, OCTs, and OCTNs
Reprinted from: *Int. J. Mol. Sci.* **2020**, *21*, 1791, doi:10.3390/ijms21051791 145

Mohammed Ali Selo, Johannes A. Sake, Carsten Ehrhardt and Johanna J. Salomon
Organic Cation Transporters in the Lung— Current and Emerging (Patho)Physiological and Pharmacological Concepts
Reprinted from: *Int. J. Mol. Sci.* **2020**, *21*, 9168, doi:10.3390/ijms21239168 169

Sophia L. Samodelov, Gerd A. Kullak-Ublick, Zhibo Gai and Michele Visentin
Organic Cation Transporters in Human Physiology, Pharmacology, and Toxicology
Reprinted from: *Int. J. Mol. Sci.* **2020**, *21*, 7890, doi:10.3390/ijms21217890 191

Zulfan Zazuli, Naut J. C. B. Duin, Katja Jansen, Susanne J. H. Vijverberg, Anke H. Maitland-van der Zee and Rosalinde Masereeuw
The Impact of Genetic Polymorphisms in Organic Cation Transporters on Renal Drug Disposition
Reprinted from: *Int. J. Mol. Sci.* **2020**, *21*, 6627, doi:10.3390/ijms21186627 213

About the Editor

Giuliano Ciarimboli (Prof. Dr.) was born in Italy. He studied Biology at Pisa University (Italy) and was a scholarship holder at the Institute of Clinical Physiology of the Italian Research Council (Consiglio Nazionale delle Ricerche, CNR) in Pisa. During this time, he was involved in the study of endogenous digitalis-like factors and pulmonary metabolism of basic amines. After this, he worked in the Hannover Medical School (Germany) and investigated the role of charge, dimension, and conformation of proteins in glomerular filtration. In 1999, the University of Hannover (Germany) awarded him a Ph.D. degree in natural sciences. He then joined the group of Experimental Nephrology at the Münster University Hospital, Germany), where Dr. Ciarimboli currently holds the position of Professor. His research interests include the regulation of organic cation transporters and their interaction with drugs. The research activity of Dr. Ciarimboli is supported by grants from the German Research Foundation. He has published 74 original refereed research papers, 12 peer-reviewed review articles, and 6 book chapters. Dr. Ciarimboli is lecturing Pharmacy students in Physiology at Munster University (Germany).

Preface to "Physiology, Biochemistry, and Pharmacology of Transporters for Organic Cations"

The Special Issue "Physiology, Biochemistry, and Pharmacology of Transporters for Organic Cations" of the *International Journal of Molecular Sciences* is dedicated to a special class of membrane transporters: transporters for organic cations. Most of these transporters belong to the solute carrier (SLC) group. Organic cations are endogenous and exogenous substances, which bear a positive charge at physiological pH. Important neurotransmitters, such as acetylcholine, dopamine, histamine, and serotonin, and metabolic products, such as creatinine, are substrates of these transporters, indicating a possible important physiological role for these transporters. On the other hand, since many drugs and xenobiotics are of a cationic nature, transporters for organic cations can have an important pharmacological and toxicological impact. Besides reviews on physiology, pharmacology, and toxicology of transporters for organic cations, which offer a concise overview of the field, the readers will find original research work focusing on specific transporter aspects.

The importance of this Special Issue derives mainly from the integration of physiological, pharmacological, and toxicological aspects of transporters for organic cations. Therefore, the Special Issue is of interest both for researchers, who are just beginning to work in this field, and also expert researchers, who would like to reach a broader understanding of the properties of transporters for organic cations.

I would like to thank all the authors and reviewers, who contributed to the Special Issue, the reviewers, and the *IJMS* Editorial Team for their expert assistance, especially Neil Ding.

Giuliano Ciarimboli
Editor

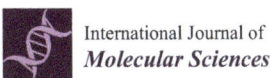

Editorial

Physiology, Biochemistry, and Pharmacology of Transporters for Organic Cations

Giuliano Ciarimboli

Experimental Nephrology, Department of Internal Medicine D, University Hospital Münster, 48149 Münster, Germany; gciari@uni-muenster.de

Received: 9 January 2021; Accepted: 1 January 2021; Published: 13 January 2021

This editorial summarizes the 13 scientific papers published in the Special Issue "Physiology, Biochemistry, and Pharmacology of Transporters for Organic Cations" of the *International Journal of Molecular Sciences*. In this Special Issue, the readers will find integrative information on transporters for organic cations. Besides reviews on physiology, pharmacology, and toxicology of these transporters [1–3], which offer a concise overview of the field, the readers will find original research work focusing on specific transporter aspects.

Specifically, the review "Organic Cation Transporters in Human Physiology, Pharmacology, and Toxicology" by Samodelov et al. [1] summarizes well the general aspects of physiology, pharmacology, and toxicology of transporter for organic cations. The other review "Organic Cation Transporters in the Lung—Current and Emerging (Patho)Physiological and Pharmacological Concepts" by Ali Selo et al. [2] focuses on these aspects of transporters for organic cations in the lung, an important but often neglected field.

In the paper "Systems Biology Analysis Reveals Eight SLC22 Transporter Subgroups, Including OATs, OCTs, and OCTNs", by performing a system biology analysis of SLC22 transporters, Engelhart et al. [4] suggest the existence of a transporter–metabolite network. They propose that, in this network, mono-, oligo-, and multi-specific SLC22 transporters interact to regulate concentrations and fluxes of many metabolites and signaling molecules. In particular, the organic cation transporters (OCT) subgroup seems to be associated with neurotransmitters and the organic cation transporters novel (OCTN) subgroup seems to be associated with ergothioneine and carnitine derivatives. Transporters of the solute carrier (SLC) 22 family may work together with transporters from other families to optimize levels of numerous metabolites and signaling molecules involved in organ crosstalk and inter-organismal communication, according to the remote sensing and signaling theory.

In the other paper by Engelhart et al. "Drosophila SLC22 Orthologs Related to OATs, OCTs, and OCTNs Regulate Development and Responsiveness to Oxidative Stress", an evolutionary analysis of putative SLC22A transporter orthologs in *Drosophila melanogaster* was performed [5]. At least 4 fruit fly transporters, probably involved in the handling of reactive oxygen species, seem to be SLC22 orthologues.

Neurotransmitters such as serotonin are important endogenous organic cations. Interestingly, the anesthetic drug ketamine has an antidepressant action. In the paper "Serotonin Transporter and Plasma Membrane Monoamine Transporter Are Necessary for the Antidepressant-Like Effects of Ketamine in Mice", Bowman et al. investigated whether this effect of ketamine is due to an influence on extracellular serotonin concentration [6]. They demonstrated that ketamine decreases serotonin clearance from the Cornu Ammonis (CA) 3 region of the murine hippocampus in vivo, probably by acting on the serotonin transporters (SERT) and the plasma membrane monoamine transporter (PMATs).

Since organic cation transporters are normally expressed in well-differentiated cells and they can be involved in the cellular uptake and/or efflux of chemotherapeutic drugs, their expression level may be related to the prognosis of cancer clinical outcome. In the communication "Identification of Prognostic Organic Cation and Anion Transporters in Different Cancer Entities by In Silico Analysis", Bayram Edemir [7] analyzed the relationship between expression of transporter mRNA and survival probability. To do this, he used data provided by The Cancer Genome Atlas (TCGA), where next-generation RNA-sequencing data for the most common tumor entities in a cohort which comprises more than 12,800 samples derived from 17 different tumor types are enclosed. In most cases, the expression level of organic cation transporters had a favorable prognostic value, suggesting that, in these cancers, tumor cells still show a certain grade of differentiation and/or better uptake of chemotherapeutic drugs.

Acute regulation of transporter activity can change the exposure of the body to drugs. While the regulation of organic cation transporters is well known, there is only scarce information on Multidrug and Toxin Extrusion Transporters (MATE) regulation. This aspect of MATE function was analyzed in detail in the paper "Rapid Regulation of Human Multidrug and Extrusion Transporters hMATE1 and hMATE2K" by Kantauskaité et al [8]. MATE activity was regulated both in uptake and in the efflux transporter configuration by several protein kinases. Some regulation pathways are common to those previously observed for OCTs, suggesting that there is the possibility to regulate hepatic and/or renal secretion of organic cations.

The activity of renal OCT2 and MATE transporters was also regulated by the transcription factor Farnesoid X receptor (FXR), for which activation increased the expression and activity of the transporters, as demonstrated in the paper "Farnesoid X Receptor Activation Stimulates Organic Cations Transport in Human Renal Proximal Tubular Cells" by Wongwan et al. [9]. On the other side, peroxisome proliferator-activated receptor alpha (PPAR-α), which is also a transcription factor, increases OCT2 and decreases MATE1 renal expression, as demonstrated in the paper "PPAR-Deletion Attenuates Cisplatin Nephrotoxicity by Modulating Renal Organic Transporters MATE-1 and OCT-2" by Freitas-Lima et al. [10]. The authors demonstrated also that genetic deletion of PPAR-α was able to protect against cisplatin-induced nephrotoxicity by decreasing OCT2 expression (OCT2 is an uptake transporter for cisplatin) and by increasing MATE1 expression (MATE1 is considered to be the secretion transporter of cisplatin).

Another mechanism by which transporter expression and function can be altered is by mutations due to the presence of single nucleotide polymorphisms (SNPs). The review "The Impact of Genetic Polymorphisms in Organic Cation Transporters on Renal Drug Disposition" by Zazuli et al. [3] illustrates the impact of OCT genetic polymorphisms on renal drug disposition and kidney injury, their clinical significances, and how to personalize therapies to minimize the risk of drug toxicity.

Focusing on the potential pharmacological role of OCT, in the paper "Tofacitinib and Baricitinib Are Taken up by Different Uptake Mechanisms Determining the Efficacy of Both Drugs in RA", Amrhein et al. [11] demonstrates that the tyrosine kinase inhibitor tofacitinib, which is approved and recommended by the European League Against Rheumatism for the treatment of rheumatoid arthritis (RA), is transported by MATE1. The expression of MATE1 is reduced under inflammatory conditions and in synovial fibroblasts from RA patients, suggesting that tofacitinib cannot exit the cells and, for this reason, has a favorable impact as RA therapeutic drug.

Rodents are used as a preclinical model to study the biological effects of drugs and xenobiotics. The paper "Functional and Pharmacological Comparison of Human, Mouse, and Rat Organic Cation Transporter 1 toward Drug and Pesticide Interaction" by Floerl et al. [12] investigates the interaction of several drugs and pesticides with mouse, rat, and human OCT1. They show that, in general, rodent and human OCT1 have the same type of interaction with these substances. However, species-specific differences can exist and should be investigated for new molecular entities. Similarly, focusing on the muscarinic receptor antagonist trospium chloride, in the investigation on "Trospium Chloride Transport by Mouse Drug Carriers of the Slc22 and Slc47 Families", Gorecki et al. [13] demonstrated that trospium is transported with similar characteristics by mouse and human OCT1, OCT2, and MATE1.

Funding: This research received no external funding.

Conflicts of Interest: The author declares no conflict of interest.

References

1. Samodelov, S.L.; Kullak-Ublick, G.A.; Gai, Z.; Visentin, M. Organic Cation Transporters in Human Physiology, Pharmacology, and Toxicology. *Int. J. Mol. Sci.* **2020**, *21*, 7890. [CrossRef] [PubMed]
2. Selo, M.A.; Sake, J.A.; Ehrhardt, C.; Salomon, J.J. Organic Cation Transporters in the Lung—Current and Emerging (Patho)Physiological and Pharmacological Concepts. *Int. J. Mol. Sci.* **2020**, *21*, 9168. [CrossRef] [PubMed]
3. Zazuli, Z.; Duin, N.J.C.B.; Jansen, K.; Vijverberg, S.J.H.; Maitland-van der Zee, A.H.; Masereeuw, R. The Impact of Genetic Polymorphisms in Organic Cation Transporters on Renal Drug Disposition. *Int. J. Mol. Sci.* **2020**, *21*, 6627. [CrossRef] [PubMed]
4. Engelhart, D.C.; Granados, J.C.; Shi, D.; Saier, M.H., Jr.; Baker, M.E.; Abagyan, R.; Nigam, S.K. Systems Biology Analysis Reveals Eight SLC22 Transporter Subgroups, Including OATs, OCTs, and OCTNs. *Int. J. Mol. Sci.* **2020**, *21*, 1791. [CrossRef] [PubMed]
5. Engelhart, D.C.; Azad, P.; Ali, S.; Granados, J.C.; Haddad, G.G.; Nigam, S.K. *Drosophila* SLC22 Orthologs Related to OATs, OCTs, and OCTNs Regulate Development and Responsiveness to Oxidative Stress. *Int. J. Mol. Sci.* **2020**, *21*, 2002. [CrossRef] [PubMed]
6. Bowman, M.A.; Vitela, M.; Clarke, K.M.; Koek, W.; Daws, L.C. Serotonin Transporter and Plasma Membrane Monoamine Transporter Are Necessary for the Antidepressant-Like Effects of Ketamine in Mice. *Int. J. Mol. Sci.* **2020**, *21*, 7581. [CrossRef] [PubMed]
7. Edemir, B. Identification of Prognostic Organic Cation and Anion Transporters in Different Cancer Entities by In Silico Analysis. *Int. J. Mol. Sci.* **2020**, *21*, 4491. [CrossRef] [PubMed]
8. Kantauskaitė, M.; Hucke, A.; Reike, M.; Ahmed Eltayeb, S.; Xiao, C.; Barz, V.; Ciarimboli, G. Rapid Regulation of Human Multidrug and Extrusion Transporters hMATE1 and hMATE2K. *Int. J. Mol. Sci.* **2020**, *21*, 5157. [CrossRef] [PubMed]
9. Wongwan, T.; Chatsudthipong, V.; Soodvilai, S. Farnesoid X Receptor Activation Stimulates Organic Cations Transport in Human Renal Proximal Tubular Cells. *Int. J. Mol. Sci.* **2020**, *21*, 6078. [CrossRef] [PubMed]
10. Freitas-Lima, L.C.; Budu, A.; Arruda, A.C.; Perilhão, M.S.; Barrera-Chimal, J.; Araujo, R.C.; Estrela, G.R. PPAR-α Deletion Attenuates Cisplatin Nephrotoxicity by Modulating Renal Organic Transporters MATE-1 and OCT-2. *Int. J. Mol. Sci.* **2020**, *21*, 7416. [CrossRef] [PubMed]
11. Amrhein, J.; Drynda, S.; Schlatt, L.; Karst, U.; Lohmann, C.H.; Ciarimboli, G.; Bertrand, J. Tofacitinib and Baricitinib Are Taken up by Different Uptake Mechanisms Determining the Efficacy of Both Drugs in RA. *Int. J. Mol. Sci.* **2020**, *21*, 6632. [CrossRef] [PubMed]
12. Floerl, S.; Kuehne, A.; Hagos, Y. Functional and Pharmacological Comparison of Human, Mouse, and Rat Organic Cation Transporter 1 toward Drug and Pesticide Interaction. *Int. J. Mol. Sci.* **2020**, *21*, 6871. [CrossRef] [PubMed]
13. Gorecki, M.; Müller, S.F.; Leidolf, R.; Geyer, J. Trospium Chloride Transport by Mouse Drug Carriers of the Slc22 and Slc47 Families. *Int. J. Mol. Sci.* **2021**, *22*, 22. [CrossRef] [PubMed]

Publisher's Note: MDPI stays neutral with regard to jurisdictional claims in published maps and institutional affiliations.

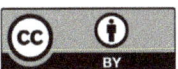

© 2021 by the author. Licensee MDPI, Basel, Switzerland. This article is an open access article distributed under the terms and conditions of the Creative Commons Attribution (CC BY) license (http://creativecommons.org/licenses/by/4.0/).

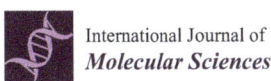

Article

Trospium Chloride Transport by Mouse Drug Carriers of the Slc22 and Slc47 Families

Matthias Gorecki, Simon F. Müller, Regina Leidolf and Joachim Geyer

Institute of Pharmacology and Toxicology, Faculty of Veterinary Medicine, Justus Liebig University Giessen, 35392 Giessen, Germany; matthiasgorecki@gmail.com (M.G.); Simon.Mueller@vetmed.uni-giessen.de (S.F.M.); Regina.Leidolf@vetmed.uni-giessen.de (R.L.)
* Correspondence: Joachim.M.Geyer@vetmed.uni-giessen.de; Tel.: +49-641-99-38404; Fax: +49-641-99-38409

Received: 2 December 2020; Accepted: 18 December 2020; Published: 22 December 2020

Abstract: Background: The muscarinic receptor antagonist trospium chloride (TCl) is used for pharmacotherapy of the overactive bladder syndrome. TCl is a hydrophilic positively charged drug. Therefore, it has low permeability through biomembranes and requires drug transporters for distribution and excretion. In humans, the organic cation transporters OCT1 and OCT2 and the multidrug and toxin extrusion MATE1 and MATE2-K carriers showed TCl transport. However, their individual role for distribution and excretion of TCl is unclear. Knockout mouse models lacking mOct1/mOct2 or mMate1 might help to clarify their role for the overall pharmacokinetics of TCl. Method: In preparation of such experiments, TCl transport was analyzed in HEK293 cells stably transfected with the mouse carriers mOct1, mOct2, mMate1, and mMate2, respectively. Results: Mouse mOct1, mOct2, and mMate1 showed significant TCl transport with Km values of 58.7, 78.5, and 29.3 µM, respectively. In contrast, mMate2 did not transport TCl but showed MPP$^+$ transport with Km of 60.0 µM that was inhibited by the drugs topotecan, acyclovir, and levofloxacin. Conclusion: TCl transport behavior as well as expression pattern were quite similar for the mouse carriers mOct1, mOct2, and mMate1 compared to their human counterparts.

Keywords: trospium; transport; OCT; MATE; drug excretion; drug transport

---

1. Introduction

Muscarinic receptor antagonists, also referred to as antimuscarinic drugs, are typically used for pharmacotherapy of the overactive bladder (OAB) syndrome, which is characterized by urinary urgency, with or without urgency urinary incontinence [1]. Licensed drugs for this indication include oxybutynin, solifenacin, fesoterodine fumarate, and trospium chloride (further referred to as trospium). Based on their physicochemical properties these compounds can be differentiated in the group of more lipophilic tertiary amines (e.g., oxybutynin and solifenacin) and the hydrophilic positively charged quaternary amine drug trospium [2]. Based on its physicochemical properties, trospium has a generally low permeability through biomembranes. As trospium is poorly metabolized in the liver, the pharmacokinetic behavior of this compound is determined mainly by the parent compound, largely involving drug transport across the plasma membrane. Its oral bioavailability is below 10% [3], and its penetration across the blood–brain barrier is highly restricted [4]. Accordingly, central nervous system (CNS) side effects, which are typical for tertiary amine antimuscarinic drugs, are less pronounced for trospium [5,6]. The active efflux of trospium at the blood–brain barrier via the ATP-binding cassette transporter P-glycoprotein (syn. MDR1, ABCB1) seems to contribute additionally to this effect [7]. In humans, trospium is largely excreted via tubular secretion into the urine and via feces, suggesting a role of drug transporters for its excretion through the liver and kidneys. In vitro studies have shown that trospium is a transport substrate of the organic cation transporters OCT1 and OCT2 [8,9], as well as of the multidrug and toxin extrusion MATE1 and MATE2-K carriers [10,11]. OCT1 (gene symbol *SLC22A1*) is primarily expressed in the basolateral membrane of enterocytes and hepatocytes, and OCT2 (gene symbol *SLC22A2*) is typically expressed in the basolateral membrane of renal proximal tubular cells [12]. In contrast, MATE2-K (gene symbol *SLC47A2*) is predominantly expressed in the apical membrane of proximal tubular cells and MATE1 (gene symbol *SLC47A1*) is additionally located in the canalicular membrane of hepatocytes [13]. In concert, these carriers enable the transcellular transport of cationic drugs via OCT-mediated uptake at the basolateral and MATE-mediated efflux at the canalicular/apical membrane in the liver (OCT1/MATE1) and kidneys (OCT2/MATE2-K and OCT2/MATE1) [14]. This cooperative transcellular drug transport was demonstrated in OCT/MATE double-transfected cell culture models [15,16]. As an example, König et al. (2011) showed significant transcellular transport of the oral antidiabetic drug metformin in OCT1/MATE1 and OCT2/MATE1 double-transfected MDCK cells, but not in respective mono-transfected cells [16]. More recently, in the same cell culture model Deutsch et al. (2019) showed significant transcellular transport of trospium in OCT1/MATE1 and OCT2/MATE1 cells that clearly exceeded that in respective single-transfected cells [11]. Based on these data, it can be suggested that OCT1/MATE1 in the liver and OCT2/MATE1 in the kidney are involved in the active excretion of trospium in OAB patients [11]. However, in vitro transport data are sometimes difficult to extrapolate to the clinical situation in patients. In order to elucidate the role of an individual drug transporter for the overall pharmacokinetics of a drug, specific transporter inhibitors can be co-applied to healthy subjects or patients and potential changes of the pharmacokinetic parameters can be analyzed. In such a setup, the OCT/MATE inhibitor ranitidine was co-applied with trospium to healthy subjects. In this study, the renal clearance of trospium was lower by ~15% in the ranitidine co-application group, most likely pointing to a drug-drug interaction at the renal tubular efflux transporters MATE1 and/or MATE2-K [3]. However, such studies have the limitation that the co-applied inhibitor may not reach all sites of carrier expression at sufficiently high concentrations for proper transport inhibition. As an alternative strategy, carrier-deficient knockout mice are often used to estimate the role of an individual drug transporter for the overall pharmacokinetics of a drug. For example, in Oct1/2$^{-/-}$ double knockout mice, deficient for mouse Oct1 and Oct2, renal secretion of tetraethylammonium (TEA) was completely abolished [17]; in Mate1$^{-/-}$ knockout mice, the urinary excretion of cephalexin and metformin was significantly reduced [18,19]; and in Abcb1a,b$^{-/-}$ double knockout mice, deficient for P-glycoprotein, brain penetration of trospium was significantly increased while its hepatobiliary excretion was reduced [7]. With a similar experimental setup, trospium distribution and excretion studies would also be of interest in respective Oct and/or Mate knockout mouse models in order to clarify the role of the deleted drug transporters for the overall pharmacokinetics of trospium. In preparation of such experiments, the present study aimed to elucidate if the mouse counterparts of human OCT1, OCT2, MATE1, and MATE2-K are also transport active for trospium. Indeed, the mouse carriers mOct1, mOct2, and mMate1 transported trospium, whereas the phylogenetically more distant mMate2 did not support trospium transport but was transport active for the cationic probe drug 1-methyl-4-phenylpyridinium (MPP$^+$).

2. Results

The mouse carriers mOct1, mOct2, and mMate1 are orthologues to their human counterparts with high protein sequence homology (Figures 1A and 2A). In contrast, mMate2 is more distant to the human MATE1 and MATE2-K carriers (Figure 2A). Of note, there seems to be no clear orthologue to human MATE2-K [20]. In order to test for trospium transport, the mouse carriers mOct1, mOct2, mMate1, and mMate2 were stably transfected into HEK293 cells and stable integration was verified by PCR expression analysis.

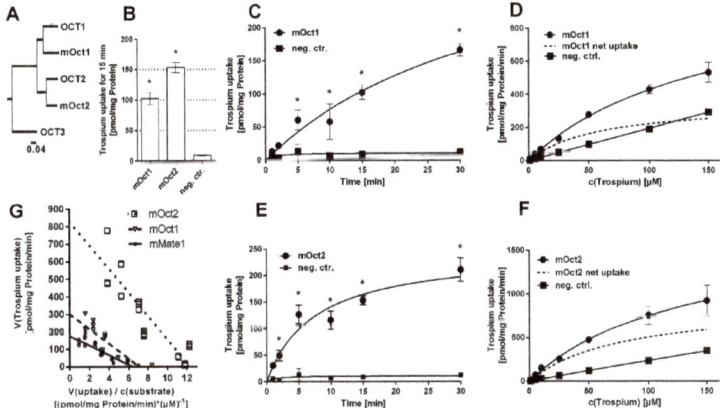

Figure 1. Trospium uptake by mOct1 and mOct2. (**A**) Phylogenetic tree of the human and mouse OCT/mOct carriers. The following GenBank accession numbers were used: NP_003048.1 for human OCT1, NP_003049.2 for human OCT2, NP_068812.1 for human OCT3, NP_033228.2 for mOct1, and NP_038695.1 for mOct2. Transport data represent means ± SD of representative experiments each with triplicate determinations. (**B**) Uptake of 1 µM trospium was analyzed in HEK293 cells stably transfected with mOct1 or mOct2 as indicated and in non-transfected control cells (neg. ctr.) over 15 min. * Significantly different from negative control with $p < 0.01$ (one-way ANOVA). Time-dependent uptake of 1 µM trospium over 1–30 min of substrate incubation via (**C**) mOct1 and (**E**) mOct2. * Significantly different from the respective time-point control with $p < 0.01$ (two-way ANOVA). Uptake at increasing trospium concentrations via (**D**) mOct1 and (**F**) mOct2. Non-transfected HEK293 cells served as control (neg. ctrl.). Carrier-specific uptake is indicated by dotted lines. Michaelis–Menten kinetic parameters were calculated from carrier-specific uptakes by nonlinear regression analysis. (**G**) Net uptake of trospium by mOct1 (Figure 1D), mOct2 (Figure 1F) and mMate1 (Figure 2D) were plotted as Eadie–Hofstee analysis. Intersection of regression lines with the y-axis indicates Vmax values; the slope indicates negative Km, and intersection with the x-axis indicates Vmax over Km.

Then, all carriers were tested for trospium transport at 1 µM compound concentration over 15 min. Whereas mOct1, mOct2 (Figure 1B), and mMate1 (Figure 2B) showed significant ($p < 0.01$) trospium transport compared with control, mMate2 was transport negative for trospium ($p > 0.01$) (Figure 2B). Next, time-dependent trospium uptake was analyzed for mOct1 (Figure 1C), mOct2 (Figure 1E), and mMate1 (Figure 2C), and showed linear uptake for all carriers over 5 min. After 30 min of transport, the trospium accumulation rates were quite similar for mOct1, mOct2, and Mate1, all being in the range of 150–200 pmol/mg protein. Michaelis–Menten parameters were determined by measuring the trospium transport over 1 min at increasing compound concentrations, ranging from 1 µM up to 150 µM for mOct1 (Figure 1D), mOct2 (Figure 1F), and mMate1 (Figure 2D). Carrier-specific uptake was calculated by subtracting uptake into untransfected HEK293 cells (indicated by dotted lines). The following transport kinetic parameters were determined: Km of 58.7 ± 15.5 µM and Vmax of 352.9 ± 39.4 pmol/mg protein/min for mOct1, Km of 78.5 ± 25.9 µM and Vmax of 899.3 ± 139.7 pmol/mg protein/min for mOct2, and Km of 29.3 ± 6.7 µM and Vmax of 184.7 ± 14.0 pmol/mg protein/min for mMate1 (Figure 1G, Table **??**). Whereas the Km values were all at comparable levels for all three carriers, mOct2 revealed by far the highest Vmax value (Figure 1F).

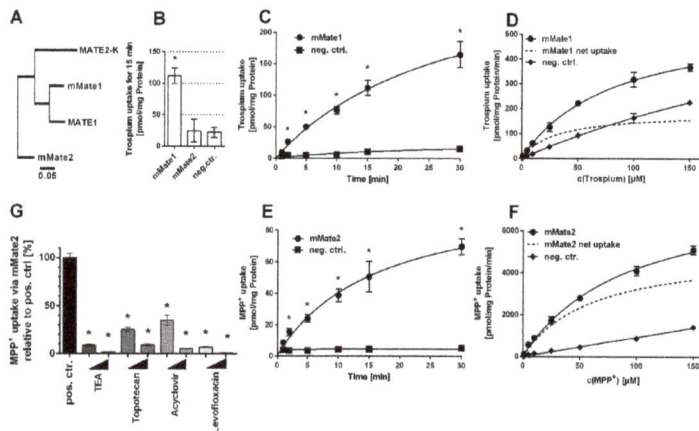

Figure 2. Trospium and MPP$^+$ uptake by mMate1 and mMate2, respectively. (**A**) Phylogenetic tree of the human and mouse MATE/Mate carriers. The following GenBank accession numbers were used: NP_060712.2 for MATE1, NP_001093116.1 for MATE2-K, NP_080459.2 for mMate1, and NP_001028714.1 for mMate2. Transport data represent means ± SD of representative experiments each with triplicate determinations. (**B**) Uptake of 1 µM trospium was analyzed in HEK293 cells stably transfected with mMate1 or mMate2 as indicated and in non-transfected control cells (neg. ctr.) over 15 min. * Significantly different from negative control with $p < 0.01$ (one-way ANOVA). Time-dependent uptake of (**C**) trospium via mMate1 and (**E**) MPP$^+$ via mMate2 over 1–30 min. * Significantly different from the respective time-point control with $p < 0.01$ (two-way ANOVA). Uptake at increasing concentrations of (**D**) trospium via mMate1 and of (**F**) MPP$^+$ via mMate2 over 1 min. Non-transfected HEK293 cells served as control (neg. ctrl.). Carrier-specific uptake is indicated by dotted lines. Michaelis–Menten kinetic parameters were calculated from carrier-specific uptakes by nonlinear regression analysis. (**G**) MPP$^+$ uptake inhibition via mMate2 at 10 µM and 100 µM inhibitor concentrations of TEA, topotecan, acyclovir, and levofloxacin, measured over 30 min. Cells not incubated with any inhibitor served as positive control (set to 100%). * Significantly different from positive control with $p < 0.01$ (one-way ANOVA).

Human Carrier	Km (µM)	Vmax (pmol/mg protein/min)	Mouse Carrier	Km (µM)	Vmax (pmol/mg protein/min)
OCT1	17 ± 5 [8] 106 ± 16 [9] 15 ± 3 [10]	93 ± 26 [8] 269 ± 18 [9] 1142 ± 157 [10]	mOct1	58.7 ± 15.5	352.9 ± 39.4
OCT2	8 ± 1 [8] 0.6 ± 0.1 [10]	92 ± 11 [8] 98 ± 22 [10]	mOct2	78.5 ± 25.9	899.3 ± 139.7
MATE1	15 ± 2 [10]	1083 ± 143 [10]	mMate1	29.3 ± 6.7	184.7 ± 14.0
MATE2-K	8 ± 2 [10]	297 ± 6 [10]	mMate2	No transport	No transport

As mMate2 did not show any transport of trospium in repeated experiments, MPP$^+$ was used as potential substrate. MPP$^+$ represents a prototypic substrate for organic cation transporters. As indicated in

Figure 2E, mMate2 showed significant time-dependent transport of MPP$^+$ with a linear phase between 1–5 min. Transport kinetics were then measured at increasing MPP$^+$ concentrations ranging from 1 µM up to 150 µM over 1 min and revealed the following Michaelis–Menten parameters: Km of 60.0 ± 5.6 µM and Vmax of 5136.0 ± 202.5 pmol/mg protein/min (Figure 2F). In order to analyze if mMate2 still represents a potential drug carrier, MPP$^+$ uptake via mMate2 was inhibited by several drugs at 10 µM and 100 µM inhibitor concentrations. As shown in Figure 2G, mMate2 was significantly inhibited by tetraethylammonium (TEA), topotecan, acyclovir, and levofloxacin.

Finally, the expression patterns of mOct1, mOct2, mMate1, and mMate2 were analyzed in liver, kidney, testis, brain, duodenum, and colon of a male C57BL/6N mouse. As indicated in Figure 3, mOct1 and mMate1 showed the highest mRNA expression levels in liver and kidney, whereas mOct2 was predominantly expressed only in the kidney. In contrast, mMate2 was highest expressed in the testis and showed only marginal expression in liver and kidney.

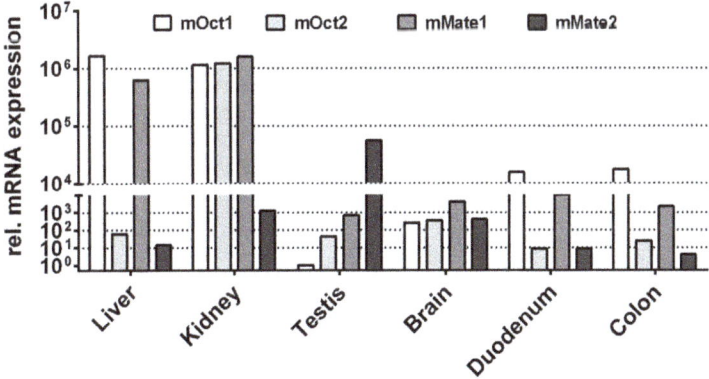

Figure 3. mRNA expression pattern of mOct1, mOct2, mMate1, and mMate2 in liver, kidney, testis, brain, duodenum, and colon of the mouse. The mRNA expression was analyzed by quantitative real-time PCR analysis using cDNAs from the indicated tissues of a male C57BL/6N mouse. Relative carrier expression was calculated by the $2^{-\Delta\Delta CT}$ method and represents carrier expression that is x times higher compared with the overall lowest expression (i.e., mOct1 testis, set as calibrator). Values represent means of duplicate determinations.

3. Discussion

The pharmacokinetics of the OAB drug trospium chloride is characterized by poor intestinal absorption, predominant elimination via the urine, and additional excretion via feces depending on the route of application [21]. Recent pharmacokinetic studies in human subjects receiving 2 mg trospium via intravenous infusion showed that 65% of the dose were eliminated into the urine and only about 3% via feces within 5 days [3]. In contrast, after oral administration of 30 mg immediate release tablets, the elimination via feces (25% of the oral dose) exceeded that of the urine excretion (6% of the oral dose). From the gut, trospium is absorbed from two distinct absorption "windows" located in the jejunum and the cecum/ascending colon [22]. However, the role of drug transporters for this process is not yet finally clear [3]. From the absorbed fraction, most of the trospium drug (~80%) appears unchanged in the urine. Thereby, elimination via the kidneys largely involves tubular secretion, as indicated by the 4-fold higher renal trospium clearance compared to the average glomerular filtration rate [21]. As a cationic drug, trospium has a generally low permeability through biomembranes, and therefore, its tubular secretion depends on membrane drug transporters. As a transcellular transport of trospium was already shown in a cell culture model expressing OCT2 and MATE1, these carriers, which are expressed at the basolateral and apical membrane of proximal tubular cells [12], respectively, are likely involved in the tubular secretion of trospium [11]. In addition, MATE2-K can be supposed to be involved in this process. MATE2-K is, like MATE1, expressed at the apical membrane of proximal tubular cells [13] and is also active in transporting trospium [10]. This assumption is supported by pharmacokinetic studies in healthy subject, which showed reduced renal clearance of trospium at co-administration with the OCT/MATE inhibitor ranitidine [3]. In the liver, OCT1 and MATE1 are co-expressed at the basolateral and canalicular membranes of hepatocytes, respectively [12,13]. Both carriers can also transport trospium when expressed in cell culture models [10] and, therefore, are supposed to be involved in the hepatobiliary excretion of this drug. In addition, based on excretion data from Abcb1a,b$^{-/-}$ knockout mice, P-glycoprotein seems to be involved in the canalicular excretion of trospium in hepatocytes [7].

In general, expression sites of mOct1, mOct2, and mMate1 reflect quite well the expression pattern of their human counterparts. Similar to human OCT2, mOct2 is predominantly expressed in the kidney [17]. However, mOct1 has a broader expression pattern and is expressed in liver (as human OCT1) and in addition in kidney and small intestine [23]. Therefore, Oct1/2$^{-/-}$ double knockout mice are used to estimate the role of Oct-mediated drug transport for the tubular secretion of drugs [17]. More complicated is the situation for the Slc47 carriers mMate1 and mMate2. Whereas mMate1 is an orthologue to human MATE1 with a similar expression pattern in the luminal membranes of renal tubular cells and bile canaliculi [24], there seems to be no mouse orthologue for human MATE2-K [20]. In contrast, mMate2 is more distant from both, MATE1 and MATE2-K, and showed predominant expression in Leydig cells of the testis [25]. However, as mMate1 is highly expressed in liver and kidney, Mate1$^{-/-}$ knockout mice are considered as an appropriate model to study the pharmacokinetic role of MATE1 and MATE2-K in vivo [18,26].

Based on the data from the present study, trospium transport data for the mouse carriers mOct1, mOct2, and mMate1 are comparable to the trospium transport data of their human counterparts. The first hints for transport of trospium via OCTs came from inhibition studies, where trospium inhibited the MPP$^+$ transport via human OCT1, OCT2, and OCT3 with IC$_{50}$ values of 6.2, 0.67, and 871 µM, respectively [27]. This was basically confirmed by a later study showing IC$_{50}$ values of 18.1, 1.36, and 710 µM for OCT1, OCT2, and OCT3, respectively, in a similar experimental setup [8]. In this study, transport of radiolabeled [^{3}H]trospium was additionally investigated and revealed K$_m$ values of 17 and 8 µM for OCT1 and OCT2, respectively, with nearly identical V$_{max}$ values of about 90 pmol/mg protein/min. In contrast, trospium transport via OCT3 was much lower, and so transport kinetics could not be determined [8]. Therefore, in the present study, trospium transport was analyzed only for mOct1 and mOct2, but not for mOct3. Even later, Bexten analyzed transport of trospium via different drug transporters but only could show trospium transport via OCT1 with K$_m$ of 106 µM and V$_{max}$ of 269 pmol/mg protein/min, but not for OCT2 [9]. In a study also including the MATE transporters, Chen et al. (2017) found IC$_{50}$ values of 15.4, 7.3, 11.5, 11.6, and 5.1 µM for trospium at the carriers OCT1, OCT2, OCT3, MATE1, and MATE2-K, respectively [10]. In addition, direct transport kinetics were determined for all these carriers and revealed K$_m$ values of 15.1, 0.6, 4.4, 15.4, and 8.2 µM for OCT1, OCT2, OCT3, MATE1, and MATE2-K, respectively [10]. Finally, transcellular transport measurements with trospium in OCT1/MATE1 and OCT2/MATE1 double-transfected cells confirmed trospium transport via OCT1, OCT2, and MATE1 [11]. Of note, transport kinetic data for the human carriers partly varied by a factor of 10, most likely due to different experimental conditions, regarding carrier transfection (transient or stable), time-point of analysis (ranging from 1–5 min), and analytical method ([^{3}H]trospium or LC-MS/MS). Against this background, it is difficult to compare directly the transport kinetics between the human and the mouse carriers. However, in direct comparison to the study by Wenge et al. [8] with comparable experimental conditions as in the present study, the Km and Vmax values were generally higher for the mouse carriers compared to their human counterparts (Table ??).

As the absolute and relative importance of a particular drug transporter can only roughly be estimated from in vitro transport data, respective mOct1/2$^{-/-}$, mMate1$^{-/-}$, or combined mOct1/2$^{-/-}$/mMate$^{-/-}$ knockout mouse models might help to elucidate the role of these drug carriers for the overall pharmacokinetics of trospium. Based on the transport data obtained in the present study and regarding the expression of mOct1, mOct2, and mMate1, these carriers are most likely involved in enteral drug absorption, hepatobiliary excretion and tubular secretion of trospium as it was also suggested for the respective human OCT and MATE carriers. Therefore, in mOct/mMate knockout mouse models, it would be particularly interesting to analyze enteral drug absorption, hepatobiliary, and tubular secretion in comparison to wild-type mice.

In contrast to mMate1, mMate2 did not transport trospium in mMate2 stably transfected HEK293 cells. Therefore, mMate2 with its highest expression in the testis does not contribute to the distribution and excretion of trospium in the mouse. However, in the present study, MPP$^+$ transport via mMate2 was demonstrated, indicating that it still represents a drug transporter. This transport was significantly inhibited by TEA, topotecan, acyclovir, and levofloxacin. This is in full agreement with a previous study that showed TEA transport via mMate2 that was significantly inhibited by cimetidine, quinidine, verapamil, and some other drugs [25].

In conclusion, the present study demonstrates for the first time transport of trospium via the mouse drug transporters mOct1, mOct2, and mMate1. Based on this data, pharmacokinetic studies with this drug can be suggested in respective mOct/mMate knockout mice in order to elucidate the role of these carriers for absorption, distribution and elimination of trospium in the mouse. Due to the similarities in the expression pattern and trospium transport behavior between the human and mouse carriers, these data then can be used for extrapolation to the situation in human patients.

4. Materials and Methods

4.1. Materials and Chemicals

All chemicals, unless otherwise stated, were obtained from Sigma-Aldrich (Taufkirchen, Germany). [^{3}H]MPP$^+$ (80 Ci/mmol) was obtained from PerkinElmer (Waltham, MA, USA) and [^{3}H]trospium trifluoroacetate (24.6 Ci/mmol) was obtained from RC Tritec AG (Teufen, Switzerland). Unlabeled trospium chloride was kindly provided by Dr. Pfleger Arzneimittel GmbH (Bamberg, Germany). For the transport experiments, [^{3}H]trospium trifluoroacetate was mixed with an excess of unlabeled trospium chloride. Due to the high excess of chloride in relation to trifluoroacetate in this preparation [^{3}H]trospium chloride is regarded as the active compound. The mixture of [^{3}H]trospium and unlabeled trospium chloride used for all transport measurements is referred to as trospium in the manuscript.

4.2. Cloning of mOct1, mOct2, mMate1, and mMate2

The full open reading frames of the mouse carriers mOct1 and mOct2 were cloned from mouse liver cDNA by RT-PCR as reported before [28]. Gene-specific forward and reverse primers were deduced from the following GenBank reference sequences: NM_009202.5 for mOct1 (*Slc22a1*) and NM_013667.3 for mOct2 (*Slc22a2*). The following gene-specific primers were used: 5'-ATT TCA AGC CAC CGC AGT TC-3' forward and 5'-CTC CCT CTT CTC TCC ACT CT-3' reverse for mOct1, as well as 5'-CAG CAT TTG CAA CCC TGT AG-3' forward and 5'-GTT GGG TTG TGT GGC TTT CG-3' reverse for mOct2. The full open reading frames of mMate1 (*Slc47a1*) and mMate2 (*Slc47a2*) were synthesized based on the reference sequences NM_026183.5 (mMate1) and NM_001033542.2 (mMate2) by BioCat GmbH (Heidelberg, Germany). All open reading frames were subcloned into the pcDNA5/FRT/TO-TOPO expression vector (Thermo Fisher Scientific, Darmstadt, Germany) under control of a CMV promoter and were sequence verified by DNA sequencing.

4.3. Generation of Stably Transfected HEK293 Cell Lines

For the generation of stably transfected cell lines, the Flp-In T-REx 293 host cell line (Thermo Fisher Scientific) was used as reported before [28]. Flp-In T-REx 293 cells contain a single, stably integrated Flp recombinase target (FRT) site at a transcriptionally active genomic locus that ensures high level gene expression from a target-integrated Flp-In expression vector. The expression vector pcDNA5/FRT/TO carries an FRT site and the hygromycin resistance gene. In the generated vectors, the cloned carrier cDNAs are under control of the cytomegalovirus (CMV) promoter and the tetracycline operator sequences ($tetO_2$). In order to establish stably transfected cell lines, the carrier pcDNA5 constructs were cotransfected with the Flp recombinase expression vector pOG44 into the Flp-In T-REx 293 host cells by Lipofectamine transfection reagent according to the manufacturer's protocol (Invitrogen, Carlsbad, CA, USA). Stable clones containing the carrier open reading frame sequences under control of the CMV/$tetO_2$ hybrid promoter were selected by culturing in selective media containing 150 µg/mL hygromycin and 50 µg/mL blasticidin. All clones were verified by quantitative mRNA expression analysis for the respective transfected carrier (see below). The stably transfected mOct1-, mOct2-, mMate1-, and mMate2-HEK293 cells were maintained in Gibco D-MEM/F12 medium (Thermo Fisher Scientific) supplemented with 10% fetal calf serum, L-glutamine (4 mM), penicillin (100 U/mL), and streptomycin (100 µg/mL) (further referred to as standard medium) at 37 °C, 5% CO_2, and 95% humidity.

4.4. Transport Measurements with MPP+ and Trospium

For transport studies, 12- or 24-well plates were coated with poly-D-lysine for better attachment of the cells, and 4.5 or 2.25×10^5 cells were plated per well, respectively. Cells were grown under standard medium, and carrier expression was induced by preincubation with tetracycline (1 µg/mL) for 72 h prior to transport experiments starting. Then, cells were washed three times with phosphate buffered saline (PBS; 137 mM NaCl, 2.7 mM KCl, 1.5 mM KH_2PO_4, 7.3 mM Na_2HPO_4, pH 7.4, 37 °C) and preincubated with sodium transport buffer containing 142.9 mM NaCl, 4.7 mM KCl, 1.2 mM $MgSO_4$, 1.2 mM KH_2PO_4, 1.8 mM $CaCl_2$, and 20 mM HEPES, adjusted to pH 7.4 for mOct and pH 8 for mMate measurements. Uptake experiments were initiated by replacing the preincubation buffer by transport buffer containing the radiolabeled test compound ([^{3}H]MPP+ or [^{3}H]trospium) and were performed at 37 °C at different time-points and substrate concentrations. For mMate2 inhibition studies, the mMate2-HEK293 cells were preincubated with transport buffer containing the inhibitor compound at 37 °C for 3 min. Then, transport measurements were started by adding the radiolabeled substrate at 37 °C over 30 min. Transport and inhibition assays were terminated by removing the transport buffer and washing five-times with ice-cold PBS. Cell monolayers were lysed in 1 N NaOH with 0.1% SDS and the cell-associated radioactivity was determined on liquid scintillation analyzer Tri-Carb 2910 TR (PerkinElmer). The protein content of the lysed cells was determined as reported before with bovine serum albumin as standard [28].

4.5. RNA Preparation and Quantitative Real-Time PCR Expression Analysis

Tissue samples were obtained from a male C57BL/6N mouse without any treatment. Housing was performed in a specific pathogen-free animal facility with a temperature-controlled environment and 12-h light/dark cycle, and standard laboratory food and water were provided ad libitum. The mouse was sacrificed with the sole purpose of using organs for scientific purposes (according to §4 para. 3 of the TierSchG) after consulting the Animal Welfare Officer (TSchB) of the Justus Liebig University Giessen (reference number: 639_M). Organs were conserved in RNAlater solution (Sigma) at −20 °C before total RNA was extracted using RNA tissue kit and Maxwell RSC (Promega, Walldorf, Germany). The RNA amount was determined using NanoDrop One (Thermo Fisher Scientific). The cDNA was synthesized using SuperScript III (Invitrogen) according to the manufacturer's instructions. For quantitative real-time PCR amplification, the following TaqMan Gene Expression Assays were used: Mm00456303_m1 for mOct1, Mm00457295_m1 for mOct2, Mm00840361_m1 for mMate1, and Mm02601013_m1 for mMate2 (Thermo Fisher Scientific). Amplification of mouse beta-actin (assay number Mm00607939_s1) was used as endogenous control. For each specimen, duplicate determinations were performed in a 96-well optical plate using 5 µl cDNA, 1.25 µl TaqMan Gene Expression Assay, 12.5 µl TaqMan Gene Expression Master Mix (Thermo Fisher Scientific), and ddH$_2$O to a final volume of 25 µl. Quantitative real-time PCR was performed on an Applied Biosystems 7300 thermal cycler. The plates were heated for 10 min at 95 °C, and subsequently, 40 cycles of 15 s at 95 °C and 60 s at 60 °C were applied. Relative carrier expression (ΔC_T) was calculated by subtracting the mean signal threshold cycle (C_T) of mouse beta-actin from the mean C_T value of the respective carrier. Subsequently, for each tissue, $\Delta\Delta C_T$ values were calculated by subtracting testis mOct1 ΔC_T (set as calibrator) from the ΔC_T of each individual tissue. After $2^{-\Delta\Delta C_T}$ transformation, data show x-fold higher carrier expression in the respective tissue.

4.6. Graphical and Statistical Analysis of Data

All graphs were created, and the respective statistical analysis was done by GraphPad Prism 6 software (GraphPad Software, La Jolla, CA, USA). Error bars within graphs represent means ± standard deviations (SD) of triplicate determinations. For single time-point uptake and uptake-inhibition experiments, one-way ANOVA with Dunnett's multiple comparison post-hoc test (one-way ANOVA) compared to respective controls was calculated and significant uptake or inhibition was indicated by * representing $p < 0.01$. For time-dependent uptake experiments, every time-point was compared to its individual time-point control by two-way ANOVA and significant uptake indicated by * represents $p < 0.01$. For calculation of K_m and V_{max} values, Michaelis–Menten equation of GraphPad Prism 6 was applied with the following parameters: least squares (ordinary) fit, no constraints, confidence interval of parameters 95%. For Eadie–Hofstee analysis, data of the concentration-dependent net uptake of trospium by mOct1 (Figure 1D), mOct2 (Figure 1F), and mMate1 (Figure 2D) were plotted together in GraphPad Prism 6. Individual [V]data (y-axis) were plotted against the mean of [V] data over respective substrate concentration [S] (V/S), and a linear regression line was fitted for each data set.

Author Contributions: Conceptualization, supervision, project administration, and funding acquisition, J.G.; methodology, investigation, data visualization and curation, M.G., S.F.M. and R.L.; draft preparation, M.G., S.F.M. and J.G.; review and editing, S.F.M. and J.G. All authors have read and agreed to the published version of the manuscript.

Funding: This research was funded by Pfleger Arzneimittel GmbH (Bamberg, Germany), grant number P337. The APC was funded by Justus Liebig University Giessen.

Acknowledgments: This study was kindly supported by Pfleger Arzneimittel GmbH (Bamberg, Germany).

Conflicts of Interest: The authors declare no conflict of interest.

Abbreviations

OCT	Organic cation transporter
MATE	Multidrug and toxin extrusion
SLC	Solute carrier
ABCB1	ATP-binding cassette transporter B1

References

1. Abrams, P.; Andersson, K.E. Muscarinic receptor antagonists for overactive bladder. *BJU Int.* **2007**, *100*, 987–1006. [CrossRef] [PubMed]
2. Wiedemann, A.; Schwantes, P.A. Antimuscarinic drugs for the treatment of overactive bladder: Are they really all the same?—A comparative review of data pertaining to pharmacological and physiological aspects. *Eur. J. Geriat.* **2001**, *9* (Suppl. 1), 29–42.
3. Abebe, B.T.; Weiss, M.; Modess, C.; Tadken, T.; Wegner, D.; Meyer, M.J.; Schwantes, U.; Neumeister, C.; Scheuch, E.; Schulz, H.U.; et al. Pharmacokinetic drug-drug interactions between trospium chloride and ranitidine substrates of organic cation transporters in healthy human subjects. *J. Clin. Pharmacol.* **2020**, *60*, 312–323. [CrossRef] [PubMed]
4. Callegari, E.; Malhotra, B.; Bungay, P.J.; Webster, R.; Fenner, K.S.; Kempshall, S.; LaPerle, J.L.; Michel, M.C.; Kay, G.G. A comprehensive non-clinical evaluation of the CNS penetration potential of antimuscarinic agents for the treatment of overactive bladder. *Br. J. Clin. Pharmacol.* **2011**, *72*, 235–246. [CrossRef] [PubMed]
5. Staskin, D.; Kay, G.; Tannenbaum, C.; Goldman, H.B.; Bhashi, K.; Ling, J.; Oefelein, M.G. Trospium chloride has no effect on memory testing and is assay undetectable in the central nervous system of older patients with overactive bladder. *Int. J. Clin. Pract.* **2010**, *64*, 1294–1300. [CrossRef] [PubMed]
6. Chancellor, M.B.; Staskin, D.R.; Kay, G.G.; Sandage, B.W.; Oefelein, M.G.; Tsao, J.W. Blood-brain barrier permeation and efflux exclusion of anticholinergics used in the treatment of overactive bladder. *Drugs Aging* **2012**, *2*, 259–273. [CrossRef]
7. Geyer, J.; Gavrilova, O.; Petzinger, E. The role of P-glycoprotein in limiting brain penetration of the peripherally acting anticholinergic overactive bladder drug trospium chloride. *Drug Metab. Dispos.* **2009**, *37*, 1371–1374. [CrossRef]
8. Wenge, B.; Geyer, J.; Bönisch, H. Oxybutynin and trospium are substrates of the human organic cation transporters. *Naunyn Schmiedebergs Arch. Pharmacol.* **2011**, *383*, 203–208. [CrossRef]
9. Bexten, M.; Oswald, S.; Grube, M.; Jia, J.; Graf, T.; Zimmermann, U.; Rodewald, K.; Zolk, O.; Schwantes, U.; Siegmund, W.; et al. Expression of drug transporters and drug metabolizing enzymes in the bladder urothelium in man and affinity of the bladder spasmolytic trospium chloride to transporters likely involved in its pharmacokinetics. *Mol. Pharm.* **2015**, *12*, 171–178. [CrossRef]
10. Chen, J.; Brockmöller, J.; Seitz, T.; König, J.; Chen, X.; Tzvetkov, M.V. Tropane alkaloids as substrates and inhibitors of human organic cation transporters of the SLC22 (OCT) and the SLC47 (MATE) families. *Biol. Chem.* **2017**, *398*, 237–249. [CrossRef]
11. Deutsch, B.; Neumeister, C.; Schwantes, U.; Fromm, M.F.; König, J. Interplay of the organic cation transporters OCT1 and OCT2 with the apically localized export protein MATE1 for the polarized transport of trospium. *Mol. Pharm.* **2019**, *1*, 510–517. [CrossRef] [PubMed]
12. Koepsell, H.; Lips, K.; Volk, C. Polyspecific organic cation transporters: Structure, function, physiological roles, and biopharmaceutical implications. *Pharm. Res.* **2007**, *24*, 1227–1251. [CrossRef]
13. Terada, T.; Inui, K. Physiological and pharmacokinetic roles of H^+/organic cation antiporters (MATE/SLC47A). *Biochem. Pharmacol.* **2008**, *75*, 1689–1696. [CrossRef] [PubMed]
14. Samodelov, S.L.; Kullak-Ublick, G.A.; Gai, Z.; Visentin, M. Organic cation transporters in human physiology, pharmacology, and toxicology. *Int. J. Mol. Sci.* **2020**, *21*, 7890. [CrossRef] [PubMed]
15. Sato, T.; Masuda, S.; Yonezawa, A.; Tanihara, Y.; Katsura, T.; Inui, K. Transcellular transport of organic cations in double-transfected MDCK cells expressing human organic cation transporters hOCT1/hMATE1 and hOCT2/hMATE1. *Biochem. Pharmacol.* **2008**, *76*, 894–903. [CrossRef]
16. König, J.; Zolk, O.; Singer, K.; Hoffmann, C.; Fromm, M.F. Double-transfected MDCK cells expressing human OCT1/MATE1 or OCT2/MATE1: Determinants of uptake and transcellular translocation of organic cations. *Br. J. Pharmacol.* **2011**, *163*, 546–555. [CrossRef] [PubMed]

17. Jonker, J.W.; Wagenaar, E.; Van Eijl, S.; Schinkel, A.H. Deficiency in the organic cation transporters 1 and 2 (Oct1/Oct2 [Slc22a1/Slc22a2]) in mice abolishes renal secretion of organic cations. *Mol. Cell. Biol.* **2003**, *23*, 7902–7908. [CrossRef]
18. Tsuda, M.; Terada, T.; Mizuno, T.; Katsura, T.; Shimakura, J.; Inui, K. Targeted disruption of the multidrug and toxin extrusion 1 (mate1) gene in mice reduces renal secretion of metformin. *Mol. Pharmacol.* **2009**, *75*, 1280–1286. [CrossRef]
19. Watanabe, S.; Tsuda, M.; Terada, T.; Katsura, T.; Inui, K. Reduced renal clearance of a zwitterionic substrate cephalexin in MATE1-deficient mice. *J. Pharmacol. Exp. Ther.* **2010**, *334*, 651–656. [CrossRef]
20. Nies, A.T.; Damme, K.; Kruck, S.; Schaeffeler, E.; Schwab, M. Structure and function of multidrug and toxin extrusion proteins (MATEs) and their relevance to drug therapy and personalized medicine. *Arch. Toxicol.* **2016**, *90*, 1555–1584. [CrossRef]
21. Doroshyenko, O.; Jetter, A.; Odenthal, K.P.; Fuhr, U. Clinical pharmacokinetics of trospium chloride. *Clin. Pharmacokinet.* **2005**, *44*, 701–720. [CrossRef] [PubMed]
22. Tadken, T.; Weiss, M.; Modess, C.; Wegner, D.; Roustom, T.; Neumeister, C.; Schwantes, U.; Schulz, H.U.; Weitschies, W.; Siegmund, W. Trospium chloride is absorbed from two intestinal "absorption windows" with different permeability in healthy subjects. *Int. J. Pharm.* **2016**, *515*, 367–373. [CrossRef] [PubMed]
23. Jonker, J.W.; Wagenaar, E.; Mol, C.A.; Buitelaar, M.; Koepsell, H.; Smit, J.W.; Schinkel, A.H. Reduced hepatic uptake and intestinal excretion of organic cations in mice with a targeted disruption of the organic cation transporter 1 (Oct1 [Slc22a1]) gene. *Mol. Cell. Biol.* **2001**, *21*, 5471–5477. [CrossRef] [PubMed]
24. Hiasa, M.; Matsumoto, T.; Komatsu, T.; Moriyama, Y. Wide variety of locations for rodent MATE1, a transporter protein that mediates the final excretion step for toxic organic cations. *Am. J. Physiol. Cell Physiol.* **2006**, *291*, C678–C686. [CrossRef]
25. Hiasa, M.; Matsumoto, T.; Komatsu, T.; Omote, H.; Moriyama, Y. Functional characterization of testis-specific rodent multidrug and toxic compound extrusion 2, a class III MATE-type polyspecific H^+/organic cation exporter. *Am. J. Physiol. Cell Physiol.* **2007**, *293*, C1437–C1444. [CrossRef]
26. Otsuka, M.; Matsumoto, T.; Morimoto, R.; Arioka, S.; Omote, H.; Moriyama, Y. A human transporter protein that mediates the final excretion step for toxic organic cations. *Proc. Natl. Acad. Sci. USA* **2005**, *102*, 17923–17928. [CrossRef]
27. Lips, K.S.; Wunsch, J.; Zarghooni, S.; Bschleipfer, T.; Schukowski, K.; Weidner, W.; Wessler, I.; Schwantes, U.; Koepsell, H.; Kummer, W. Acetylcholine and molecular components of its synthesis and release machinery in the urothelium. *Eur. Urol.* **2007**, *51*, 1042–1053. [CrossRef]
28. Geyer, J.; Döring, B.; Meerkamp, K.; Ugele, B.; Bakhiya, N.; Fernandes, C.F.; Godoy, J.R.; Glatt, H.; Petzinger, E. Cloning and functional characterization of human sodium-dependent organic anion transporter (SLC10A6). *J. Bio. Chem.* **2007**, *282*, 19728–19741. [CrossRef]

Publisher's Note: MDPI stays neutral with regard to jurisdictional claims in published maps and institutional affiliations.

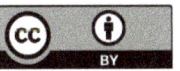

© 2020 by the authors. Licensee MDPI, Basel, Switzerland. This article is an open access article distributed under the terms and conditions of the Creative Commons Attribution (CC BY) license (http://creativecommons.org/licenses/by/4.0/).

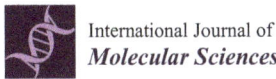

Article

Serotonin Transporter and Plasma Membrane Monoamine Transporter Are Necessary for the Antidepressant-Like Effects of Ketamine in Mice

Melodi A. Bowman [1], Melissa Vitela [1], Kyra M. Clarke [1,2], Wouter Koek [2,3] and Lynette C. Daws [1,2,*]

[1] Department of Cellular and Integrative Physiology at University of Texas Health, San Antonio, TX 78229, USA; bowmanma@livemail.uthscsa.edu (M.A.B.); vitela@uthscsa.edu (M.V.); kyraclarke@mac.com (K.M.C.)
[2] Department of Pharmacology at University of Texas Health, San Antonio, TX 78229, USA; koek@uthscsa.edu
[3] Department of Psychiatry at University of Texas Health, San Antonio, TX 78229, USA
* Correspondence: daws@uthscsa.edu

Received: 29 September 2020; Accepted: 12 October 2020; Published: 14 October 2020

Abstract: Major depressive disorder is typically treated with selective serotonin reuptake inhibitors (SSRIs), however, SSRIs take approximately six weeks to produce therapeutic effects, if any. Not surprisingly, there has been great interest in findings that low doses of ketamine, a non-competitive N-methyl-D-aspartate (NMDA) receptor antagonist, produce rapid and long-lasting antidepressant effects. Preclinical studies show that the antidepressant-like effects of ketamine are dependent upon availability of serotonin, and that ketamine increases extracellular serotonin, yet the mechanism by which this occurs is unknown. Here we examined the role of the high-affinity, low-capacity serotonin transporter (SERT), and the plasma membrane monoamine transporter (PMAT), a low-affinity, high-capacity transporter for serotonin, as mechanisms contributing to ketamine's ability to increase extracellular serotonin and produce antidepressant-like effects. Using high-speed chronoamperometry to measure real-time clearance of serotonin from CA3 region of hippocampus in vivo, we found ketamine robustly inhibited serotonin clearance in wild-type mice, an effect that was lost in mice constitutively lacking SERT or PMAT. As expected, in wild-type mice, ketamine produced antidepressant-like effects in the forced swim test. Mapping onto our neurochemical findings, the antidepressant-like effects of ketamine were lost in mice lacking SERT or PMAT. Future research is needed to understand how constitutive loss of either SERT or PMAT, and compensation that occurs in other systems, is sufficient to void ketamine of its ability to inhibit serotonin clearance and produce antidepressant-like effects. Taken together with existing literature, a critical role for serotonin, and its inhibition of uptake via SERT and PMAT, cannot be ruled out as important contributing factors to ketamine's antidepressant mechanism of action. Combined with what is already known about ketamine's action at NMDA receptors, these studies help lead the way to the development of drugs that lack ketamine's abuse potential but have superior efficacy in treating depression.

Keywords: serotonin transporter; plasma membrane monoamine transporter; ketamine; isoflurane; serotonin clearance; antidepressant-like activity; chronoamperometry; tail suspension test; forced swim test

1. Introduction

Suicide rates have increased dramatically in recent years [1], and treatment resistant depression is a leading cause of suicide [2]. Treatment resistant depression affects up to 30% of people with depression, and, as its name implies, cannot be treated with traditional antidepressant medications such as selective serotonin reuptake inhibitors (SSRIs) [3], underscoring a dire need for novel medications that are effective in treating *all* individuals suffering from depression. Great interest has been generated from clinical studies showing that a single dose of ketamine produces rapid, dramatic, and sustained depression symptom relief, even in individuals suffering from treatment resistant depression [4–6]. Recently, the Federal Drug Administration approved (S)-Ketamine use exclusively in patients with treatment resistant depression [7]. However, the mechanism(s) by which ketamine exerts its pronounced and consistent antidepressant effects are not yet fully understood. Ketamine is a noncompetitive N-methyl-D-aspartate (NMDA) receptor antagonist. Not surprisingly, most preclinical studies have therefore focused on how blockade of NMDA receptors can exert antidepressant-like effects [8]. Ketamine triggers intracellular signaling pathways, including eukaryotic elongation factor 2 (eEF2) kinase, resulting in rapid increases in brain derived neurotrophic factor (BDNF) protein translation [8,9]. This increase in BDNF activates the mammalian target of rapamycin (mTOR) pathway, which in turn induces rapid synaptogenesis. Currently this is viewed as the primary mechanism underlying ketamine's antidepressant-like effects in preclinical studies [8,10]. However, growing attention is turning to ketamine's ability to increase extracellular serotonin.

The antidepressant effect of SSRIs is initiated by blockade of the serotonin transporter (SERT) and ensuing increase in extracellular serotonin [11,12]. Like SSRIs, ketamine also causes robust increases in extracellular serotonin in brain regions important in the pathophysiology of mood disorders [13–15]. Underscoring the importance of serotonin in ketamine's antidepressant action, recent studies showed that ketamine was without antidepressant-like activity in rodents treated with parachlorophenylalanine (PCPA) to deplete serotonin [16–19]. However it is unclear whether ketamine's ability to increase extracellular serotonin is mediated through glutamatergic control of serotonin release and/or via direct actions at SERT [20], the high-affinity, low-capacity (i.e., "uptake-1") transporter for serotonin.

In addition to SERT, our lab, and others, found that low-affinity, high-capacity (i.e., "uptake-2") transporters play a prominent role in regulating serotonin transmission [21–25]. Examples of "uptake-2" transporters include the plasma membrane monoamine transporter (PMAT) and organic cation transporters (OCTs). PMAT and OCTs are inhibited by decynium-22 (D22) and are collectively known as D22-sensitive transporters. Since PMAT is the most efficient transporter of serotonin among D22-sensitive "uptake-2" transporters, and is widely expressed in human brain, including limbic regions important in controlling mood [25], the possibility is raised that inhibition of PMAT-mediated serotonin uptake may also contribute to ketamine's antidepressant actions. Therefore, we hypothesized that SERT and/or PMAT may contribute to the antidepressant-like effects of ketamine.

To explore this possibility, we used in vivo high-speed chronoamperometry to measure ketamine's local effects on clearance of exogenously applied serotonin in CA3 region of hippocampus, a brain region important in regulating mood and for the actions of SSRIs [26], in wild-type and constitutive SERT knockout (−/−) and PMAT−/− mice. In parallel, we determined how ketamine's effects on serotonin clearance mapped onto behavior in the tail suspension test (TST) and forced swim test (FST), commonly used behavioral assays that detect drugs with antidepressant potential [27,28]. To our knowledge, this is the first study to directly explore SERT and PMAT involvement in ketamine's mechanism of action in vivo, and the first study to examine serotonin clearance in constitutive PMAT−/− mice. We also examined the effects of isoflurane anesthesia on serotonin release and clearance, prior to using this anesthetic for these in vivo high-speed chronoamperometry studies.

2. Results

2.1. Isoflurane Does Not Evoke Serotonin Release or Inhibit Serotonin Clearance at Concentrations Needed to Maintain Anesthesia

In the past, we have routinely used a mixture of alpha-chloralose and urethane to anesthetize rodents for chronoamperometric recordings. This was the anesthetic of choice because it reportedly does not interfere with monoamine transporters [29,30]. However, isoflurane has advantages over alpha-chloralose urethane, primary among them the ability to control the surgical plane of anesthesia more precisely and consistently. Isoflurane does not impact the dopamine transporter (DAT) [31] but has been reported to impact serotonin release in vitro and in vivo [32–35], although results are inconsistent. Therefore, before using isoflurane in our experiments, we confirmed that at concentrations needed to maintain anesthesia, isoflurane does not cause serotonin release or impact serotonin clearance in CA3 region of hippocampus. To this end, we carried out a concentration-response study using in vivo high-speed chronoamperometry in C57BL/6 male mice.

We found no evidence of measurable endogenous serotonin release following administration of any of the isoflurane concentrations, as evidenced by the baseline signal remaining stable (data not shown). Clearance of exogenously applied serotonin from extracellular fluid of the CA3 region of hippocampus was analyzed after each concentration of isoflurane ranging from 1.0–3.0% and given in 0.5% increments in a randomized order among mice. Peak signal amplitude (µM), time to clear between 20% and 60% (T_{20}-T_{60}, in s) of peak signal amplitude, and time to clear 80% (T_{80}, in s) of peak signal amplitude were analyzed (Figure 1A). Serotonin was pressure-ejected into CA3 region of hippocampus to achieve signals of approximately 0.5 µM (Figure 1B). The amount (in pmol) of serotonin required to achieve signals of this amplitude did not vary as a function of isoflurane concentration and averaged 1.8 ± 0.3 pmol (one-way ANOVA: $F(3,17) = 0.24$, $p = 0.89$). We found that clearance times for serotonin were not different from those we have previously recorded using alpha-chloralose urethane anesthesia, with T_{20}-T_{60} (Figure 1C) and T_{80} (Figure 1D) clearance values for signals of ~0.5 µM serotonin most commonly ranging from 100–200 s and 200–300 s, respectively. One-way ANOVA of T_{20}-T_{60} and T_{80} serotonin clearance times revealed no significant difference among isoflurane concentrations (T_{20}-T_{60}: $F(3,17) = 1.08$, $p = 0.38$; T_{80}: $F(3,17) = 1.34$, $p = 0.29$) (Figure 1C,D), with the highest concentration (2.5%) trending to increase serotonin clearance time, i.e., to inhibit serotonin clearance. Concentrations of isoflurane higher than 2.5% were not examined due to mice not surviving at 3.0% isoflurane. During our experiments, we maintained mice at an anesthetic plane using 1.0–1.5% isoflurane, as higher concentrations tend to interfere with respiration. Thus, these studies confirm that isoflurane, at doses required for maintenance of a surgical plane of anesthesia, do not evoke detectable serotonin release or interfere with serotonin clearance in vivo.

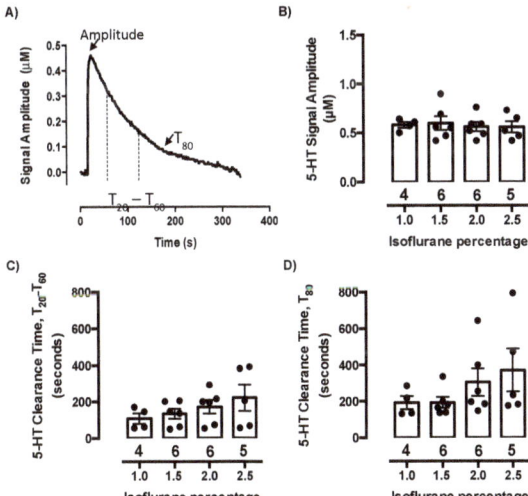

Figure 1. Isoflurane does not impact serotonin clearance at low concentrations. (**A**) Representative trace with signal parameters defined; (**B**) Serotonin signal amplitude did not change as a function of isoflurane percentage; (**C**) Serotonin clearance time (T_{20}-T_{60}) and (**D**) (T_{80}) in seconds at varying concentrations of isoflurane (1.0–2.5%). There was no statistically significant difference in serotonin clearance time among the isoflurane concentrations. Circles represent individual mice. Data are mean ± S.E.M.

2.2. Comparison of Serotonin Clearance among SERT and PMAT Genotypes

We found no difference among genotypes in the pmol amount of serotonin required to achieve signal amplitudes of ~0.5 µM (2.0 ± 0.3, 1.8 ± 0.2, 1.8 ± 0.2 and 1.6 ± 0.1 pmol for SERT+/+, SERT−/−, PMAT+/+ and PMAT−/− mice, respectively). Representative serotonin signals for each genotype are shown in Figure 2A. Since a significant difference in variance for each of the serotonin signal parameters was detected among genotypes, we applied a Welch's one-way ANOVA to the analyses of these data, which does not assume that all groups were sampled from populations with equal variances. Welch's one-way ANOVA revealed that signal amplitudes did not differ among genotypes ($F(3,11.8) = 0.56$, $p = 0.65$) (Figure 2B), however there was a significant effect of genotype for T_{20}-T_{60} serotonin clearance time ($F(3,10.1) = 3.81$, $p = 0.05$) but not for T_{80} clearance time ($F(3,11.0) = 2.4$, $p = 0.12$) (Figure 2D). Tukey's post-hoc comparisons showed this difference in T_{20}-T_{60} to be driven by PMAT+/+ mice clearing serotonin more slowly than SERT+/+ mice ($p = 0.03$) (Figure 2C). Given both lines are bred on a C57BL/6 background this finding was unexpected. That PMAT−/− mice clear serotonin as efficiently as SERT+/+ mice (Figure 2C,D) suggests that there is no consequence of constitutive PMAT knockout for serotonin clearance, at least at the concentration of serotonin used in these studies, and that this apparent difference between SERT+/+ and PMAT+/+ mice is peculiar to this cohort of PMAT+/+ mice. It is important to emphasize that the genotypes of all mice were double-checked to rule out the possibility that PMAT genotypes had been recorded inaccurately. We found this not to be the case, with all genotypes being confirmed as correct.

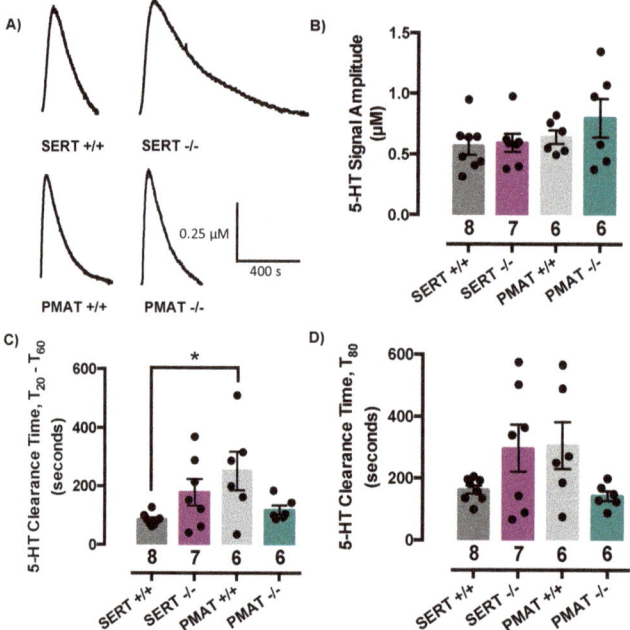

Figure 2. Comparison of serotonin clearance among serotonin transporter (SERT) and plasma membrane monoamine transporter (PMAT) genotypes. (**A**) Representative traces of basal serotonin clearance in SERT+/+, SERT−/−, PMAT+/+, and PMAT−/− mice. (**B**) Basal serotonin signal amplitude, and (**D**) T_{80} clearance time did not differ significantly among genotypes. There was an effect of genotype in basal T_{20}-T_{60} serotonin clearance time (**C**) where PMAT+/+ cleared serotonin more slowly than SERT+/+ mice (but see Figure 3). Welch's one-way ANOVA with Tukey's post-hoc comparisons. * $p < 0.05$. Circles represent individual mice. Data are mean ± S.E.M.

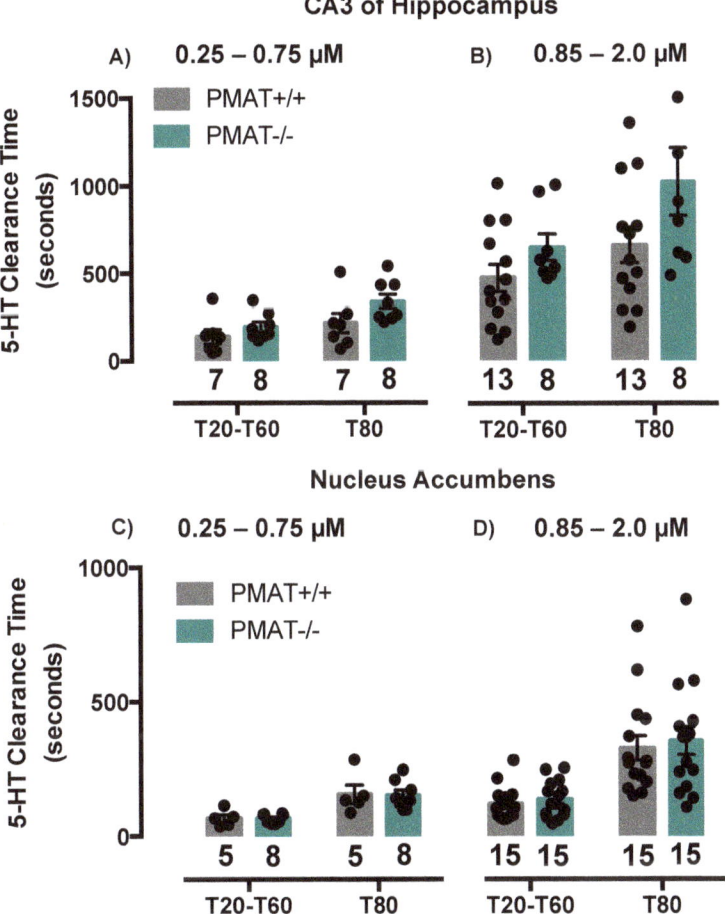

Figure 3. Serotonin clearance time (T_{20}-T_{60} and T_{80}) does not differ between PMAT+/+ and PMAT−/− mice, regardless of serotonin concentration. (**A**) There was no statistically significant difference between PMAT+/+ and PMAT−/− mice in serotonin clearance time (T_{20}-T_{60} and T_{80}) in CA3 of hippocampus at "low" concentration of serotonin (0.25 µM to 0.75 µM) or (**B**) "high" concentrations of serotonin (0.85 µM to 2.0 µM). (**C**) There was no statistically significant difference between PMAT+/+ and PMAT−/− mice in serotonin clearance time (T_{20}-T_{60} and T_{80}) in nucleus accumbens at "low" concentration of serotonin (0.25 µM to 0.75 µM) and (**D**) "high" concentrations of serotonin (0.85 µM to 2.0 µM). Note that the ordinates differ between CA3 region of hippocampus (panels A and B), and NAcc (panels C and D). Circles represent individual mice. Data are as mean ± S.E.M.

To investigate this apparent paradox further, we conducted additional experiments in two separate cohorts of PMAT+/+ and PMAT−/− mice and varied the concentration of serotonin delivered. In the first cohort, we measured serotonin clearance in the same brain region, CA3 region of hippocampus. In this cohort of PMAT+/+ mice, both T_{20}-T_{60} and T_{80} clearance times were consistent with those of SERT+/+ mice for signals of similar amplitude and were ~100 s and 200 s, respectively (compare Figure 3A with Figure 2C,D). Figure 3A shows that for the lower serotonin concentrations tested (0.25 to 0.75 µM) there was no difference in clearance time from extracellular fluid of CA3 region of hippocampus for either T_{20}-T_{60} ($t(13) = 1.18$, $p = 0.26$) or T_{80} ($t(13) = 1.82$, $p = 0.09$), between PMAT+/+

and PMAT−/− mice. As expected, at higher serotonin concentrations (0.85 to 2.0 µM), T_{20}-T_{60} and T_{80} clearance times were longer than those of lower serotonin concentrations, and in PMAT+/+ mice were ~500 s and 650 s, respectively (compare grey bars in Figure 3A,B). Similar to the results obtained with low serotonin concentrations (0.25 to 0.75 µM), at higher serotonin concentrations (0.85 to 2.0 µM) there was no difference in serotonin clearance time for either T_{20}-T_{60} ($t(19) = 1.50$, $p = 0.15$) or T_{80} ($t(19) = 1.84$, $p = 0.08$) between PMAT+/+ and PMAT−/− mice, although in PMAT−/− mice clearance trended to be slower than in PMAT+/+ mice, consistent with loss of the low-affinity, high-capacity PMAT (Figure 3B).

Using a separate cohort of mice, we examined serotonin clearance in the nucleus accumbens (NAcc) in order to determine if the lack of difference in serotonin clearance time in CA3 region of hippocampus between PMAT+/+ and PMAT−/− mice generalized to other brain regions. We found that serotonin clearance in NAcc was faster than in CA3 region of hippocampus, with T_{20}-T_{60} and T_{80} clearance times of ~50 s and 150 s, respectively, for lower serotonin concentrations (0.25 to 0.75 µM), and ~100 s and 350 s, respectively, for higher serotonin concentrations (0.85 to 2.0 µM) (Figure 3C,D). As in hippocampus, there was no difference in serotonin clearance time between genotypes at either low (0.25 to 0.75 µM) serotonin concentrations (T_{20}-T_{60}: ($t(11) = 0.02$, $p = 0.98$) or T_{80}: ($t(11) = 0.11$, $p = 0.91$)) or higher (0.85 to 2.0 µM) serotonin concentrations (T_{20}-T_{60}: ($t(28) = 0.70$, $p = 0.49$) or T_{80}: ($t(28) = 0.39$, $p = 0.70$)) (Figure 3C,D). Based on findings from these more extensive investigations of serotonin clearance in PMAT+/+ and PMAT−/− mice, together with confirmation of mouse genotypes, we conclude that constitutive knockout of PMAT does not significantly impact serotonin clearance at the concentrations of serotonin tested. Moreover, we therefore conclude that the longer serotonin clearance in PMAT+/+ mice, relative to SERT+/+ mice reported in Figure 2, is exclusively due to sampling variation.

Consistent with our previous findings [21,36,37], serotonin clearance trended to be slower in SERT−/− mice than their wild-type counterparts (T_{20}-T_{60}: ($t(13) = 2.15$, $p = 0.05$); T_{80}: ($t(13) = 1.85$, $p = 0.09$).

2.3. Ketamine Inhibits Serotonin Clearance in Wild-Type Mice, but Not in SERT−/− or PMAT−/− Mice

To test the hypothesis that ketamine increases extracellular serotonin by inhibiting its clearance via SERT and/or PMAT, we used in vivo high-speed chronoamperometry to measure clearance of exogenous serotonin from the extracellular fluid of CA3 region of hippocampus of anesthetized mice before and after local application of ketamine or phosphate buffered saline (PBS) vehicle in SERT+/+, PMAT+/+, SERT−/−, and PMAT−/− mice (Figure 4). Representative traces for serotonin clearance after ketamine in each genotype are shown in Figure 4A. Ketamine did not influence signal amplitude in any genotype ($F(2,35) = 0.79$, $p = 0.46$) (Figure 4A,B, Table 1), but significantly increased serotonin clearance time in both SERT+/+ and PMAT+/+ mice. As there was no statistically significant difference in the percent increase in serotonin clearance time following ketamine between SERT+/+ (T_{20}-T_{60}: 83 ± 38%; T_{80}: 92 ± 25%) and PMAT+/+ (T_{20}-T_{60}: 59 ± 24%; T_{80}: 58 ± 24%) mice [T_{20-60}, $t(9) = 0.55$, $p = 0.60$; T_{80}, $t(10) = 0.97$, $p = 0.36$], wild-type percent change data were pooled. Two-way ANOVA of the percent change in T_{20}-T_{60} serotonin clearance time from pre-treatment (PBS vs. ketamine) values revealed a main effect of ketamine to prolong serotonin clearance time (main effect of treatment: ($F(1,35) = 5.65$, $p = 0.02$), main effect of genotype: ($F(2,35) = 3.27$, $p = 0.05$)), and interaction ($F(2,35) = 2.88$, $p = 0.07$) (Figure 4C). As per recommendations by Hsu et al. [38] and Maxwell et al. [39], post-hoc analyses were conducted even though the interaction was not statistically significant at the 5% level. PBS had no effect on serotonin clearance (in any genotype), whereas ketamine prolonged T_{20}-T_{60} serotonin clearance in wild-type mice ($p = 0.01$), but not in SERT−/− ($p = 0.98$) or PMAT−/− mice ($p = 0.99$), as also evidenced by post-hoc comparisons of the effects of ketamine among genotypes (wild-type vs. SERT−/−, $p = 0.05$; wild-type vs. PMAT−/−, $p = 0.03$).

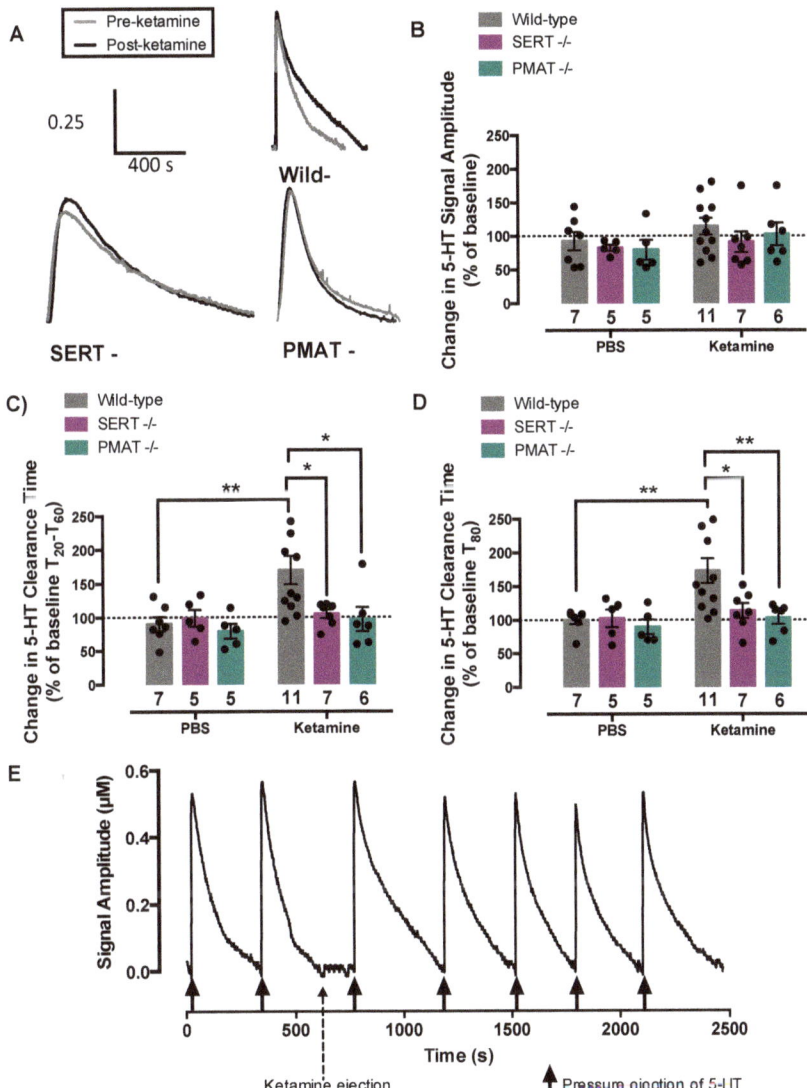

Figure 4. Ketamine significantly inhibited serotonin clearance in wild-type mice, but not in mice lacking SERT or PMAT. (**A**) Representative oxidation currents produced by pressure-ejecting serotonin into CA3 region of hippocampus before (grey) and after (black) local application of ketamine. Traces are superimposed for ease of comparison. (**B**) Percent change in serotonin signal amplitude did not differ between treatments and across genotypes. Percent change in serotonin clearance time (**C**) T_{20}-T_{60}, and (**D**) T_{80} increased in wild-type mice, but was unchanged in SERT−/− and PMAT−/− mice. (**E**) Representative time course for serotonin clearance in a wild-type mouse following ketamine ejection. Note that pressure-ejection of ketamine did not perturb baseline oxidation current, indicating that ketamine did not evoke detectable release of endogenous serotonin. * $p < 0.05$ ** $p < 0.01$. Circles represent individual mice. Data are mean ± S.E.M.

Table 1. Summary of pre- and post-serotonin signal amplitudes and time course (T_{20}-T_{60} and T_{80}) for serotonin clearance 2 min following pressure-ejection of phosphate buffered saline (PBS) or ketamine into CA3 region of hippocampus.

Genotype		SERT+/+	SERT+/+	SERT−/−	SERT−/−	PMAT+/+	PMAT+/+	PMAT−/−	PMAT−/−
Drug		PBS	Ketamine	PBS	Ketamine	PBS	Ketamine	PBS	Ketamine
N		4	5	5	7	3	6	5	6
Amp (μM)	Pre	0.44 ± 0.08	0.62 ± 0.09	0.46 ± 0.06	0.59 ± 0.07	0.56 ± 0.11	0.64 ± 0.06	0.74 ± 0.16	0.77 ± 0.15
	Post	0.47 ± 0.16	0.66 ± 0.18	0.37 ± 0.32	0.59 ± 0.19	0.48 ± 0.15	0.74 ± 0.08	0.62 ± 0.18	0.72 ± 0.11
T_{20}-T_{60} (s)	Pre	109 ± 13	83 ± 6	173 ± 39	178 ± 45	361 ± 99	251 ± 66	138 ± 54	171 ± 51
	Post	114 ± 22	149 ± 28 #	186 ± 56	188 ± 50	282 ± 102	326 ± 55 #	109 ± 46	171 ± 60
T_{80} (s)	Pre	194 ± 20	155 ± 18	273 ± 56	297 ± 77	475 ± 173	306 ± 76	183 ± 55	193 ± 49
	Post	202 ± 19	278 ± 21 **	305 ± 86	321 ± 78	487 ± 221	422 ± 81 *	165 ± 60	206 ± 67

Pre- and post-drug values for peak signal amplitude and clearance time (T_{20}-T_{60} and T_{80}) 2 min after local application of PBS or ketamine. ** $p < 0.01$ * $p < 0.05$ significantly different from pre-drug value (paired t-test), # $p = 0.08$, Mean ± S.E.M.

Similarly, two-way ANOVA of the percent change in T_{80} serotonin clearance time from pre-treatment values revealed a main effect of ketamine to increase serotonin clearance time ($F(1,35) = 6.54$, $p = 0.02$), main effect of genotype ($F(2,35) = 4.01$, $p = 0.03$), and interaction ($F(2,35) = 2.92$, $p = 0.07$) (Figure 4D). Post-hoc analysis showed PBS had no effect on serotonin clearance (in any genotype), whereas ketamine prolonged T_{80} serotonin clearance in wild-type mice ($p = 0.01$), but not in SERT−/− (= 0.98) or PMAT−/− ($p > 0.99$) mice, as also evidenced by post-hoc comparisons of the effects of ketamine among genotypes (wild-type vs. SERT−/−, $p = 0.05$; wild-type vs. PMAT−/−, $p = 0.02$). The effect of intrahippocampally applied ketamine to inhibit serotonin clearance persisted for approximately 20 min in both SERT+/+ and PMAT+/+ mice, returning to pre-drug clearance times by 30 min (Figure 4E). Average pre- and 2-min post-treatment signal amplitude, T_{20}-T_{60}, and T_{80} values are reported in Table 1, where paired t-test analyses revealed similar statistically-significant outcomes.

Taken together, these results suggest that loss of either SERT or PMAT is sufficient to eliminate ketamine's ability to inhibit serotonin clearance. To determine if inhibition of serotonin clearance via SERT and/or PMAT is necessary for the antidepressant-like effects of ketamine we turned to the TST and FST.

2.4. Antidepressant-Like Effects of Ketamine Are Lost in Mice Lacking SERT or PMAT

To test the hypothesis that SERT and/or PMAT are necessary for the antidepressant-like effect of ketamine, we measured immobility time in the TST and FST in SERT+/+, PMAT+/+, SERT−/− and PMAT−/− mice. However, first we used wild-type (C57BL/6) mice to confirm, in our hands, that 32 mg/kg ketamine produced robust (near maximal) antidepressant-like effects, as reported by others [16,40,41]. Since the TST is the most used test for antidepressant-like activity in mice, we used this test first. We found that none of the ketamine doses tested (3.2, 10, or 32 mg/kg) produced antidepressant-like effects in wild-type mice ($F(3,42) = 0.36$, $p = 0.78$) (Figure 5A). These findings agree with those of others [42].

We turned to the FST, which has been shown to provide more consistent results when examining the antidepressant-like effects of ketamine [43]. Consistent with this literature, we found that ketamine produced dose-dependent and significant antidepressant-like effects in wild-type mice ($F(3,29) = 4.15$, $p = 0.02$). Tukey's post hoc multiple comparisons test showed that 32.0 mg/kg ketamine was statistically different from saline ($p = 0.03$) (Figure 5B) and produced an effect of similar magnitude to that reported in the literature [16,40,41]. Therefore, for all subsequent experiments, 32.0 mg/kg ketamine was used to assess the antidepressant-like effect of ketamine using the FST.

We also looked for climbing behavior, which is routinely recorded during the FST when using rats as it aids in determining if the antidepressant-like actions of a drug are more strongly influenced by serotonergic or noradrenergic and dopaminergic systems; drugs that act to increase serotonin increase swimming, whereas drugs that act to increase norepinephrine and/or dopamine increase climbing [44,45]. We found that climbing behavior was essentially non-existent in mice given ketamine, suggesting that effects of ketamine were unlikely mediated by increased norepinephrine or dopamine signaling.

Replicating our findings in wild-type C57BL/6 mice, ketamine produced a robust antidepressant-like effect in SERT+/+ mice, which was absent in SERT−/− mice. Two-way ANOVA of time spent immobile revealed a statistically significant ketamine by genotype interaction ($F(1,44) = 5.72$, $p = 0.02$) (main effect of ketamine: $F(1,44) = 6.27$, $p = 0.02$; main effect of genotype: $F(1,44) = 2.42$, $p = 0.13$). Post-hoc analysis showed that 32.0 mg/kg ketamine significantly decreased immobility time in SERT+/+ mice compared to saline treated SERT+/+ mice ($p = 0.003$) and compared to saline treated SERT−/− mice ($p = 0.03$), however there was no effect of ketamine in SERT−/− mice ($p > 0.99$) (Figure 5C).

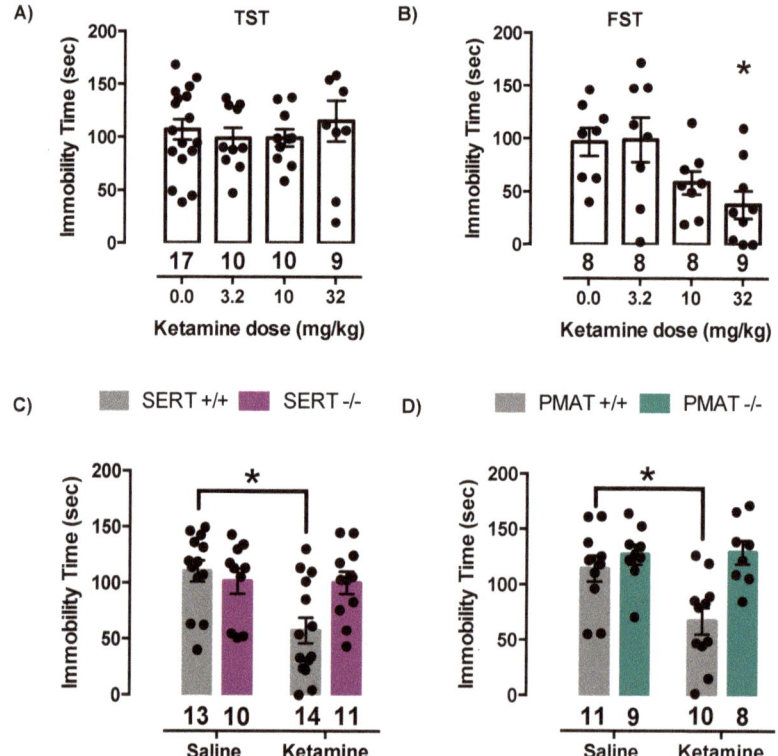

Figure 5. Ketamine lacks antidepressant-like effects in constitutive SERT or PMAT knockout mice. (**A**) Immobility time (s) in the tail suspension test and (**B**) Immobility time (s) in the forced swim test, in C57BL/6 mice given ketamine (3.2, 10, or 32 mg/kg) or saline. * $p < 0.05$ represents 32.0 mg/kg ketamine significantly different from saline. Tukey's post-hoc test for multiple comparisons. (**C**) Immobility time in the FST after 32.0 mg/kg ketamine or saline administered one hour prior to testing in SERT+/+ or SERT−/− mice. * $p < 0.05$ represents 32.0 mg/kg ketamine significantly different from saline; Tukey's post-hoc test for multiple comparisons. (**D**) Immobility time in the FST after 32.0 mg/kg ketamine or saline administered one hour prior to testing in PMAT+/+ or PMAT−/− mice. * $p < 0.05$ represents 32.0 mg/kg ketamine significantly different from saline. Tukey's post-hoc test for multiple comparisons. Circles represent individual mice. Data are mean ± S.E.M.

Similarly, ketamine produced an antidepressant-like effect in PMAT+/+ mice, which was absent in PMAT−/− mice. Two-way ANOVA of time spent immobile revealed a statistically significant ketamine by genotype interaction ($F(1,34) = 4.82$, $p = 0.04$) (main effect of ketamine: ($F(1,34) = 4.03$, $p = 0.05$); main effect of genotype: ($F(1,34) = 11.14$, $p = 0.002$). Post-hoc analysis showed that 32.0 mg/kg ketamine significantly decreased immobility time in PMAT+/+ mice compared to saline treated PMAT+/+ mice ($p = 0.02$) and compared to saline treated PMAT−/− mice ($p = 0.002$), however there was no effect of ketamine in PMAT−/− mice ($p = 0.99$) (Figure 5D). Taken together, these results indicate that elimination of either SERT or PMAT voids ketamine of its antidepressant-like effects.

2.5. Ketamine Does Not Influence Locomotor Activity of SERT+/+, SERT−/−, PMAT+/+, or PMAT−/− Mice

Locomotor activity of mice was not impacted by ketamine (32 mg/kg). In SERT+/+ and SERT−/− mice, there was no statistically significant interaction between ketamine treatment and genotype in locomotor activity of the mice ($F(1,28) = 0.27$, $p = 0.61$). There was also no main effect of ketamine treatment (F(1,28) = 0.003, p = 0.9) nor main effect of genotype (F(1,28) = 0.67, p = 0.42) (Figure 6A). Similarly, in PMAT+/+ and PMAT−/− mice, there was no statistically significant interaction between ketamine treatment and genotype (F(1,40) = 1.01, p = 0.32). There was also no main effect of ketamine treatment (F(1,40) = 0.008, p = 0.93) nor main effect of genotype (F(1,40) = 0.10, p = 0.75) (Figure 6B). Therefore, it is unlikely that effects of ketamine on locomotor activity affected outcomes in the FST.

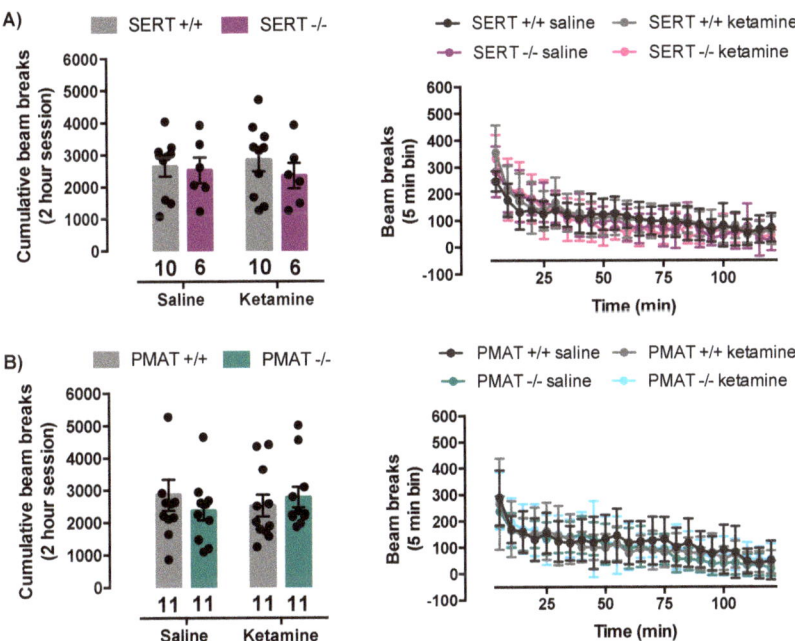

Figure 6. Ketamine did not significantly impact locomotor activity of SERT+/+, SERT−/−, PMAT+/+, or PMAT−/− mice. (**A**) There was no significant difference in locomotor activity of SERT+/+ and SERT−/−, or (**B**) PMAT+/+ and PMAT−/− mice, when given ketamine or saline. Bar graphs show total number of beam breaks in the two-hour recording period. Panels on the right show beam breaks in 5 min bins as a function of time. Circles represent individual mice. Data are mean ± S.E.M.

3. Discussion

The key findings from this study are that ketamine inhibits serotonin clearance in the CA3 region of the hippocampus (Figure 4) and produces antidepressant-like effects (Figure 5) in a SERT- and PMAT-dependent manner. These data support an important role of serotonin in the antidepressant actions of ketamine through interaction with SERT and PMAT. Puzzling, however, is the finding that elimination of either SERT or PMAT was sufficient to render ketamine devoid of its serotonin clearance-inhibiting and antidepressant-like effects. Given that SERT−/− mice have a full complement of PMAT, and PMAT−/− mice have a full complement of SERT, it is surprising that ketamine's ability to inhibit serotonin clearance and to produce antidepressant-like effects was lost, rather than diminished, suggesting a more complex interplay between ketamine and these transporters than previously thought. That these are constitutive knockouts likely comes into play, given that compensation in other systems is probable (discussed later). However, because SERT and PMAT overlap in their neuronal distribution, it is tempting to speculate that they may exist as heteromers, and only when in this configuration can ketamine exert inhibitory actions on serotonin clearance. Clearly, future research is needed to understand how constitutive loss of either SERT or PMAT, and compensation that occurs in other systems, is sufficient to abolish ketamine's ability to inhibit serotonin clearance and produce antidepressant-like effects.

Although much research to date has focused on ketamine's action as an antagonist at NMDA receptors, our findings add to increasing evidence showing a critical role for serotonin in the antidepressant effects of ketamine. The importance of serotonin is perhaps best exemplified by reports from several groups who found that the antidepressant-like effect of ketamine is lost when serotonin is depleted via PCPA treatment [16–18]. Consistent with an important role for serotonin in the antidepressant effects of ketamine, multiple studies have shown that ketamine increases extracellular serotonin, yet the mechanism(s) by which this occurs remains unclear [15,18,46–50]. Our studies point to ketamine-induced inhibition of serotonin clearance via SERT and PMAT as potential mechanisms.

The idea that ketamine blocks uptake of serotonin via SERT has been hypothesized since the 1970s. From that time to present day, investigators have used a variety of approaches to test this hypothesis, including measuring the ability of ketamine to inhibit uptake of tritiated ($[^3H]$)-serotonin into synaptosomes prepared from rodent brain [51], cell lines expressing murine or human SERT [52,53], and human platelets, which are rich in SERT [53]. Inhibition values (IC_{50} or Ki) range from ~50 to 230 µM, no doubt varying based on the system used to measure inhibition of $[^3H]$-serotonin uptake. In 1982, Martin and colleagues [54] leveraged p-chloroamphetamine (PCA), a substrate for SERT that leads to depletion of serotonin, to gain insight into ketamine's actions in vivo. They found that rats pre-treated with anesthetic doses of ketamine (80, 120, or 160 mg/kg), but not lower doses, were protected from the serotonin depleting effect of PCA, suggesting that ketamine blocks transport of PCA into serotonin neurons via SERT. While studies such as these have provided support for actions of ketamine at SERT, they suggest that inhibition of SERT by ketamine only occurs at concentrations much greater than those needed for antidepressant (or anesthetic) action. For example, in humans, plasma concentrations of ketamine needed for anesthesia are reported to be ~9 µM [55], while subanesthetic doses of ketamine used for treatment of depression result in plasma concentrations less than 1 µM [56–58]. Due to this, controversy has remained regarding the importance of blockade of serotonin uptake in the clinical efficacy of ketamine.

To gain a better understanding of the relationship between plasma and brain concentrations of ketamine and antidepressant-like effect in rodents, Can and colleagues [20] measured plasma and brain tissue concentrations of ketamine and its metabolites after systemic administration of 10 mg/kg ketamine in mice, a sub-anesthetic dose, which they found to have antidepressant-like effects [41]. Ketamine concentration peaked 10 min post injection at approximately 4 nmol/mL in plasma and 7 nmol/g in brain tissue, corresponding to approximately 4 µM and 7 µM, respectively. Using in vitro binding assays, they found that ketamine did not inhibit binding to SERT up to concentrations of 10 µM, and concluded that ketamine does not inhibit SERT at "therapeutically" relevant concentrations in mice [20]. These findings are in contrast to positron emission tomography (PET) studies in rhesus monkeys, where a subanesthetic dose of ketamine (1.5 mg/kg) was found to reduce binding of $[^{11}C]$-3-amino-4-(2-dimethylaminomethyl-phenylsulfanyl)benzonitrile ($[^{11}C]$DASB) to SERT [50]. More recently, Spies and colleagues [59] used PET imaging in humans to examine the effects of 0.5 mg/kg ketamine, a commonly used therapeutic dose in the treatment of depression. Though they did not find significant inhibition of $[^{11}C]$DASB binding to SERT, they found a positive correlation between ketamine plasma levels and SERT occupancy, which trended to statistical significance. Since higher doses of ketamine are also used clinically, these studies encourage further investigation of ketamine's action at SERT.

Our chronoamperometry studies are consistent with inhibition of serotonin uptake being an important mechanism of action of ketamine. Although we cannot know the precise concentration of ketamine reaching the recording electrode following pressure-ejection of drug locally into brain, we can estimate the concentration relatively accurately based on earlier studies (see Methods). We designed these studies so as to deliver approximately 2 µM in the area surrounding the recording electrode, a concentration less than the peak ketamine concentration (~7 µM) reported to reach brain in mice after a dose of 10 mg/kg [20]. Importantly, pressure-ejection of ketamine directly into brain has the advantage of allowing study of ketamine's actions in vivo, in the absence of its metabolites. We found that in wild-type mice, ketamine robustly inhibited serotonin clearance in CA3 region of hippocampus, a brain region important for mood and therapeutic effects of antidepressants [26]. Consistent with an important role for SERT, this effect of ketamine was lost in mice constitutively lacking SERT. Moreover, this effect of ketamine was also lost in mice constitutively lacking PMAT. These data add support to findings that ketamine inhibits SERT at therapeutically relevant concentrations and brings a new player to the table: inhibition of PMAT.

The conclusion that ketamine inhibits serotonin uptake via SERT and PMAT at concentrations that produce antidepressant-like effects in mice is justified based on the clear-cut absence of this effect in SERT−/− and PMAT−/− mice. However, these data raise several questions, the most obvious being, why is elimination of either SERT or PMAT sufficient to render ketamine devoid of its serotonin clearance-inhibiting action? Given that both are constitutive knockouts, compensation in other systems (including other transporters or regulatory mechanisms) is likely at play. For example, it is known that OCT3 expression (mRNA and protein) is upregulated in SERT−/− mice [21]. It is possible that inhibitory actions of ketamine on serotonin clearance via PMAT in SERT−/− mice are masked by accelerated serotonin uptake via OCT3. A similar argument could be applied to PMAT−/− mice. To our knowledge, this is the first study to measure serotonin clearance in hippocampus and NAcc of PMAT−/− mice in vivo. To date, the only study investigating compensation in other transporters in PMAT−/− mice found no increase in mRNA expression of SERT, NET, DAT, OCT1, OCT2, and OCT3 in choroid plexus [60], however, protein levels were not measured and the possibility of functional upregulation of one or more of these transporters in PMAT−/− mice cannot be ruled out. In terms of functional studies, [^{3}H]serotonin uptake into in vitro preparations of choroid plexus showed slower uptake in PMAT−/− mice compared to PMAT+/+ mice [60], however, it is difficult to ascertain the physiological relevance since the concentration(s) of substrate were not reported. Regardless, our in vivo findings suggest that at the serotonin concentrations studied here, serotonin clearance is not different between PMAT+/+ and PMAT−/− mice, indicating that compensatory mechanisms for serotonin clearance might be at play in constitutive PMAT−/− mice. This idea is further supported by PMAT−/− mice displaying normal behavior in a battery of tests, with only subtle differences in anxiety-like and coping behaviors compared to PMAT+/+ mice reported [61].

Importantly, our findings on the effects of ketamine to inhibit serotonin clearance correlated with the ability of ketamine to produce antidepressant-like effects. Ketamine produced robust antidepressant-like effects in wild-type mice, which were lost in SERT−/− and PMAT−/− mice. Antidepressant-like effects of ketamine in mice are consistently reported, yet the conditions under which this is detected varies. Unlike Can et al. [20] we did not find antidepressant-like effects of 10 mg/kg in either the TST or FST. However, this is in keeping with findings of others who have also found this dose to be ineffective in these tests [16,42,62,63]. Although there are some reports of ketamine producing antidepressant-like effects in mice in the TST [62,64], our data support those of others who find the TST insensitive to detecting antidepressant-like effects of ketamine [42]. Importantly, we found that ketamine dose-dependently reduced immobility time in the FST to a magnitude similar to reports of others [16,42,62,63], and this effect was clearly lost in SERT−/− and PMAT−/− mice.

Of course, because ketamine was delivered systemically in these behavioral studies, a role for metabolites of ketamine cannot be ruled out [20,41,46,49]. For example, Zanos and colleagues [41] found that (2R,6R)-hydroxynorketamine (HNK) has antidepressant-like effects similar to those of ketamine, and others found HNK to increase extracellular serotonin similar to ketamine [46,49]. We therefore cannot rule out the possibility that behavioral results from our study are due, at least in part, to HNK. However, data generated from chronoamperometry experiments, where ketamine was locally applied to CA3 region of hippocampus, suggest that the behavioral effects of ketamine were strongly driven by the parent compound, and not by its metabolites. That said, it will be important for future studies to interrogate the role of ketamine's metabolites in inhibition of serotonin clearance in vivo.

While the antidepressant actions of ketamine have been the focus of this study, our results raise the possibility that SERT and/or PMAT might also be mechanisms involved in the addictive properties of ketamine, as well as its anesthetic actions. For example, it is well known that SERT is an important target for drugs of abuse, including psychostimulants such as 3, 4 methylenedioxymethamphetamine (MDMA, Ecstasy), and synthetic cathinones, known as bath salts, which inhibit transport of serotonin and/or cause reverse transport of serotonin via SERT. Ketamine at anesthetic doses is reported to increase serotonin, which may be involved in the psychotic-like symptoms occurring during ketamine emergence [58]. Along these lines, there are numerous other downsides to ketamine, including the possibility of hallucinations and dissociative effects, hypertension, tachycardia, and respiratory depression [58]. Whether SERT and/or PMAT are involved in these actions of ketamine remains unknown. Clearly, the mechanisms contributing to ketamine's effects are complex, given its well-known action at NMDA receptors, its myriad effects on monoamine neurotransmission, and the recently reported dependency of ketamine on the opioid system for its antidepressant properties [65]. The avenues for future research dissecting these mechanisms of action are rich.

In sum, these studies provide evidence for an important role of SERT and PMAT in the serotonin clearance inhibiting and antidepressant actions of ketamine, and pave the way for future studies to understand the seemingly paradoxical loss of these effects in mice lacking either SERT or PMAT.

4. Materials and Methods

4.1. Animals

Naïve adult male SERT+/+, SERT−/−, PMAT+/+, and PMAT−/− mice bred on a C57BL/6 background, or C57BL/6 mice, from our in-house colonies were used for all experiments. Genotype comparisons were made among littermates, bred by +/− intercross to produce all three genotypes within a litter. Mice are backcrossed (+/+ × −/− to yield +/−) every 6th generation. Sex differences in the antidepressant-like effect of ketamine have been previously reported, where female animals were found to be more sensitive [66–68]. For the present studies we selected a dose of ketamine (32 mg/kg) known to produce (near maximal) antidepressant-like effects in males, and used only male mice so as to reduce the number of animals needed for this initial study. However future studies in females will be necessary to determine the generality of present findings. We confirmed that this dose produced robust antidepressant-like effects in our hands by carrying out dose-response studies in wild-type (C57BL/6) mice before commencing studies to compare the antidepressant-like effects of ketamine in SERT+/+, SERT−/−, PMAT +/+, and PMAT −/− mice. Mice were between 3 and 12 months of age for all experiments. Mice were housed in plastic cages (29 cm × 18 cm × 13 cm) containing 7090 Teklad sani-chip bedding (Envigo, East Millstone, NJ) and maintained on a 12/12 hr light/dark cycle (lights on at 7:00 am) in a temperature-controlled (24 °C) vivarium. Mice were weaned at postnatal day 21 and housed with same sex littermates with no more than 5 mice per cage. Mice were given free access to food (Teklad LM-485 mouse/rat sterilizable diet 7012 chow (Envigo, East Millstone, NJ)) and water. All procedures were conducted in accordance with the National Institute of Health Guide for the Care and Use of Laboratory Animals (Institute of Laboratory Animal, Resources, Commission of Life Sciences, National Research Council, https://grants.nih.gov/grants/olaw/Guide-for-the-Care-and-use-of-laboratory-animals.pdf), and with the approval of the Institutional Animal Care and Use Committee, The University of Texas Health Science Center at San Antonio (protocol number: 20020014AR; Originally approved in 2002, current expiration 30 Sept. 2021).

4.2. High-Speed Chronoamperometry

In vivo high-speed chronoamperometry was used to examine transporter efficiency by recording real-time serotonin clearance. Experiments were conducted using methods adapted from Daws and Toney [21,24,69,70]. Carbon fiber electrodes were fabricated based on methods from Gerhardt [71,72] and described in Daws and Toney, and Williams et al. [70,73]. In brief, a single carbon fiber (30 μm diameter) was sealed in fused silica tubing (Schott North America, Elmsford, NY, USA). Nafion coating (5% solution; Sigma-Aldrich, St. Louis, MO, USA) was applied to carbon fiber electrodes to prevent anions in extracellular fluid from coming in contact with the carbon fiber [69,70]. Sensitivity to serotonin and its metabolite 5-hydroxyindoleacetic acid (5-HIAA) were measured by calibrating electrodes to increasing concentrations of serotonin (0.2 to 1.0 μM in 0.2 μM increments) in the presence of 5-HIAA (250 μM). Only those electrodes with a selectivity ratio for serotonin over 5-HIAA greater than 100:1 and a linear response ($r^2 \geq 0.9$) to serotonin were used.

The Nafion-coated carbon fiber electrode was attached to a four-barrel glass micropipette (FHC, Bowdoin, ME, USA) with their tips separated by 200 μm. Barrels of the micropipette were filled with either serotonin (200 μm), ketamine (400 μm), or phosphate-buffered saline (PBS). Note that the concentration of neurotransmitter and drug reaching the recording electrode is estimated to be ~200-fold less than the barrel concentration, based on our routine findings that pressure-ejection of ~20 nL of 200 μM serotonin, 200 μm away from the recording electrode, results in signal amplitudes of ~0.5–1.0 μM [69,70]. Thus, in these experiments, the concentration of ketamine reaching the electrode is estimated to be ~2 μM.

The electrode assembly was lowered into either the CA3 region of the hippocampus (anteroposterior −1.93 and mediolateral +2.0 from bregma; −2.0 from dura; [74]) or nucleus accumbens (anteroposterior +1.36 and mediolateral +1.85 from bregma; −5.0 from dura at 10° angle from midline; [74]) of an anesthetized mouse. Isoflurane (5%) was used to initially anesthetize the mouse and 1.0–1.5% isoflurane was used throughout the experiment to maintain anesthesia. Body temperature was maintained at 36–37 °C by a water circulated heating pad.

FAST-16 system (Quanteon, Nicholasville, KY, USA) was used for the high-speed chronoamperometric recordings. Oxidation potentials consisted of 100 ms pulses of +0.55 V alternated with 900 ms intervals during which the resting potential was maintained at 0 V. The active electrode voltage was applied with respect to a silver chloride reference electrode placed in the contralateral superficial cortex. Oxidation and reduction currents were digitally integrated during the last 80 ms of each 100 ms voltage pulse.

Exogenous serotonin was pressure ejected into the CA3 region of the hippocampus. Once reproducible serotonin signals (~0.5 μM, ~2 pmol in 15 nL) were obtained, ketamine (54 pmol in 136 nl) or an equivalent volume of PBS was pressure ejected locally into the CA3 region of the hippocampus. Following ketamine or PBS pressure ejection, serotonin was pressure ejected every 5 min until serotonin clearance time returned to pre-drug values. The T_{80} time course (time it takes for the signal to decline by 80% of the peak signal amplitude), T_{20}-T_{60} time course (time it takes for the signal to decline by 20–60% of the peak signal amplitude), and peak signal amplitude were analyzed (Figure 1A).

At the completion of the experiment, an electrolytic lesion was made to mark the placement of the electrode tip. Brains were removed, frozen, and stored at −80 °C for histological analysis. Brains were thawed to −18 °C and sliced into 20 μm thick sections and stained with thionin for verification of electrode placement. Two animals were eliminated from the analyses due to electrode placement outside of CA3 region of hippocampus.

4.3. Effects of Isoflurane on Serotonin Clearance

Male C57BL/6 mice were placed into a Plexiglas chamber (25 cm × 10 cm × 10 cm) and 5% isoflurane was applied to the chamber via a precision vaporizer (Protech International Inc., TX, USA). Once completely anesthetized, mice were moved to the stereotaxic frame with their nose placed inside the anesthesia mask. During surgery isoflurane was maintained at 2%, but once the electrode was lowered into the brain isoflurane was set to 1.5% and subsequently maintained at 1.5% or 1.0% for approximately 30 min before the start of the experiment.

During the experiment, mice were administered varying concentrations of isoflurane in a randomized order to examine the effect of isoflurane on serotonin clearance. Each concentration of isoflurane (ranging from 1.0–3.0%, given in 0.5% increments) was administered for 5 min before pressure ejecting serotonin. Five minutes was chosen to allow adequate time for the effects of the new concentration to occur, and to detect any release of endogenous serotonin that may be elicited by isoflurane.

4.4. Tail Suspension Test

Tail suspension test (TST) experiments were performed as described by Steru et al. [75,76]. Mice received either saline, 3.2, 10.0, or 32.0 mg/kg ketamine intraperitoneally (i.p.) one hour prior to testing. These doses of ketamine were chosen based on previous studies examining the antidepressant-like effect of ketamine in mice in the TST [77]. Before testing, an aluminum bar (2 cm x 0.3 cm x 10 cm) was fastened to the tail of the mouse using adhesive tape and was placed at a 90° angle to the longitudinal axis of the tail with 3–4 cm between the base of the tail and the end of the bar. Opposite the tail taped end of the bar was a hole that was used to secure the bar to a hook in the top of a visually isolated box (40 cm × 40 cm × 40 cm). Mice were suspended for six minutes with the ventral surface and front and hind limbs of the mouse facing a digital video camera outside of the box. After the six-minute recording session ended, mice were removed from the bar and returned to their home cage. Moments of immobility were defined by the absence of initiated movement and included passive swaying. Total immobility was recorded by observers blinded to treatment conditions. A mouse was excluded from the study if it climbed its tail for 3 or more seconds. Seven mice were excluded on these grounds, with mice from all genotypes being involved. Mice were randomly assigned to treatment conditions and were tested only once.

4.5. Forced Swim Test

Forced swim test (FST) experiments were performed as described by Lucki [78]. A separate cohort of mice were used in the FST. Mice received either saline or 3.2, 10.0, or 32.0 mg/kg ketamine i.p. 60 min before testing. During testing, mice were confined in transparent cylindrical Plexiglas containers (19 cm diameter, 25.4 cm height, and 15 cm water level) containing water (23–25 °C). The test lasted for 6 min and the entire swim session was recorded. Once the test ended, mice were removed from the water and dried off with paper towels before being placed into a holding cage on a heating pad to aid in drying. Once dry, mice were returned to their home cages. Digital recording cameras were placed above the Plexiglas containers to record the mice from above. This vantage point was used in order to view all four limbs during the test. Moments of swimming and immobility were scored by an observer blinded to treatment. Immobility was defined as absence of active behaviors and remaining passively floating or making minor limb movements to stay afloat. Behaviors during the last four minutes of the swim session were scored [79].

4.6. Locomotor Activity

As ketamine has been shown to affect locomotor activity [80–82], it was important to assess whether ketamine impacted locomotor activity to rule out possible decreases in immobility time being due to ketamine-induced hyperactivity. We examined the effect of 32 mg/kg ketamine on locomotor activity as we found this to be the only dose to significantly reduce immobility time in the FST. None of the doses influenced immobility time in the TST. Locomotor boxes (30 cm × 15 cm × 15 cm), located within sound-attenuating ventilated chambers (MED Associates Inc., St. Albans, VT, USA), were equipped with infrared emitters and receivers (Multi-Varimex, Columbus Instruments, Columbus, OH, USA). Naïve mice received an i.p. injection of either saline or 32.0 mg/kg ketamine and immediately placed into a locomotor box. Locomotor activity of mice was examined for 2 h post injection with locomotion measured as infrared beam breaks per 5 min period.

4.7. Drugs

Ketamine hydrochloride (Sigma-Aldrich, St. Louis, MO, USA) was dissolved in physiologic saline and injected i.p. at doses expressed as salt weight per kilogram of body weight. The injection volume was 10 mL/kg.

4.8. Data Analysis

Data were analyzed using Prism 6.0 (GraphPad, San Diego, CA, USA). Data are expressed as mean ± S.E.M. $p \leq 0.05$ was considered statistically significant for all analyses.

4.8.1. High-Speed Chronoamperometry

For isoflurane studies, effects on pmol amount serotonin delivered to achieve signal amplitudes of ~0.5 µM and on serotonin clearance parameters (T_{20}-T_{60} and T_{80} in seconds) in C57BL/6 mice were analyzed using a one-way ANOVA (isoflurane concentration), with Tukey's post-hoc multiple comparisons. Amount of serotonin pressure-ejected, signal amplitude, and basal time course parameters among SERT and PMAT genotypes were analyzed using a Welch's one-way ANOVA (genotype), as variances were found to differ significantly among groups. Tukey's post-hoc comparisons were made when relevant. Changes in serotonin signal parameters (amplitude, T_{20}-T_{60}, and T_{80}) induced by ketamine or PBS vehicle were expressed as a percent change from pre-drug/vehicle values, and analyzed using a two-way ANOVA (treatment x genotype) followed by Tukey's post-hoc multiple comparisons test. Raw data for pre- and post-drug/vehicle values shown in Table 1 were analyzed by paired t-tests.

4.8.2. Tail Suspension Test and Forced Swim Test

The dose-dependency of ketamine's antidepressant-like effects was first examined in C57BL/6 mice using the TST and FST. Dose-response data were analyzed using a one-way ANOVA (dose) followed by Tukey's post hoc multiple comparisons test. Since there were no significant effects of ketamine (at any dose) in the TST, the antidepressant-like effect of ketamine in SERT+/+, SERT−/−, PMAT+/+, and PMAT−/− mice was examined using the FST. The antidepressant-like effect of the highest dose of ketamine (32 mg/kg) was compared with saline across the different genotypes using a two-way ANOVA (treatment x genotype) followed by Tukey's post hoc multiple comparisons test.

4.8.3. Locomotor Activity

Locomotor activity was assessed following saline or 32 mg/kg ketamine injection across all genotypes of mice (SERT+/+, SERT−/−, PMAT+/+, and PMAT−/−) using two-way ANOVA (treatment x genotype) followed by Tukey's multiple comparisons test.

5. Conclusions

At "therapeutically" relevant concentrations in mice, ketamine inhibited serotonin clearance and produced antidepressant-like effects in wild-type mice, but not in SERT−/− and PMAT−/− mice. Taken together with existing literature [15–19,45,47–50], a critical role for serotonin and its inhibition of uptake via SERT and PMAT cannot be ruled out as important contributing factors to ketamine's antidepressant mechanism of action. These findings pave the way for future experiments to interrogate the role, and mechanism of action, of SERT and PMAT in the antidepressant actions of ketamine, which will add to literature suggesting that concurrent blockade of SERT and "uptake-2" transporters, such as PMAT, has greater antidepressant efficacy than SSRIs alone [21,23,24]. Combined with what is already known about ketamine's action at NMDA receptors, these studies will help lead the way to development of drugs that lack ketamine's abuse potential but have superior efficacy in treating depression.

Author Contributions: Conceptualization, M.A.B., and L.C.D.; methodology, M.A.B., and L.C.D.; validation, M.A.B., M.V., and K.M.C.; formal analysis, M.A.B., W.K., and L.C.D.; investigation, M.A.B., M.V., and K.M.C.; resources, L.C.D.; data curation, M.A.B.; writing—original draft preparation, M.A.B.; writing—review and editing, L.C.D., W.K.; visualization, M.A.B., and L.C.D.; supervision, L.C.D.; project administration, M.A.B.; funding acquisition, L.C.D. All authors have read and agreed to the published version of the manuscript.

Funding: This research was funded by National Institutes of Health, grant numbers R01MH093320 and R01 MH106978.

Acknowledgments: We are grateful to Joanne Wang, University of Washington, School of Pharmacy, Department of Pharmaceutics, Seattle, WA, for providing us with PMAT knockout mice. We are thankful to the late Dennis Murphy, National Institutes of Mental Health, for providing us with founders to begin our colony of SERT knockout mice. We thank T. Lee Gilman, for her contributions to studies of serotonin clearance in nucleus accumbens of PMAT wild-type and knockout mice.

Conflicts of Interest: The authors declare no conflict of interest.

Abbreviations

+/+	Wild-type
−/−	Knockout
[^{11}C]DASB	[^{11}C]-3-amino-4-(2-dimethylaminomethyl-phenylsulfanyl)benzonitrile
5-HIAA	5-hydroxyindoleacetic acid
ANOVA	Analysis of variance
BDNF	Brain derived neurotrophic factor
DAT	Dopamine transporter
FST	Forced swim test
HNK	(2R,6R)-hydroxynorketamine
NMDA	N-methyl-D-aspartate
NAcc	Nucleus accumbens
NET	Norepinephrine transporter
OCT1	Organic cation transporter 1
OCT2	Organic cation transporter 2
OCT3	Organic cation transporter 3
PBS	Phosphate buffered saline
PCA	p-Chloroamphetamine
PCPA	Parachlorophenylalanine
PET	Positron emission tomography
PMAT	Plasma membrane monoamine transporter
SERT	Serotonin transporter
SSRI	Selective serotonin reuptake inhibitor
TST	Tail suspension test

References

1. Center for Behavioral Health Statistics and Quality. Key Substance Use and Mental Health Indicators in the United States: Results from the 2015 National Survey on Drug Use and Health 2016, HHS Publication No. SMA 16-4984, NSDUH Series H-51. Available online: http://www.samhsa.gov/data (accessed on 28 April 2020).
2. Mathys, M.; Mitchell, B.G. Targeting treatment-resistant depression. *J. Pharm. Pract.* **2011**, *24*, 520–533. [CrossRef] [PubMed]
3. McIntyre, R.S.; Filteau, M.-J.; Martin, L.; Patry, S.; Carvalho, A.; Cha, D.S.; Barakat, M.; Miguelez, M. Treatment-resistant depression: Definitions, review of the evidence, and algorithmic approach. *J. Affect. Disord.* **2014**, *156*, 1–7. [CrossRef] [PubMed]
4. Mathew, S.J.; Shah, A.; Lapidus, K.; Clark, C.; Jarun, N.; Ostermeyer, B.; Murrough, J.W. Ketamine for treatment-resistant unipolar depression. *CNS Drugs* **2012**, *26*, 189–204. [CrossRef] [PubMed]

5. Mathews, D.C.; Henter, I.D.; Zarate, C.A., Jr. Targeting the glutamatergic system to treat major depressive disorder. *Drugs* **2012**, *72*, 1313–1333. [CrossRef] [PubMed]
6. Monteggia, L.M.; Zarate, C., Jr. Antidepressant actions of ketamine: From molecular mechanisms to clinical practice. *Curr. Opin. Neurol.* **2015**, *30*, 139–143. [CrossRef]
7. U.S. Food and Drug Administration. FDA Approves New Nasal Spray Medication for Treatment-Resistant Depression; Available Only at Certified Doctor's Office or Clinic [Press Release] 2019. Available online: https://www.fda.gov/news-events/press-announcements/fda-approves-new-nasal-spray-medication-treatment-resistant-depression-available-only-certified (accessed on 28 April 2020).
8. Kavalali, E.T.; Monteggia, L.M. Targeting homeostatic synaptic plasticity for treatment of mood disorders. *Neuron* **2020**, *106*, 715–726. [CrossRef]
9. Autry, A.E.; Adachi, M.; Nosyreva, E.; Na, E.S.; Los, M.F.; Cheng, P.-F.; Kavalali, E.T.; Monteggia, L.M. NMDA receptor blockade at rest triggers rapid behavioural antidepressant responses. *Nature* **2011**, *475*, 91–97. [CrossRef]
10. Li, N.; Lee, B.; Liu, R.-J.; Banasr, M.; Dwyer, J.M.; Iwata, M.; Li, X.-Y.; Aghajanian, G.; Duman, R.S. mTOR-dependent synapse formation underlies the rapid antidepressant effects of NMDA antagonists. *Science* **2010**, *329*, 959–964. [CrossRef]
11. Angoa-Pérez, M.; Kane, M.J.; Briggs, D.I.; Herrera-Mundo, N.; Sykes, C.E.; Francescutti, D.M.; Kuhn, D.M. Mice genetically depleted of brain serotonin do not display a depression-like behavioral phenotype. *ACS Chem. Neurosci.* **2014**, *5*, 908–919. [CrossRef]
12. Lucki, I. The spectrum of behaviors influenced by serotonin. *Biol. Psychiatry* **1998**, *44*, 151–162. [CrossRef]
13. Lindefors, N.; Barati, S.; O'Connor, W.T. Differential effects of single and repeated ketamine administration on dopamine, serotonin, and GABA transmission in rat medial prefrontal cortex. *Brain Res.* **2014**, *759*, 205–212. [CrossRef]
14. Iravani, M.M.; Muscat, R.; Kruk, Z.L. MK-801 interaction with the 5-HT transporter: A real-time study in brain slices using fast cyclic voltammetry. *Synapse* **1999**, *32*, 212–224. [CrossRef]
15. Amargós-Bosch, M.; Lopez-Gil, X.; Artigas, F.; Adell, A. Clozapine and olanzapine, but not haloperidol, suppress serotonin efflux in the medial prefrontal cortex elicited by phencyclidine and ketamine. *Int. J. Neuropsychopharmacol.* **2006**, *9*, 565–573. [CrossRef] [PubMed]
16. Fukumoto, K.; Iijima, M.; Chaki, S. The antidepressant effects of an mGlu2/3 receptor antagonist and ketamine require AMPA receptor stimulation in the mPFC and subsequent activation of the 5-HT neurons in the DRN. *Neuropsychopharmacology* **2016**, *41*, 1046–1056. [CrossRef]
17. Gigliucci, V.; O'Dowd, G.; Casey, S.; Egan, D.; Gibney, S.; Harkin, A. Ketamine elicits sustained antidepressant-like activity via a serotonin-dependent mechanism. *Psychopharmacology* **2013**, *228*, 157–166. [CrossRef]
18. Pham, T.H.; Mendez-David, I.; Defaix, C.; Guiard, B.P.; Tritschler, L.; David, D.J.; Gardier, A.M. Ketamine treatment involves medial prefrontal cortex serotonin to induce a rapid antidepressant-like activity in BALB/cJ mice. *Neuropharmacology* **2017**, *112*, 198–209. [CrossRef]
19. Gaarn du Jardin, K.; Liebenberg, N.; Müller, H.K.; Elfving, B.; Sanchez, C.; Wegener, G. Differential interaction with the serotonin system by S-ketamine, vortioxetine, and fluoxetine in a genetic rat model of depression. *Psychopharmacology* **2016**, *233*, 2813–2825. [CrossRef]
20. Can, A.; Zanos, P.; Moaddel, R.; Kang, H.J.; Dossou, K.S.S.; Wainer, I.W.; Cheer, J.F.; Frost, D.O.; Huang, X.-P.; Gould, T.D. Effects of ketamine and ketamine metabolites on evoked striatal dopamine release, dopamine receptors, and monoamine transporters. *J. Pharmacol. Exp. Ther.* **2016**, *359*, 159–170. [CrossRef]
21. Baganz, N.L.; Horton, R.E.; Calderon, A.S.; Owens, W.A.; Munn, J.L.; Watts, L.T.; Koldzic-Zivanovic, N.; Jeske, N.A.; Koek, W.; Toney, G.M.; et al. Organic cation transporter 3: Keeping the brake on extracellular serotonin in serotonin-transporter-deficient mice. *Proc. Natl. Acad. Sci. USA* **2008**, *105*, 18976–18981. [CrossRef]
22. Baganz, N.; Horton, R.; Martin, K.; Holmes, A.; Daws, L.C. Repeated swim impairs serotonin clearance via a corticosterone-sensitive mechanism: Organic cation transporter 3, the smoking gun. *J. Neurosci.* **2010**, *30*, 15185–15195. [CrossRef]
23. Daws, L.C. Unfaithful neurotransmitter transporters: Focus on serotonin uptake and implications for antidepressant efficacy. *Pharmacol. Ther.* **2009**, *121*, 89–99. [CrossRef] [PubMed]

24. Horton, R.E.; Apple, D.M.; Owens, W.A.; Baganz, N.L.; Cano, S.; Mitchell, N.C.; Vitela, M.; Gould, G.G.; Koek, W.; Daws, L.C. Decynium-22 enhances SSRI-induced antidepressant-like effects in mice: Uncovering novel targets to treat depression. *J. Neurosci.* **2013**, *33*, 10534–10543. [CrossRef]
25. Zhou, M.; Engel, K.; Wang, J. Evidence for significant contribution of a newly identified monoamine transporter (PMAT) to serotonin uptake in the human brain. *Biochem. Pharmacol.* **2007**, *73*, 147–154. [CrossRef] [PubMed]
26. Campbell, S.; MacQueen, G. The role of the hippocampus in the pathophysiology of major depression. *J. Psychiatry Neurosci.* **2004**, *29*, 417–426.
27. Bowman, M.A.; Daws, L.C. Targeting serotonin transporters in the treatment of juvenile and adolescent depression. *Front. Neurosci.* **2019**, *13*. [CrossRef] [PubMed]
28. Cryan, J.F.; Holmes, A. The ascent of mouse: Advances in modeling human depression and anxiety. *Nat. Rev. Drug Discov.* **2005**, *4*, 775–790. [CrossRef]
29. Garris, P.A.; Budygin, E.A.; Phillips, P.E.M.; Venton, B.J.; Robinson, D.L.; Bergstrom, B.P.; Rebec, G.V.; Wightman, R.M. A role for presynaptic mechanisms in the actions of nomifensine and haloperidol. *Neuroscience* **2003**, *118*, 819–829. [CrossRef]
30. Sabeti, J.; Gerhardt, G.A.; Zahniser, N.R. Chloral hydrate and ethanol, but not urethane, alter the clearance of exogenous dopamine recorded by chronoamperometry in striatum of unrestrained rats. *Neurosci. Lett.* **2003**, *343*, 9–12. [CrossRef]
31. Brodnik, Z.D.; España, R.A. Dopamine uptake dynamics are preserved under isoflurane anesthesia. *Neurosci. Lett.* **2015**, *606*, 129–134. [CrossRef]
32. Johansen, S.L.; Iceman, K.E.; Iceman, C.R.; Taylor, B.E.; Harris, M.B. Isoflurane causes concentration-dependent inhibition of medullary raphe 5-HT neurons in situ. *Auton. Neurosci.* **2015**, *193*, 51–56. [CrossRef]
33. Martin, D.C.; Adams, D.J.; Aronstam, R.S. The influence of isoflurane on the synaptic activity of 5-Hydroxytryptamine. *Neurochem. Res.* **1990**, *15*, 969–973. [CrossRef]
34. Mukaida, K.; Shichino, T.; Koyanagi, S.; Himukashi, S.; Fukuda, K. Activity of the serotonergic system during isoflurane anesthesia. *Anesth. Analg.* **2007**, *104*, 836–839. [CrossRef]
35. Whittington, R.A.; Virág, L. Isoflurane decreases extracellular serotonin in the mouse hippocampus. *Anesth. Analg.* **2006**, *103*, 92–98. [CrossRef] [PubMed]
36. Daws, L.C.; Montañez, S.; Munn, J.L.; Owens, W.A.; Baganz, B.L.; Boyce-Rustay, J.M.; Millstein, R.A.; Wiedholz, L.M.; Murphy, D.L.; Holmes, A. Ethanol inhibits clearance of brain serotonin by a serotonin transporter-independent mechanism. *J. Neurosci.* **2006**, *26*, 6431–6438. [CrossRef] [PubMed]
37. Montañez, S.; Owens, W.A.; Gould, G.G.; Murphy, D.L.; Daws, L.C. Exaggerated effect of fluvoxamine in heterozygote serotonin transporter knockout mice. *J. Neurochem.* **2003**, *86*, 210–219. [CrossRef] [PubMed]
38. Hsu, J.C. Multiple Comparisons. In *Theory and Methods*; Chapman & Hall/CRC: Boca Raton, FL, USA, 1996.
39. Maxwell, S.E.; Delaney, H.D.; Kelley, K. Designing Experiments and Analyzing Data. In *A Model Comparison Perspective*, 3rd ed.; Routledge: New York, NY, USA, 2018.
40. Fukumoto, K.; Iijima, M.; Chaki, S. Serotonin-1A receptor stimulation mediates effects of a metabotropic glutamate 2/3 receptor antagonist, 2S-2-amino-2-(1S,2S-2-carboxycycloprop-1-yl)-3-(xanth-9-yl) propanoic acid (LY341495), and an N-methyl-D-aspartate receptor antagonist, ketamine, in the novelty-suppressed feeding test. *Psychopharmacology* **2014**. [CrossRef]
41. Zanos, P.; Moaddel, R.; Morris, P.J.; Georgiou, P.; Fischell, J.; Elmer, G.I.; Alkondon, M.; Yuan, P.; Pribut, H.J.; Singh, N.S.; et al. NMDAR inhibition-independent antidepressant actions of ketamine metabolites. *Nature* **2016**, *533*, 481–486. [CrossRef] [PubMed]
42. Popik, P.; Kos, T.; Sow-Kucma, M.; Nowak, G. Lack of persistent effects of ketamine in rodent models of depression. *Psychopharmacology* **2008**, *198*, 421–430. [CrossRef]
43. Polis, A.J.; Fitzgerald, P.J.; Hale, P.J.; Watson, B.O. Rodent ketamine depression-related research: Finding patterns in a literature of variability. *Behav. Brain Res.* **2019**, *376*, 112153. [CrossRef]
44. Cryan, J.F.; Valentino, R.J.; Lucki, I. Assessing substrates underlying the behavioral effects of antidepressants using the modified rat forced swimming test. *Neurosci. Biobehav. Rev.* **2005**, *29*, 547–569. [CrossRef]
45. Bogdanova, O.V.; Kanekar, S.; D'Anci, K.E.; Renshaw, P.F. Factors influencing behavior in the forced swim test. *Physiol. Behav.* **2013**, *118*, 227–239. [CrossRef] [PubMed]
46. Ago, Y.; Tanabe, W.; Higuchi, M.; Tsukada, S.; Tanaka, T.; Yamaguchi, T.; Igarashi, H.; Yokoyama, R.; Seiriki, K.; Kasai, A.; et al. (R)-ketamine induces a greater increase in prefrontal 5-HT release

than (S)-ketamine and ketamine metabolites via an AMPA receptor-independent mechanism. *Int. J. Neuropsychopharmacol.* **2019**, *22*, 665–674. [CrossRef] [PubMed]

47. Kinoshita, H.; Nishitani, N.; Nagai, Y.; Andoh, C.; Asaoka, N.; Kawai, H.; Shibui, N.; Nagayasu, K.; Shirakawa, H.; Nakagawa, T.; et al. Ketamine-induced prefrontal serotonin release is mediated by cholinergic neurons in the pedunculopontine tegmental nucleus. *Int. J. Neuropharmacol.* **2018**, *21*, 305–310. [CrossRef] [PubMed]

48. López-Gil, X.; Jiménez-Sánchez, L.; Campa, L.; Castro, E.; Frago, C.; Adell, A. Role of serotonin and noradrenaline in the rapid antidepressant action of ketamine. *ACS Chem. Neurosci.* **2019**, *10*, 3318–3326. [CrossRef]

49. Pham, T.H.; Defaix, C.; Xu, X.; Deng, S.-X.; Fabresse, N.; Alvarez, J.-C.; Landry, D.W.; Brachman, R.A.; Denny, C.A.; Gardier, A.M. Common neurotransmission recruited in (R,S)-ketamine and (2R,2S)-hydroxynorketamine-induced sustained antidepressant-like effects. *Biol. Psychiatry* **2018**, *84*, e3–e6. [CrossRef]

50. Yamamoto, S.; Ohba, H.; Nishiyama, S.; Harada, N.; Kakiuchi, T.; Tsukada, H.; Domino, E.F. Subanesthetic doses of ketamine transiently decrease serotonin transporter activity: A PET study in conscious monkeys. *Neuropsychopharmacology* **2013**, *38*, 2666–2674. [CrossRef]

51. Azzaro, A.J.; Smith, D.J. The inhibitory action of ketamine hcl on [^{3}H]5-hydroxytryptamine accumulation by rat brain synaptosomal-rich fractions: Comparison with [^{3}H]catecholamine and [^{3}H]gamma-aminobutyric acid uptake. *Neuropharmacology* **1977**, *16*, 349–356. [CrossRef]

52. Nishimura, M.; Sato, K.; Okada, T.; Yoshiya, I.; Schloss, P.; Shimada, S.; Tohyama, M. Ketamine inhibits monoamine transporters expressed in human embryonic kidney 293 cells. *Anesthesiology* **1998**, *88*, 768–774. [CrossRef]

53. Barann, M.; Stamer, U.M.; Lyutenska, M.; Stüber Bönisch, H.; Urban, B. Effects of opioids on human serotonin transporters. *Naunyn-Schmiedeberg's Arch. Pharmacol.* **2015**, *388*, 43–49. [CrossRef]

54. Martin, L.L.; Bouchal, R.L.; Smith, D.J. Ketamine inhibits serotonin uptake in vivo. *Neuropharmacology* **1982**, *21*, 113–118. [CrossRef]

55. Idvall, J.; Ahlgren, I.; Aronsen, K.R.; Stenberg, P. Ketamine infusions: Pharmacokinetics and clinical effects. *Br. J. Anesth.* **1979**, *51*, 1167–1173. [CrossRef]

56. Zarate, C.A., Jr.; Brutsche, N.E.; Ibrahim, L.; Franco-Chaves, J.; Diazgranados, N.; Cravchik, A.; Selter, J.; Marquardt, C.A.; Liberty, V.; Luckenbaugh, D.A. Replication of ketamine's antidepressant efficacy in bipolar depression: A randomized controlled add-on trial. *Biol. Psychiatry* **2012**, *71*, 939–946. [CrossRef] [PubMed]

57. Loo, C.K.; Gálvez, V.; O'Keefe, E.; Mitchell, P.B.; Hadzi-Pavlovic, D.; Leyden, J.; Harper, S.; Somogyi, A.A.; Lai, R.; Weickert, C.S.; et al. Placebo-controlled pilot trial testing dose titration and intravenous, intramuscular and subcutaneous routes for ketamine in depression. *Acta Psychiatr. Scand.* **2016**, *134*, 48–56. [CrossRef]

58. Zanos, P.; Moaddel, R.; Morris, P.J.; Riggs, L.M.; Highland, J.N.; Georgiou, P.; Pereira, E.F.R.; Albuquerque, E.X.; Thomas, C.J.; Zarate, C.A., Jr.; et al. Ketamine and ketamine metabolite pharmacology: Insights into therapeutic mechanisms. *Pharmacol. Rev.* **2018**, *70*, 621–660. [CrossRef] [PubMed]

59. Spies, M.; James, G.M.; Berroterán-Infante Ibeschitz, H.; Kranz, G.S.; Unterholzner, J.; Godbersen, M.; Gryglewski, G.; Hienert, M.; Jungwirth, J.; Pichler, V.; et al. Assessment of ketamine binding of the serotonin transporter in humans with positron emission tomography. *Int. J. Neuropharmacol.* **2018**, *21*, 145–153. [CrossRef] [PubMed]

60. Duan, H.; Wang, J. Impaired monoamine and organic cation uptake in choroid plexus in mice with targeted disruption of the plasma membrane monoamine transporter (Slc29a4) gene. *J. Biol. Chem.* **2013**, *288*, 3535–3544. [CrossRef]

61. Gilman, T.L.; George, C.M.; Vitela, M.; Herrera-Rosales, M.; Basiouny, M.S.; Koek, W.; Daws, L.C. Constitutive plasma membrane monoamine transporter (PMAT, Slc29a4) deficiency subtly affects anxiety-like and coping behaviours. *Eur. J. Neurosci.* **2018**, *48*, 1706–1716. [CrossRef]

62. Fukumoto, K.; Toki, H.; Iijima, M.; Hashihayata, T.; Yamaguchi, J.-I.; Hashimoto, K.; Chaki, S. Antidepressant potential of (R)-ketamine in rodent models: Comparison with (S)-ketamine. *J. Pharmacol. Exper. Ther.* **2017**, *361*, 9–16. [CrossRef]

63. Lindholm, J.S.O.; Autio, H.; Vesa, L.; Antila, H.; Lindemann, L.; Hoener, M.C.; Skolnick, P.; Rantamaki, T.; Castren, E. The antidepressant-like effects of glutamatergic drugs ketamine and AMPA receptor potentiator LY 451646 are preserved in *bdnf+/-* heterozygous null mice. *Neuropharmacology* **2012**, *62*, 391–397. [CrossRef]

64. Yamaguchi, J.I.; Toki, H.; Qu, Y.; Yang, C.; Koike, H.; Hashimoto, K.; Mizuno-Yasuhira, A.; Chaki, S. (2R,6R)-Hydroxynorketamine is not essential for the antidepressant actions of (R)-ketamine in mice. *Neuropsychopharmacology* **2018**, *43*, 1900–1907. [CrossRef]
65. Klein, M.E.; Chandra, J.; Sheriff, S.; Malinow, R. Opioid system is necessary but not sufficient for antidepressive actions of ketamine in rodents. *Proc. Natl. Acad. Sci. USA* **2020**, *117*, 2656–2662. [CrossRef] [PubMed]
66. Carrier, N.; Kabbaj, M. Sex differences in the antidepressant-like effects of ketamine. *Neuropharmacology* **2013**, *70*, 27–34. [CrossRef] [PubMed]
67. Franceschelli, A.; Sens, J.; Herchick, S.; Thelen, C.; Pitychoutis, M. Sex differences in the rapid and the sustained antidepressant-like effects of ketamine in stress-naïve and "depressed" mice exposed to chronic mild stress. *Neuroscience* **2015**, *290*, 49–60. [CrossRef] [PubMed]
68. Thelen, C.; Sens, J.; Mauch, J.; Pandit, R.; Pitychoutis, P.M. Repeated ketamine treatment induces sex-specific behavioral and neurochemical effects in mice. *Behav. Brain Res.* **2016**, *312*, 305–312. [CrossRef] [PubMed]
69. Daws, L.C.; Owens, W.A.; Toney, G.M. High-speed chronoamperometry to measure biogenic amine release and uptake in vivo. In *Neurotransmitter Transporters–Investigate Methods*; Sitte, H., Bonisch, H., Eds.; Humana Press: Totowa, NJ, USA, 2016; pp. 53–81.
70. Daws, L.C.; Toney, G.M. High-speed chronoamperometry to study kinetics and mechanisms for serotonin clearance in vivo. In *Electrochemical Methods for Neuroscience*; Michael, A.C., Borland, L.M., Eds.; CRC Press/Taylor & Francis: Boca Raton, FL, USA, 2007.
71. Gerhardt, G.A. Rapid chronocoulometric measurements of norepinephrine overflow and clearance in CNS tissues. In *Voltammetric Methods in Brain Systems, Neuromethods*; Boulton, A.A., Baker, G.B., Adams, R.N., Eds.; Humana Press: Totowa, NJ, USA, 1995; Volume 27. [CrossRef]
72. Perez, X.A.; Andrews, A.M. Chronoamperometry to determine differential reductions in uptake in brain synaptosomes from serotonin transporter knockout mice. *Anal. Chem.* **2005**, *77*, 818–826. [CrossRef]
73. Williams, J.M.; Owens, W.A.; Turner, G.H.; Saunders, C.; Dipace, C.; Blakely, R.D.; France, C.P.; Gore, J.C.; Daws, L.C.; Avison, M.J.; et al. Hypoinsulinemia regulates amphetamine-induced reverse transport of dopamine. *PLoS Biol.* **2007**, *5*, e274. [CrossRef]
74. Franklin, K.B.J.; Paxinos, G. *The Mouse Brain in Stereotaxic Coordinates*; Academic: Syndey, Australia, 1997.
75. Steru, L.; Chermat, R.; Thierry, B.; Simon, P. The tail suspension test: A new method for screening antidepressants in mice. *Psychopharmacology* **1985**, *85*, 367–370. [CrossRef]
76. Castagné, V.; Moser, P.; Roux, S.; Porsolt, R.D. Rodent models of depression: Forced swim and tail suspension behavioral despair tests in rats and mice. *Curr. Protoc. Neurosci.* **2011**, *8*. [CrossRef]
77. Koike, H.; Iijima, M.; Chaki, S. Involvement of AMPA receptor in both the rapid and sustained antidepressant-like effects of ketamine in animal models of depression. *Behav. Brain Res.* **2011**, *224*, 107–111. [CrossRef]
78. Lucki, I. The forced swimming test as a model for core and component behavioral effects of antidepressant drugs. *Behav. Pharmacol.* **1997**, *8*, 523–532. [CrossRef]
79. Lucki, I.; Dalvi, A.; Mayorga, A.J. Sensitivity to the effects of pharmacologically selective antidepressants in different strains of mice. *Psychopharmacology* **2001**, *155*, 315–322. [CrossRef]
80. Imre, G.; Fokkema, D.S.; Den Boer, J.A.; Ter Horst, G.J. Dose-response characteristics of ketamine effect on locomotion, cognitive function and central neuronal activity. *Brain Res. Bull.* **2005**, *69*, 338–345. [CrossRef] [PubMed]
81. Trujillo, K.A.; Zamora, J.J.; Warmoth, K.P. Increased response to ketamine following treatment at long intervals: Implications for intermittent use. *Biol. Psychiatry* **2008**, *63*, 178–183. [CrossRef] [PubMed]
82. Parise, E.M.; Alcantara, L.F.; Warren, B.L.; Wright, K.N.; Hadad, R.; Sial, O.K.; Kroeck, K.G.; Iñiguez, S.D.; Bolaños-Guzmán, C.A. Repeated ketamine exposure induces an enduring resilient phenotype in adolescent and adult rats. *Biol. Psychiatry* **2013**, *74*, 750–759. [CrossRef] [PubMed]

Publisher's Note: MDPI stays neutral with regard to jurisdictional claims in published maps and institutional affiliations.

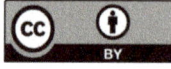

© 2020 by the authors. Licensee MDPI, Basel, Switzerland. This article is an open access article distributed under the terms and conditions of the Creative Commons Attribution (CC BY) license (http://creativecommons.org/licenses/by/4.0/).

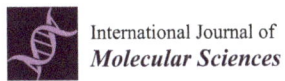

Article

PPAR-α Deletion Attenuates Cisplatin Nephrotoxicity by Modulating Renal Organic Transporters MATE-1 and OCT-2

Leandro Ceotto Freitas-Lima [1], Alexandre Budu [1], Adriano Cleis Arruda [1,2], Mauro Sérgio Perilhão [1,2], Jonatan Barrera-Chimal [3,4], Ronaldo Carvalho Araujo [1,2] and Gabriel Rufino Estrela [2,5,*]

[1] Departamento de Biofísica, Universidade Federal de São Paulo, Sao Paulo 04039032, Brazil; lcf.lima@gmail.com (L.C.F.-L.); alexandre.budu@unifesp.br (A.B.); arruda_adriano@hotmail.com (A.C.A.); maurospersonal3@gmail.com (M.S.P.); araujo.ronaldo@unifesp.br (R.C.A.)
[2] Departamento de Medicina, Disciplina de Nefrologia, Universidade Federal de São Paulo, São Paulo 04039032, Brazil
[3] Instituto de Investigaciones Biomédicas, Universidad Nacional Autónoma de México, Mexico City 04510, Mexico; jbarrera@biomedicas.unam.mx
[4] Unidad de Investigación UNAM-INC, Instituto Nacional de Cardiología Ignacio Chávez, Mexico City 14080, Mexico
[5] Departamento de Oncologia Clínica e Experimental, Disciplina de Hematologia e Hematoterapia, Universidade Federal de São Paulo, São Paulo 04037002, Brazil
* Correspondence: g.estrela@unifesp.br; Tel.: +55-11-5576-4859

Received: 10 August 2020; Accepted: 25 September 2020; Published: 8 October 2020

Abstract: Cisplatin is a chemotherapy drug widely used in the treatment of solid tumors. However, nephrotoxicity has been reported in about one-third of patients undergoing cisplatin therapy. Proximal tubules are the main target of cisplatin toxicity and cellular uptake; elimination of this drug can modulate renal damage. Organic transporters play an important role in the transport of cisplatin into the kidney and organic cations transporter 2 (OCT-2) has been shown to be one of the most important transporters to play this role. On the other hand, multidrug and toxin extrusion 1 (MATE-1) transporter is the main protein that mediates the extrusion of cisplatin into the urine. Cisplatin nephrotoxicity has been shown to be enhanced by increased OCT-2 and/or reduced MATE-1 activity. Peroxisome proliferator-activated receptor alpha (PPAR-α) is the transcription factor which controls lipid metabolism and glucose homeostasis; it is highly expressed in the kidneys and interacts with both MATE-1 and OCT-2. Considering the above, we treated wild-type and PPAR-α knockout mice with cisplatin in order to evaluate the severity of nephrotoxicity. Cisplatin induced renal dysfunction, renal inflammation, apoptosis and tubular injury in wild-type mice, whereas PPAR-α deletion protected against these alterations. Moreover, we observed that cisplatin induced down-regulation of organic transporters MATE-1 and OCT-2 and that PPAR-α deletion restored the expression of these transporters. In addition, PPAR-α knockout mice at basal state showed increased MATE-1 expression and reduced OCT-2 levels. Here, we show for the first time that PPAR-α deletion protects against cisplatin nephrotoxicity and that this protection is via modulation of the organic transporters MATE-1 and OCT-2.

Keywords: cisplatin nephrotoxicity; PPAR-alpha; organic transporters

1. Introduction

Cisplatin is a very effective drug against solid tumors. However, severe side effects have been reported [1,2]. Cisplatin-induced nephrotoxicity, which is usually dose-dependent, affects about one-third of patients undergoing cisplatin treatment [1,2]. Some animal studies have shown that cisplatin accumulates in the kidney more than in other organs [3–5]. It affects the proximal tubules of the kidneys by different mechanisms, such as oxidative stress, inflammation, DNA damage and apoptosis [1,2]. The initial step for cisplatin nephrotoxicity is entering the cells; some authors have suggested that the cellular uptake of cisplatin is mediated, in part, by transport proteins [6,7]. Thus, organic cation transporters (OCTs) play a role in cisplatin transport into the kidneys [8]. OCTs are located at basolateral membranes and are highly expressed in the kidneys [8,9]. Cisplatin interacts preferably with OCT-2 [10], and the inhibition or deletion of OCT-2 attenuates cisplatin nephrotoxicity [11–13]. Multidrug and toxin extrusion 1 (MATE-1) transporter is a protein involved in cisplatin secretion into the urine, which is localized at apical membrane [14,15]. MATE-1 deletion in mice exacerbates cisplatin nephrotoxicity [16], whereas increased MATE-1 expression decreases platinum accumulation in renal cells after cisplatin treatment [17]. Peroxisome proliferator-activated receptor alpha (PPAR-α) is a transcription factor that controls fatty acid oxidation and glucose homeostasis, and it is highly expressed in the liver and kidneys [18,19]. Our group recently showed that PPAR-α interacts with both *MATE-1* and *OCT-2* [20]. Considering that the modulation of organic transporters is an important mechanism to either increase or attenuate cisplatin nephrotoxicity, we investigated the effect of PPAR-α deletion on cisplatin nephrotoxicity severity and whether these effects are mediated by modulation of organic transporters.

2. Results

2.1. PPAR-α Deletion Attenuates Cisplatin-Induced Renal Injury

We treated C57BL6 and PPAR-α-deficient mice with a single dose of cisplatin (20 mg/kp i.p). Ninety-six hours after cisplatin (CP) treatment, the wild-type mice showed increased serum creatinine and urea levels, while PPAR-α knockout mice (CP PPARKO) avoided the increase of these parameters (Table 1. Moreover, real-time PCR was performed in the kidney to assess renal injury markers. Cisplatin treatment (CP) upregulated the mRNA levels of NGAL and KIM-1 and PPAR-α ablation (CP PPARKO) attenuated the upregulation of these molecules (Table 1).

Table 1. Effects of peroxisome proliferator-activated receptor alpha (PPAR-α) deletion on renal injury and function.

Title	VEH	CP	CP PPARKO
Parameters	Mean ± SEM	Mean ± SEM	Mean ± SEM
Creatinine (mg/dL)	0.591 ± 0.023	3.639 ± 0.611 ***	0.853 ± 0.063 ###
Urea (mg/dL)	62.62 ± 1.512	575.6 ± 48.39 ***	109.4 ± 17.50 ###
NGAL mRNA expression	1.105 ± 0.235	308.1 ± 55.39 ***	71.04 ± 24.56 ##
KIM-1 mRNA expression	1.160 ± 0.311	732.8 ± 88.50 **	163.2 ± 54.69 #

Data are presented as mean ± SEM. ** $p < 0.01$, *** $p < 0.001$. compared to the VEH group. # $p < 0.05$; ## $p < 0.01$; ### $p < 0.001$. compared to the CP group.

2.2. PPAR-α Deletion Blunts Renal Expression of Inflammatory and Apoptosis-Related Genes

Several studies have evidenced that inflammation contributes to cisplatin-induced nephrotoxicity [1,2]. Proinflammatory cytokines are produced mainly by activated macrophages and are tightly involved in augmenting inflammatory reactions [21]. CP exponentially increased renal expression of *TNF-α*, *IL-1β* and *IL-6*, while CP PPARKO blunted these increases (Figure 1A–C). Cisplatin-induced renal cell death involves several pathways, including apoptosis. We performed qPCR for *TNFR-2*, which is related to apoptosis extrinsic pathway and *Bax/Bcl-2*, which is related to apoptosis intrinsic pathway. CP upregulated *TNFR-2* and *Bax/Bcl-2* in renal tissue and CP PPARKO avoided the upregulation of these apoptosis-related genes (Figure 1D–E).

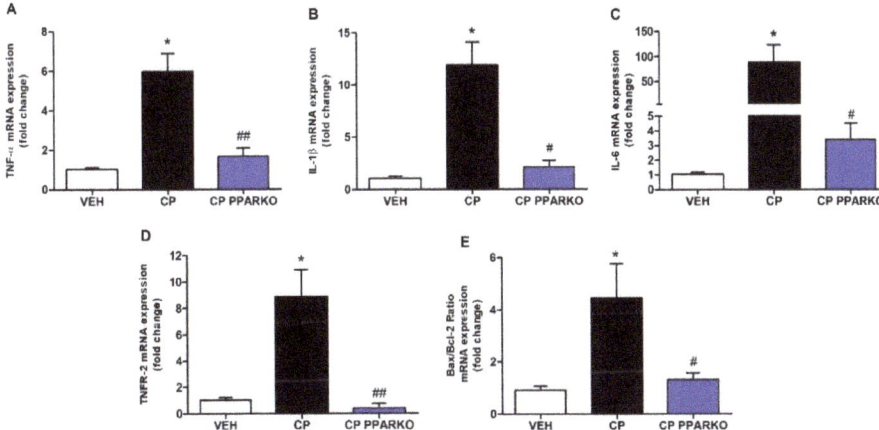

Figure 1. PPAR-α deletion attenuates cisplatin-induced increased pro-inflammatory cytokines and apoptosis related genes. Cisplatin treatment (CP) increased mRNA levels of pro-inflammatory cytokines, (**A**) *TNF-α*, (**B**) *IL-1β* and (**C**) *IL-6* in renal tissue; PPAR-α knockout mice (CP PPARKO) prevented this increase. Apoptosis-related genes (**D**) *TNFR-2* and (**E**) *Bax/Bcl-2* ratio were also increased by cisplatin (CP) and PPAR-α deletion (CP PPARKO) avoided this increase. n = 5–6 per group. One-way ANOVA followed by post hoc Tukey's test. * $p < 0.05$ compared to the VEH group. # $p < 0.05$; ## $p < 0.01$ compared to the CP group.

2.3. PPAR-α Ablation Protects against Cisplatin-Induced Apoptosis and Tubular Injury

Cisplatin affects the proximal tubules of the kidneys through several mechanisms, including tubular necrosis. In the histological analysis, we observed a large increase of tubular injury in cisplatin-treated mice, while PPAR-α knockout mice showed tubular cells protected against cisplatin-induced nephrotoxicity (Figure 2A–B). Cisplatin administration leads to increased apoptosis in the kidney. Caspase-3 is the main executioner caspase and is activated in the apoptotic cell, by both intrinsic and extrinsic pathways. Immunofluorescence was performed to identify apoptosis in renal tissue. Cisplatin treatment increased caspase-3 in wild-type mice and PPAR-α ablation prevented the increase of this protein (Figure 2B).

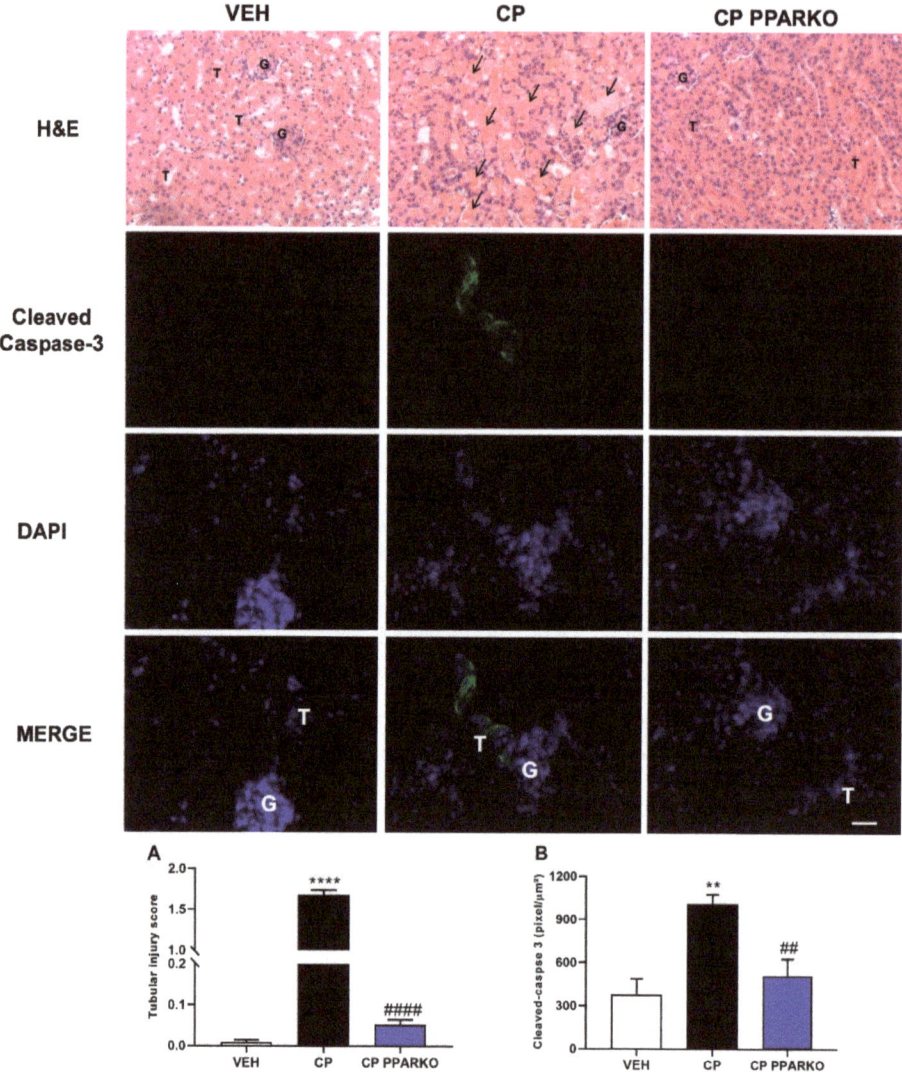

Figure 2. PPAR-α deletion attenuates tubular injury and apoptosis induced by cisplatin after 96 h. Representative photomicrography of H&E staining. (**A**) CP treatment increases tubular injury while PPAR-α deletion attenuates it. (**B**) Immunofluorescence was performed to assess apoptosis. CP increases cleaved caspase-3 staining and CP PPARKO reverses this increase. In arrows is indicated tubules with the tubular lumen obstructed by the tubular casts and cell detachment from the tubular basement membrane. G to indicate glomeruli and a T for examples of tubules with normal structure, no cell detachment and free tubular lumen. $n = 5$ per group. Scale bar = 100 µm. One-way ANOVA followed by post hoc Tukey's test. ** $p < 0.01$, **** $p < 0.0001$. compared to the VEH group. ## $p < 0.01$, #### $p < 0.0001$; compared to the CP group.

2.4. PPAR-α Deletion Prevents Downregulation of Organic Transporters Induced by Cisplatin

Organic Transporters, such as OCT-2 and MATE-1, are of great importance in cisplatin nephrotoxicity: the first one is the main transporter of cisplatin into kidney cells, and the second one is responsible for cisplatin extrusion from the kidney into the urine. Cisplatin treatment induced the downregulation of OCT-2 and MATE-1 in the renal tissue, while PPAR-α deletion prevented cisplatin-induced downregulation of MATE-1 (Figure 3A–B) and OCT-2 (Figure 4A–B).

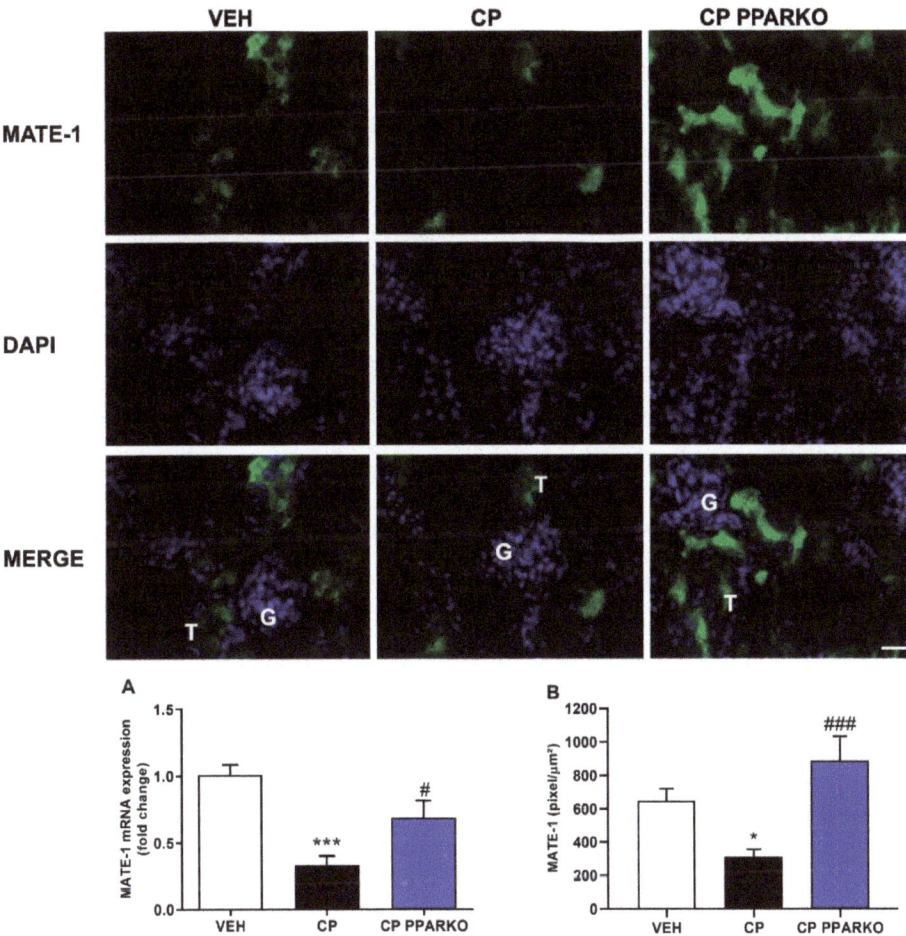

Figure 3. PPAR-α knockout mice mitigate the decreased mRNA and protein expression by immunofluorescence of MATE-1. Ninety-six hours after cisplatin treatment (CP) downregulates (**A**) mRNA and (**B**) protein levels of MATE-1. PPAR-α knockout mice (CP PPARKO) prevented this downregulation. G to indicate glomeruli and a T to indicate tubules. $n = 5$ per group. One-way ANOVA followed by post hoc Tukey's test. Scale bar = 100 μm. * $p < 0.05$, *** $p < 0.001$ compared to the VEH group. # $p < 0.05$, ### $p < 0.001$ compared to the CP group.

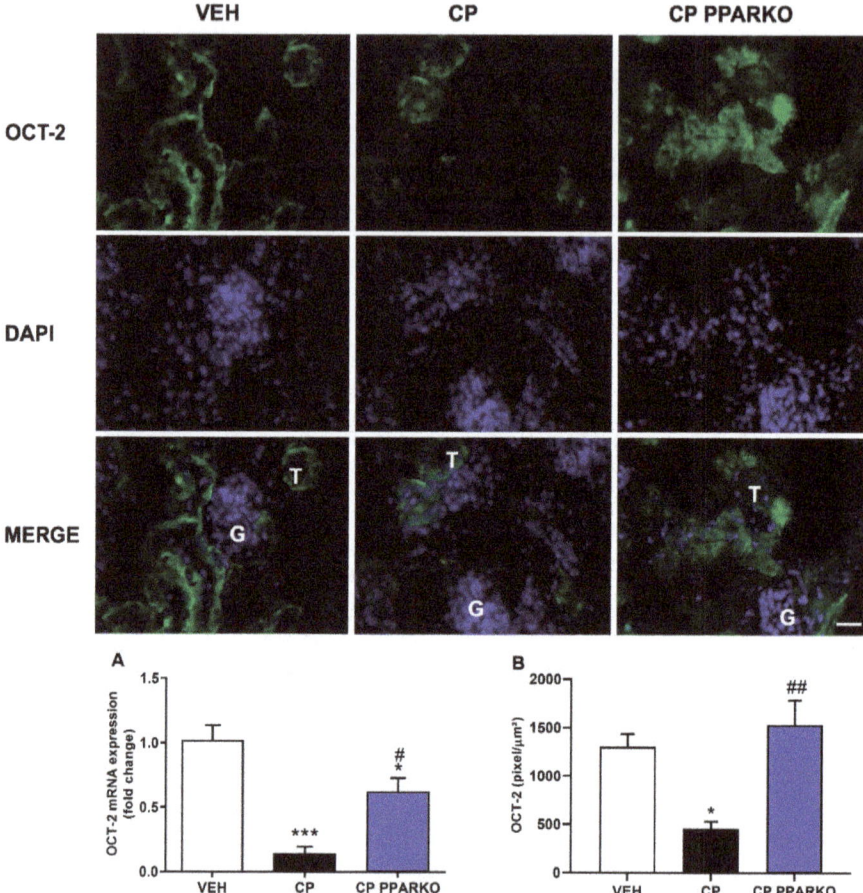

Figure 4. PPAR-α ablation attenuates downregulation of mRNA and protein expression by immunofluorescence of organic cations transporter 2 (OCT-2). Ninety-six hours after cisplatin treatment (CP) downregulates (**A**) mRNA and (**B**) protein (levels of OCT-2. PPAR-α knockout mice (CP PPARKO) attenuated this downregulation. G to indicate glomeruli and a T to indicate tubules. $n = 5$ per group. One-way ANOVA followed by post hoc Tukey's test. Scale bar = 100 μm. * $p < 0.05$, *** $p < 0.001$ compared to the VEH group. # $p < 0.05$, ## $p < 0.01$; compared to the CP group.

2.5. PPAR-α Knockout Modulates Organic Transporters

Immunofluorescence and real-time PCR were performed to check organic transporters protein and mRNA levels at the basal state. PPAR-α absence did not alter MATE-1 mRNA expression (Figure 5A); however, PPARKO mice showed increased MATE-1 protein levels observed in immunofluorescence (Figure 5B). In addition, organic cations transporter 2 (OCT-2) mRNA expression and protein levels were decreased in PPAR-α knockout mice (Figure 6A,B).

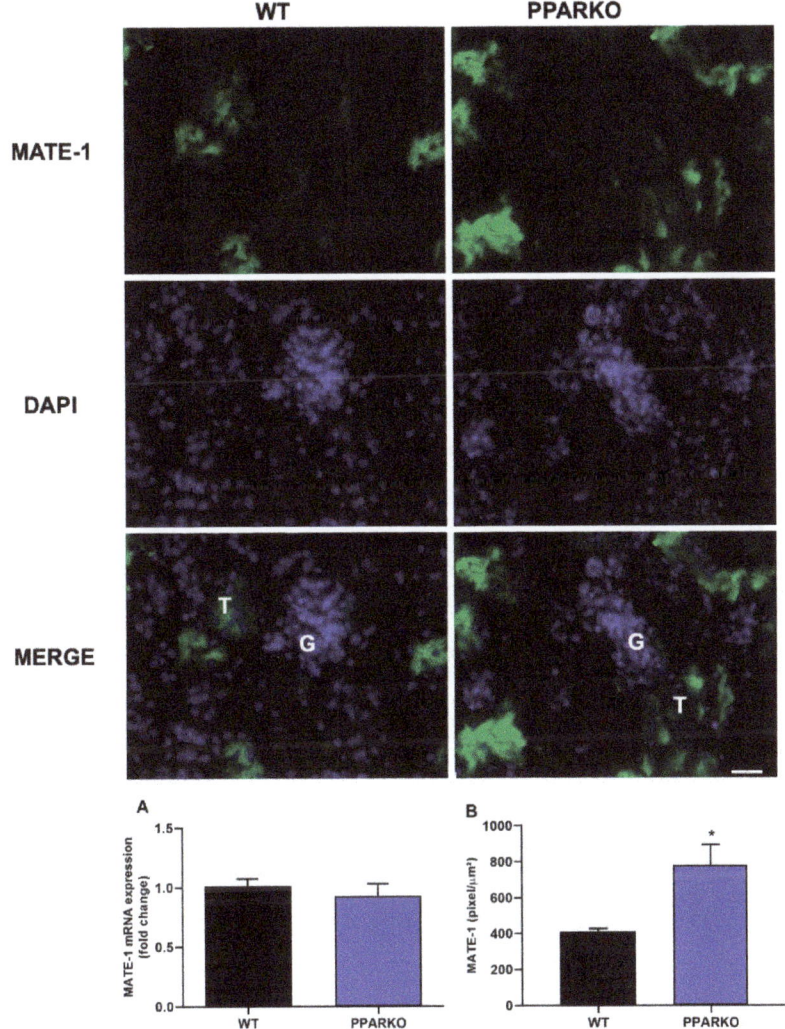

Figure 5. PPAR-α absence enhances protein expression by immunofluorescence of multidrug and toxin extrusion 1 (MATE-1). (**A**) No differences between WT and PPARKO mice were found in *MATE-1* mRNA levels. (**B**) However, PPAR-α knockout mice enhanced MATE-1 protein levels. G to indicate glomeruli and a T to indicate tubules. $n = 5$ per group. Scale bar = 100 μm. Two-tailed Student's t-test. * $p < 0.05$, compared to the WT group.

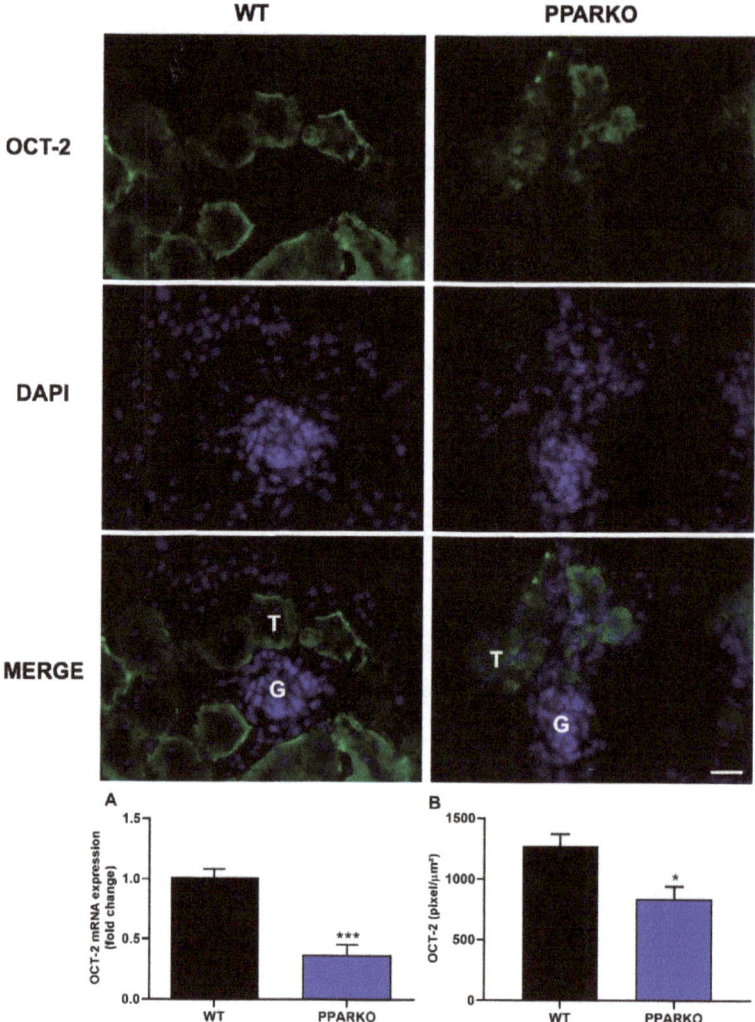

Figure 6. PPAR-α absence decreases mRNA and protein expression by immunofluorescence of organic cations transporter 2 (OCT-2). PPAR-α knockout mice presented reduced (**A**) mRNA and (**B**) protein levels of renal OCT-2. G to indicate glomeruli and a T to indicate tubules. $n = 5$ per group. Two-tailed Student's t-test. Scale bar = 100 μm. * $p < 0.05$, *** $p < 0.001$ compared to the WT group.

3. Discussion

Cisplatin is one of the most potent chemotherapy drugs used against solid tumors. It has a high success rate after treatment, although nephrotoxicity affects about one-third of patients treated with it [22]. Membrane transporters, such as MATE-1 and OCT-2, are of great importance for mediating cellular transport of cisplatin [6]. Our group has recently shown that PPAR-α, a transcription factor highly expressed in the kidneys, which controls lipid metabolism and glucose homeostasis, interacts with both MATE-1 and OCT-2 [20]. The modulation of both membrane transporters should be better explored for the use of therapies that can reduce nephrotoxicity in cisplatin-treated patients.

Our data shows that PPAR-α deletion attenuates cisplatin-induced nephrotoxicity, mainly by modulating the expression of the membrane transporter responsible for cisplatin extrusion from the kidneys. We have previously shown that restoration of MATE-1 expression after cisplatin nephrotoxicity is very important to decrease platinum accumulation in renal tissue [17].

Here, we show that PPAR-α deficiency was capable of reversing renal dysfunction by decreasing serum creatinine and urea levels induced by cisplatin treatment. Kidney injury molecule-1 (KIM-1) is known to be a biomarker of renal proximal tubular injury and is markedly upregulated after acute kidney injury [23–25]. The production and release of neutrophil gelatinase-associated lipocalin (NGAL) from tubular cells after renal damage are increased and it has been a useful biomarker for assessing the severity of kidney injury [26,27]. In order to confirm that PPAR-α deletion protects against renal damage, we performed qPCR for KIM-1 and NGAL and found that cisplatin treatment exponentially increased these markers in renal tissue, while PPAR-α knockout mice attenuated the increasement of this kidney damage markers after cisplatin exposure. In addition to direct cellular toxicity, inflammation plays an important role in cisplatin nephrotoxicity. Over the years, a number of mediators of inflammatory renal injury have been identified, and inflammatory cytokines have shown to be increased after cisplatin toxicity [28–30]. TNF-α plays an important role in many infectious and inflammatory diseases. TNF-α inhibition and deletion reduced cisplatin-induced renal injury and increased survival rates after its administration [28]. In our study, we observed that cisplatin treatment increased proinflammatory cytokines and that PPAR-α knockout mice can reverse it.

Multiple pathways and molecules are involved in cisplatin-induced nephrotoxicity and apoptosis is observed after cisplatin administration [31,32]. Apoptosis may occur in cisplatin treatment by activation of apoptotic pathways, such as intrinsic mitochondrial pathway and extrinsic pathway activated by death receptors [1,33,34]. TNFR-2 mediates apoptosis in cisplatin-induced injury and is one of the death receptors of the extrinsic pathway [35]. Moreover, the Bax/Bcl-2 ratio can be used to determine the intrinsic pathway of apoptosis [33,34]. Cisplatin treatment induced upregulation of TNFR-2 and Bax/Bcl-2 ratio, while PPAR-α knockout mice are protected against this upregulation. We confirmed apoptosis by analysis of cleaved caspase-3, which is the executioner caspase. In addition to apoptosis, necrosis is commonly observed with cisplatin treatment. Indeed, our cisplatin treatment presented huge histological changes of acute tubular necrosis, while PPAR-α deletion was able to avoid it.

As PPAR-α ablation attenuates renal dysfunction, renal injury, inflammatory- and apoptosis-related markers, we further investigated if organic transporters may be involved in PPAR-α deficiency protection. We found that cisplatin induced downregulation of both MATE-1 and OCT-2 in renal tissue, while PPAR-α knockout mice restored the expression of both membrane transporters, important to note that this effect in WT mice may also be related with destruction and loss of tubules. MATE-1 is an important membrane transporter, responsible for cisplatin extrusion from the kidney into the urine [7,14], and its deletion exacerbates cisplatin nephrotoxicity [16]. Indeed, our data corroborates the study by Oda et al. who observed decreased OCT-2 and MATE-1 protein levels in renal tissue after cisplatin treatment. Decreased OCT-2 expression can delay platinum incorporation and diminished MATE-1 expression can increase platinum accumulation in renal cells; therefore, reduced expression of both transporters appears to enhance cisplatin accumulation in renal tissue [36]. We have previously shown that restored MATE-1 expression in renal tissue is important to decrease the renal toxicity induced by platinum accumulation [17]. In silico prediction of binding sites provides evidence that PPAR-α response elements (PPRE) regulate MATE-1 [37]. In addition, PPAR-α has been shown to regulate the transcription of OCT-2 gene: co-transfection of OCT-2 luciferase reporter construct with PPRE leads to a 10-fold increase in transcriptional activity [36]. Moreover, we found that PPAR-α knockout mice present reduced expression of OCT-2 and increased expression of MATE-1, which lead to less cisplatin available to enter renal cells and increase the capacity to extrude cisplatin from cells into urine.

Interestingly past works show that PPAR-α activation promotes protection in different models of kidney injury [33,38–44]. Indeed, its well stablish that increasement of lipid metabolism is beneficial in several models of diseases [45–47]. However, not much is discussed regarding other metabolic pathways compensation due to impaired lipid metabolism in PPAR-α deficiency. Further studies are required to better elucidated these mechanisms of metabolic compensation that drive PPAR-α deletion to promote protection against cisplatin nephrotoxicity.

Here, we show for the first time that PPAR-α deletion is capable of attenuating cisplatin-induced nephrotoxicity and that this is due to the restoration of both MATE-1 and OCT-2 expression, thus suggesting that increases cisplatin extrusion from the kidneys into the urine and decreases the direct toxicity caused by cisplatin accumulation in renal cells.

4. Materials and Methods

4.1. Animals

Littermates wild-type (WT, C57/BL6J) and PPAR-α knockout (PPARα KO, B6; 129S4-Pparatm1Gonz/J, Jackson laboratory) male mice weighing 23–27 g and aged 10–14 weeks were used for these experiments. The animals were obtained from the Animal Care Facility of the Federal University of São Paulo (UNIFESP). All animals were housed in individual, standard cages and had free access to water and food. All procedures were previously reviewed and approved by the internal ethics committee of the Federal University of São Paulo (CEUA 6823010319 issued on 5 June 2019).

4.2. Experimental Protocol

The mice were divided into 3 groups for each experiment: vehicle group (VEH), cisplatin (CP)-treated group and PPARα KO + cisplatin (CP PPARKO)-treated group. We used n = 5–6 for each experiment and condition, experiments were repeated 2 to 3 times.

4.3. Cisplatin Treatment

Single doses of cisplatin (20 mg/kg—Bergamo, Taboão da Serra, Brazil) were injected intraperitoneally. Tissues and blood were collected 96 h after injection. Vehicle group animals received 0.9% NaCl intraperitoneally at same volume as cisplatin.

4.4. Blood Sampling and Kidney Collection

The mice were anesthetized with ketamine (91 mg/kg) and xylazine (9.1 mg/kg) intraperitoneally and blood was collected via heart puncture. Blood was allowed to clot for 2 h at room temperature and then centrifuged for 20 min at 2000× g. The samples were stored at −20 °C. Kidney tissue was collected, and renal capsule was removed. Transversal cuts were performed, and the kidneys were stored at −80 °C.

4.5. Renal Function

Serum creatinine and urea levels were used to determine renal function. Samples were analyzed using commercially available colorimetric assay kits (Labtest, Lagoa Santa, Brazil).

4.6. RNA Extraction and RT-qPCR

Whole kidney total RNA was isolated using TRIzol Reagent (Invitrogen, Carlsbad, CA, USA). The RNA integrity was assessed by electrophoresis on an agarose gel. cDNA was synthesized using the "High Capacity cDNA Reverse Transcription Kit" (Applied Biosystems, Foster City, CA, USA). Standard curves were plotted to determine the amplification efficiency for each primer pair. Real-time PCR was performed using two systems: TaqMan system (Applied Biosystems, Carlsbad, CA) using probes for IL-6 (mm00446190-m1), YWHAZ (mm03950126-s1) and GAPDH (mm99999915-g1); and SYBR Green system (Thermo Scientific, Waltham, MA, USA) using specific primers for β-actin, 18s, IL-1β, NGAL, KIM-1, BAX, BCL-2, TNFR-2, TNF-α, OCT-2 and MATE-1; the primers were designed using primer3 web and their specificity was confirmed using NCBI primer-BLAST; their sequences are shown in Table 2. The cycling conditions for both TaqMan and SYBR Green reactions were as follows:

10 min. at 95 °C, followed by 45 cycles of 30 s at 95 °C, 30 s at 60 °C and 30 s at 72 °C. Target mRNA expression was normalized to both housekeeping genes, β-actin and 18s for SYBR and to YHWHAZ and GAPDH for TaqMan and expressed as a relative value using the comparative threshold cycle (Ct) method ($2^{-\Delta\Delta Ct}$). The expression levels of the genes of interest were normalized to the vehicle group and presented as fold change.

Table 2. Sequences of the primers used for real-time PCR assays.

Primers for RT–PCR	xxx	xxx
Gene	Forward 5′-3′	Reverse 5′-3′
18S	CGC CGC TAG AGG TGA AAT TC	TCT TGG CAA ATG CTT TCG C
β-actin	CTG GCC TCA CTG TCC ACC TT	CGG ACT CAT CGT ACT CCT GCT T
BAX	CGG CGA ATT GGA GAT GAA CTG	GCA AAG TAG AAG AGG GCA ACC
BCL-2	ACC GTC GTG ACT TCG CAG AG	GGT GTG CAG ATG CCG GTT CA
IL-1β	AGG AGA ACC AAG CAA CGA CA	CGT TTT TCC ATC TTC TTC TTT G
KIM-1	TGT CGA GTG GAG ATT CCT GGA TGG T	GGT CTT CCT GTA GCT GTG GGC C
MATE-1	AGG CCA AGA AGT CCT CAG CTA TT	ACG CAG AAG GTC ACA GCA AA
NGAL	ATG TGC AAG TGG CCA CCA CG	CGC ATC CCA GTC AGC CAC AC
OCT-2	AGC CTG CCT AGC TTC GGT TT	TGC CCA TTC TAC CCA AGC A
TNF-α	GCC TCT TCT CAT TCC TGC TTG	CTG ATG AGA GGG AGG CCA TT
TNFR-2	GTC GCG CTG GTC TTC GAA CTG	GGT ATA CAT GCT TGC CTC ACA GTC

4.7. Tubular Injury Analyses

The kidneys were fixed in 10% formaldehyde and then dehydrated and embedded in paraffin. Sections (4 µm) were cut and stained with hematoxylin–eosin. At least six subcortical fields were visualized and analyzed for each mouse using a (Zeiss, Oberkochen, Germany) microscope at a 200× magnification. Tubular injury score was determined based on the percentage of tubules showing luminal casts, cell detachment or dilation and assigned according to the following scale: 0 = 0 to 5%, 1 = 6 to 25%, 2 = 26 to 50%, 3 = 51 to 75% and 4 > 75%.

4.8. Kidney Extraction and Sectioning

The kidney was harvested and then cryoprotected for additional 2 days by immersion in 30% sucrose at −20 °C. Acetone-fixed cryosections (7 µm; Cryostat-Leica Biosystem, Wetzlar, Germany)) were mounted for immunofluorescence analysis.

4.9. Immunofluorescence

The immunofluorescence was performed according to Cavalcante et al. 2019 [48]. Briefly, after fixed with −20 °C acetone the kidney sections were incubated with primary mouse anti-cleaved caspase-3 antibody (1:300, Cell Signaling, Danvers, MA, USA #9661S), anti-MATE-1 antibody (1:200, Santa Cruz, Dallas, TX, USA, sc-138983) or anti-OCT-2 antibody (1:250, Boster Bio, Pleasanton, CA, USA, PB9394) overnight at 4 °C. Nonspecific binding was controlled by replacing a negative control with the primary antibody. After this, the sections were incubated with Alexa Fluor 488 anti-rabbit (1:300, Thermo Fisher, #A11034) during 2 h. The nuclei were stained with DAPI (1:2000, Thermo Fisher, #D1306). Finally, the slices were coverslipped in Mowiol (Sigma-Aldrich, San Luis, MO, USA) mounting media. Sections were imaged in Zeiss fluorescence microscope (Zeiss, Oberkochen, Germany) using a 488 nm excitation. During the microscopic analysis, an overview was performed to qualify the slides, then 10 images were acquired employing a 10× objective, and finally, a representative image was acquired using a 20× objective. The fluorescence intensity was analyzed using ImageProPlus software (version 4.0) and the results were presented as fluorescence intensity/area. Pictures were taking using exactly the same illumination conditions. It is worth to note that all these procedures were performed in a double-blind manner.

4.10. Statistical Analysis

All data are presented as mean ± SEM. Intergroup differences significance was assessed by one-way analysis of variance (ANOVA) with the Tukey's correction for multiple comparisons. The value for statistical significance was established at $p < 0.05$. All statistical analyses were performed using GraphPad Prism 8 (GraphPad, La Jolla, CA, USA).

Author Contributions: G.R.E. and R.C.A. designed the study. G.R.E., L.C.F.-L., A.B., A.C.A., M.S.P. and J.B.-C. performed the experiments. G.R.E., L.C.F.-L., A.B., J.B.-C. and R.C.A. analyzed the data. G.R.E., L.C.F.-L., J.B.-C. and R.C.A. wrote the study. All authors have read and agreed to the published version of the manuscript.

Funding: This work was supported by grants from the Fundação de Amparo a Pesquisa do Estado de São Paulo (FAPESP grant 2015/20082-7 and 2017/23599-6) and National Autonomous University of Mexico-DGAPA-PAPIIT (IN202919 to JBC).

Conflicts of Interest: The authors declare that the research was conducted in the absence of any commercial or financial relationships that could be construed as a potential conflict of interest. The funders had no role in the design of the study; in the collection, analyses or interpretation of data; in the writing of the manuscript or in the decision to publish the results.

Abbreviations

CP	Cisplatin
GAPDH	Glyceraldehyde 3-phosphate dehydrogenase
IL-1β	Interleukin-1 beta
IL-6	Interleukin-6
KIM-1	Kidney injury molecule-1
MATE-1	Multidrug and toxin extrusion protein 1
NGAL	Neutrophil gelatinase-associated lipocalin
OCT-2	Organic cation transporter-2
PPAR-α	Peroxisome-proliferator-activated receptor alpha
PPARKO	Peroxisome-proliferator-activated receptor alpha knockout
PPRE	Peroxisome-proliferator-activated receptor alpha response elements
TNF-α	Tumor necrosis factor alpha
TNFR-2	Tumor necrosis factor alpha receptor-2
VEH	Vehicle control group
BAX	B-cell lymphoma 2 associated x protein
BCL-2	B-cell lymphoma 2
WT	Wild-type
YWHAZ	14-3-3 protein zeta/delta

References

1. Miller, R.P.; Tadagavadi, R.K.; Ramesh, G.; Reeves, W.B. Mechanisms of Cisplatin nephrotoxicity. *Toxins (Basel)* **2010**, *2*, 2490–2518. [CrossRef] [PubMed]
2. Pabla, N.; Dong, Z. Cisplatin nephrotoxicity: Mechanisms and renoprotective strategies. *Kidney Int.* **2008**, *73*, 994–1007. [CrossRef] [PubMed]
3. Litterst, C.L.; Gram, T.E.; Dedrick, R.L.; Leroy, A.F.; Guarino, A.M. Distribution and disposition of platinum following intravenous administration of cis-diamminedichloroplatinum(II) (NSC 119875) to dogs. *Cancer Res.* **1976**, *36*, 2340–2344. [PubMed]
4. Kodama, A.; Watanabe, H.; Tanaka, R.; Kondo, M.; Chuang, V.T.; Wu, Q.; Endo, M.; Ishima, Y.; Fukagawa, M.; Otagiri, M.; et al. Albumin fusion renders thioredoxin an effective anti-oxidative and anti-inflammatory agent for preventing cisplatin-induced nephrotoxicity. *Biochim. Biophys. Acta* **2014**, *1840*, 1152–1162. [CrossRef] [PubMed]

5. Kuhlmann, M.K.; Burkhardt, G.; Köhler, H. Insights into potential cellular mechanisms of cisplatin nephrotoxicity and their clinical application. *Nephrol Dial Transplant.* **1997**, *12*, 2478–2480. [CrossRef] [PubMed]
6. Ciarimboli, G. Membrane transporters as mediators of cisplatin side-effects. *Anticancer Res.* **2014**, *34*, 547–550. [CrossRef]
7. Ciarimboli, G. Membrane transporters as mediators of Cisplatin effects and side effects. *Scientifica (Cairo)* **2012**, *2012*, 473829. [CrossRef]
8. Ciarimboli, G. Organic cation transporters. *Xenobiotica* **2008**, *38*, 936–971. [CrossRef]
9. Koepsell, H. Polyspecific organic cation transporters: Their functions and interactions with drugs. *Trends Pharmacol. Sci.* **2004**, *25*, 375–381. [CrossRef]
10. Ciarimboli, G.; Ludwig, T.; Lang, D.; Pavenstädt, H.; Koepsell, H.; Piechota, H.J.; Haier, J.; Jaehde, U.; Zisowsky, J.; Schlatter, E. Cisplatin nephrotoxicity is critically mediated via the human organic cation transporter 2. *Am. J. Pathol.* **2005**, *167*, 1477–1484. [CrossRef]
11. Pabla, N.; Gibson, A.A.; Buege, M.; Ong, S.S.; Li, L.; Hu, S.; Du, G.; Sprowl, J.A.; Vasilyeva, A.; Janke, L.J.; et al. Mitigation of acute kidney injury by cell-cycle inhibitors that suppress both CDK4/6 and OCT2 functions. *Proc. Natl. Acad. Sci. USA* **2015**, *112*, 5231–5236. [CrossRef] [PubMed]
12. Sprowl, J.A.; Lancaster, C.S.; Pabla, N.; Hermann, E.; Kosloske, A.M.; Gibson, A.A.; Li, L.; Zeeh, D.; Schlatter, E.; Janke, L.J.; et al. Cisplatin-induced renal injury is independently mediated by OCT2 and p53. *Clin. Cancer Res.* **2014**, *20*, 4026–4035. [CrossRef] [PubMed]
13. Ciarimboli, G.; Deuster, D.; Knief, A.; Sperling, M.; Holtkamp, M.; Edemir, B.; Pavenstädt, H.; Lanvers-Kaminsky, C.; am Zehnhoff-Dinnesen, A.; Schinkel, A.H.; et al. Organic cation transporter 2 mediates cisplatin-induced oto- and nephrotoxicity and is a target for protective interventions. *Am. J. Pathol.* **2010**, *176*, 1169–1180. [CrossRef] [PubMed]
14. Yokoo, S.; Yonezawa, A.; Masuda, S.; Fukatsu, A.; Katsura, T.; Inui, K. Differential contribution of organic cation transporters, OCT2 and MATE1, in platinum agent-induced nephrotoxicity. *Biochem. Pharmacol.* **2007**, *74*, 477–487. [CrossRef]
15. Harrach, S.; Ciarimboli, G. Role of transporters in the distribution of platinum-based drugs. *Front. Pharmacol.* **2015**, *6*, 85. [CrossRef]
16. Nakamura, T.; Yonezawa, A.; Hashimoto, S.; Katsura, T.; Inui, K. Disruption of multidrug and toxin extrusion MATE1 potentiates cisplatin-induced nephrotoxicity. *Biochem. Pharmacol.* **2010**, *80*, 1762–1767. [CrossRef]
17. Estrela, G.R.; Wasinski, F.; Felizardo, R.J.F.; Souza, L.L.; Câmara, N.O.S.; Bader, M.; Araujo, R.C. MATE-1 modulation by kinin B1 receptor enhances cisplatin efflux from renal cells. *Mol. Cell Biochem.* **2017**, *428*, 101–108. [CrossRef]
18. Kersten, S. Peroxisome proliferator activated receptors and lipoprotein metabolism. *PPAR Res.* **2008**, *2008*, 132960. [CrossRef]
19. Kersten, S.; Seydoux, J.; Peters, J.M.; Gonzalez, F.J.; Desvergne, B.; Wahli, W. Peroxisome proliferator-activated receptor alpha mediates the adaptive response to fasting. *J Clin Investig.* **1999**, *103*, 1489–1498. [CrossRef]
20. Arruda, A.C.; Perilhão, M.S.; Santos, W.A.; Gregnani, M.F.; Budu, A.; Neto, J.C.R.; Estrela, G.R.; Araujo, R.C. PPARα-Dependent Modulation by Metformin of the Expression of OCT-2 and MATE-1 in the Kidney of Mice. *Molecules* **2020**, *25*, 392. [CrossRef]
21. Arango Duque, G.; Descoteaux, A. Macrophage cytokines: Involvement in immunity and infectious diseases. *Front. Immunol.* **2014**, *5*, 491. [CrossRef] [PubMed]
22. Florea, A.M.; Büsselberg, D. Cisplatin as an anti-tumor drug: Cellular mechanisms of activity, drug resistance and induced side effects. *Cancers (Basel)* **2011**, *3*, 1351–1371. [CrossRef] [PubMed]
23. Ichimura, T.; Brooks, C.R.; Bonventre, J.V. Kim-1/Tim-1 and immune cells: Shifting sands. *Kidney Int.* **2012**, *81*, 809–811. [CrossRef] [PubMed]
24. Han, W.K.; Bailly, V.; Abichandani, R.; Thadhani, R.; Bonventre, J.V. Kidney Injury Molecule-1 (KIM-1): A novel biomarker for human renal proximal tubule injury. *Kidney Int.* **2002**, *62*, 237–244. [CrossRef] [PubMed]
25. Ichimura, T.; Bonventre, J.V.; Bailly, V.; Wei, H.; Hession, C.A.; Cate, R.L.; Sanicola, M. Kidney injury molecule-1 (KIM-1), a putative epithelial cell adhesion molecule containing a novel immunoglobulin domain, is up-regulated in renal cells after injury. *J. Biol. Chem.* **1998**, *273*, 4135–4142. [CrossRef] [PubMed]

26. Bolignano, D.; Donato, V.; Coppolino, G.; Campo, S.; Buemi, A.; Lacquaniti, A.; Buemi, M. Neutrophil gelatinase-associated lipocalin (NGAL) as a marker of kidney damage. *Am. J. Kidney Dis.* **2008**, *52*, 595–605. [CrossRef]
27. Mori, K.; Nakao, K. Neutrophil gelatinase-associated lipocalin as the real-time indicator of active kidney damage. *Kidney Int.* **2007**, *71*, 967–970. [CrossRef]
28. Ramesh, G.; Reeves, W.B. TNF-alpha mediates chemokine and cytokine expression and renal injury in cisplatin nephrotoxicity. *J. Clin. Investig.* **2002**, *110*, 835–842. [CrossRef]
29. Lu, L.H.; Oh, D.J.; Dursun, B.; He, Z.; Hoke, T.S.; Faubel, S.; Edelstein, C.L. Increased macrophage infiltration and fractalkine expression in cisplatin-induced acute renal failure in mice. *J. Pharmacol. Exp. Ther.* **2008**, *324*, 111–117. [CrossRef]
30. Faubel, S.; Lewis, E.C.; Reznikov, L.; Ljubanovic, D.; Hoke, T.S.; Somerset, H.; Oh, D.J.; Lu, L.; Klein, C.L.; Dinarello, C.A.; et al. Cisplatin-induced acute renal failure is associated with an increase in the cytokines interleukin (IL)-1beta, IL-18, IL-6, and neutrophil infiltration in the kidney. *J. Pharmacol. Exp. Ther.* **2007**, *322*, 8–15. [CrossRef]
31. Zhu, S.; Pabla, N.; Tang, C.; He, L.; Dong, Z. DNA damage response in cisplatin-induced nephrotoxicity. *Arch. Toxicol.* **2015**, *89*, 2197–2205. [CrossRef] [PubMed]
32. Shiraishi, F.; Curtis, L.M.; Truong, L.; Poss, K.; Visner, G.A.; Madsen, K.; Nick, H.S.; Agarwal, A. Heme oxygenase-1 gene ablation or expression modulates cisplatin-induced renal tubular apoptosis. *Am. J. Physiol. Renal. Physiol.* **2000**, *278*, F726–F736. [CrossRef] [PubMed]
33. Estrela, G.R.; Wasinski, F.; Batista, R.O.; Hiyane, M.I.; Felizardo, R.J.; Cunha, F.; de Almeida, D.C.; Malheiros, D.M.; Câmara, N.O.; Barros, C.C.; et al. Caloric Restriction Is More Efficient than Physical Exercise to Protect from Cisplatin Nephrotoxicity via PPAR-Alpha Activation. *Front. Physiol.* **2017**, *8*, 116. [CrossRef] [PubMed]
34. Estrela, G.R.; Wasinski, F.; Almeida, D.C.; Amano, M.T.; Castoldi, A.; Dias, C.C.; Malheiros, D.M.; Almeida, S.S.; Paredes-Gamero, E.J.; Pesquero, J.B.; et al. Kinin B1 receptor deficiency attenuates cisplatin-induced acute kidney injury by modulating immune cell migration. *J. Mol. Med. (Berl)* **2014**, *92*, 399–409. [CrossRef] [PubMed]
35. Ramesh, G.; Reeves, W.B. TNFR2-mediated apoptosis and necrosis in cisplatin-induced acute renal failure. *Am. J. Physiol. Renal. Physiol.* **2003**, *285*, F610–F618. [CrossRef] [PubMed]
36. Oda, M.; Koyanagi, S.; Tsurudome, Y.; Kanemitsu, T.; Matsunaga, N.; Ohdo, S. Renal circadian clock regulates the dosing-time dependency of cisplatin-induced nephrotoxicity in mice. *Mol. Pharmacol.* **2014**, *85*, 715–722. [CrossRef] [PubMed]
37. Fang, L.; Zhang, M.; Li, Y.; Liu, Y.; Cui, Q.; Wang, N. PPARgene: A Database of Experimentally Verified and Computationally Predicted PPAR Target Genes. *PPAR Res.* **2016**, *2016*, 6042162. [CrossRef]
38. Li, S.; Mariappan, N.; Megyesi, J.; Shank, B.; Kannan, K.; Theus, S.; Price, P.M.; Duffield, J.S.; Portilla, D. Proximal tubule PPARα attenuates renal fibrosis and inflammation caused by unilateral ureteral obstruction. *Am. J. Physiol. Renal. Physiol.* **2013**, *305*, F618–F627. [CrossRef]
39. Li, S.; Nagothu, K.K.; Desai, V.; Lee, T.; Branham, W.; Moland, C.; Megyesi, J.K.; Crew, M.D.; Portilla, D. Transgenic expression of proximal tubule peroxisome proliferator-activated receptor-alpha in mice confers protection during acute kidney injury. *Kidney Int.* **2009**, *76*, 1049–1062. [CrossRef]
40. Negishi, K.; Noiri, E.; Maeda, R.; Portilla, D.; Sugaya, T.; Fujita, T. Renal L-type fatty acid-binding protein mediates the bezafibrate reduction of cisplatin-induced acute kidney injury. *Kidney Int.* **2008**, *73*, 1374–1384. [CrossRef]
41. Li, S.; Gokden, N.; Okusa, M.D.; Bhatt, R.; Portilla, D. Anti-inflammatory effect of fibrate protects from cisplatin-induced ARF. *Am. J. Physiol. Renal. Physiol.* **2005**, *289*, F469–F480. [CrossRef] [PubMed]
42. Nagothu, K.K.; Bhatt, R.; Kaushal, G.P.; Portilla, D. Fibrate prevents cisplatin-induced proximal tubule cell death. *Kidney Int.* **2005**, *68*, 2680–2693. [CrossRef]
43. Li, S.; Basnakian, A.; Bhatt, R.; Megyesi, J.; Gokden, N.; Shah, S.V.; Portilla, D. PPAR-alpha ligand ameliorates acute renal failure by reducing cisplatin-induced increased expression of renal endonuclease G. *Am. J. Physiol. Renal. Physiol.* **2004**, *287*, F990–F998. [CrossRef] [PubMed]
44. Li, S.; Wu, P.; Yarlagadda, P.; Vadjunec, N.M.; Proia, A.D.; Harris, R.A.; Portilla, D. PPAR alpha ligand protects during cisplatin-induced acute renal failure by preventing inhibition of renal FAO and PDC activity. *Am. J. Physiol. Renal. Physiol.* **2004**, *286*, F572–F580. [CrossRef]

45. Calkin, A.C.; Giunti, S.; Jandeleit-Dahm, K.A.; Allen, T.J.; Cooper, M.E.; Thomas, M.C. PPAR-alpha and -gamma agonists attenuate diabetic kidney disease in the apolipoprotein E knockout mouse. *Nephrol. Dial. Transplant.* **2006**, *21*, 2399–2405. [CrossRef] [PubMed]
46. Collino, M.; Aragno, M.; Mastrocola, R.; Benetti, E.; Gallicchio, M.; Dianzani, C.; Danni, O.; Thiemermann, C.; Fantozzi, R. Oxidative stress and inflammatory response evoked by transient cerebral ischemia/reperfusion: Effects of the PPAR-alpha agonist WY14643. *Free Radic. Biol. Med.* **2006**, *41*, 579–589. [CrossRef]
47. Yue, T.L.; Bao, W.; Jucker, B.M.; Gu, J.L.; Romanic, A.M.; Brown, P.J.; Cui, J.; Thudium, D.T.; Boyce, R.; Burns-Kurtis, C.L.; et al. Activation of peroxisome proliferator-activated receptor-alpha protects the heart from ischemia/reperfusion injury. *Circulation* **2003**, *108*, 2393–2399. [CrossRef]
48. Cavalcante, P.A.M.; Alenina, N.; Budu, A.; Freitas-Lima, L.C.; Alves-Silva, T.; Agudelo, J.S.H.; Qadri, F.; Camara, N.O.; Bader, M.; Araújo, R.C. Nephropathy in Hypertensive Animals Is Linked to M2 Macrophages and Increased Expression of the YM1/Chi3l3 Protein. *Mediat. Inflamm.* **2019**, *2019*, 9086758. [CrossRef]

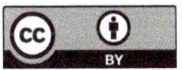

© 2020 by the authors. Licensee MDPI, Basel, Switzerland. This article is an open access article distributed under the terms and conditions of the Creative Commons Attribution (CC BY) license (http://creativecommons.org/licenses/by/4.0/).

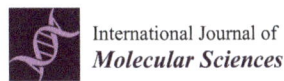

Article

Functional and Pharmacological Comparison of Human, Mouse, and Rat Organic Cation Transporter 1 toward Drug and Pesticide Interaction

Saskia Floerl, Annett Kuehne and Yohannes Hagos *

PortaCellTec Biosciences GmbH, 37075 Goettingen, Germany; floerl@portacelltec.de (S.F.); kuehne@portacelltec.de (A.K.)
* Correspondence: hagos@portacelltec.de; Tel.: +49-551-30966440

Received: 20 July 2020; Accepted: 18 September 2020; Published: 19 September 2020

Abstract: Extrapolation from animal to human data is not always possible, because several essential factors, such as expression level, localization, as well as the substrate selectivity and affinity of relevant transport proteins, can differ between species. In this study, we examined the interactions of drugs and pesticides with the clinically relevant organic cation transporter hOCT1 (SLC22A1) in comparison to the orthologous transporters from mouse and rat. We determined K_m-values (73 ± 7, 36 ± 13, and 57 ± 5 µM) of human, mouse and rat OCT1 for the commonly used substrate 1-methyl-4-phenylpyridinium (MPP) and IC_{50}-values of decynium22 (12.1 ± 0.8, 5.3 ± 0.4, and 10.5 ± 0.4 µM). For the first time, we demonstrated the interaction of the cationic fungicides imazalil, azoxystrobin, prochloraz, and propamocarb with human and rodent OCT1. Drugs such as ketoconazole, clonidine, and verapamil showed substantial inhibitory potential to human, mouse, and rat OCT1 activity. A correlation analysis of hOCT1 versus mouse and rat orthologs revealed a strong functional correlation between the three species. In conclusion, this approach shows that transporter interaction data are in many cases transferable between rodents and humans, but potential species differences for other drugs and pesticides could not be excluded, though it is recommendable to perform functional comparisons of human and rodent transporters for new molecular entities.

Keywords: solute carrier (SLC) family; OCT1; SLC22A1; species differences; drugs; pesticides

---

1. Introduction

Numerous hydrophilic compounds require membrane transporters to surmount the plasma membrane of cells. Members of the ATP-binding cassette (ABC) as well as transporters belonging to the solute carrier (SLC) transporter superfamily facilitate the cellular entry or exit of small organic molecules. The driving force for ABC transporter-mediated efflux is provided by ATP hydrolysis, classifying the ABC transporters as primary active. The SLC transporters translocate their substrate through the plasma membrane by electrochemical gradients. Thus, they are secondary or tertiary active transporter. The organic cation transporter 1 (OCT1) is the first member of the SLC22 subfamily (SLC22A1). In 1994, rOct1 was initially identified from rat kidney and encoded 556 amino acids [1,2]. In the following years, several mammalian OCT1 orthologs from human, mouse and rabbit were identified [3,4]. Human OCT1 consists of 554 amino acids and shares 78% sequence identity with both mouse and rat Oct1. Human OCT1 is highly expressed in the liver [3,4], where it is located in the sinusoidal membrane of hepatocytes [5]. In rodents, Oct1 is expressed not only in the liver but also highly in the kidney, small intestine, and lung [6]. In the small intestine, OCT1 is localized at the luminal membrane of enterocytes [7,8], in contrast to the basolateral expression of OCT1 in hepatocytes. In the human liver, the highest expression of membrane transporters was demonstrated for hOCT1 [9]. OCT1 mediates the uptake of cationic substrates from the sinusoid into hepatocytes and contributes to the first step of hepatic excretion of endogenous as well as exogenous cationic compounds. In humans, OCT1 enables the reabsorption of organic cations from primary urine, unlike rodent Oct1, which is expressed on the basolateral membrane of proximal tubule cells [10]. As a multi-specific transporter, OCT1 translocates structurally different endogenous as well as exogenous substrates such as choline, corticosterone, acetylcholine, guanidine, and drugs such as metformin, atropine, ranitidine, cisplatin derivates, sumatriptan, morphine, as well as toxins, such as aflatoxin B1, monocrotaline, and ethidiumbromide [8,9,11,12].

Human OCT1 is one of around ten SLC and ABC transporters selected by the Food and Drug Administration (FDA) and European Medicines Agency (EMA) [13] to be tested as part of drug approval, because of their clinical relevance as drug and toxin transporters and the possible involvement in drug–drug interactions (DDI). The initial toxicity as well as pharmacokinetic studies in early drug development are accomplished mainly in laboratory animals, particularly in rodents. Generally, mice and rats are the species of first choice in drug development, since their organisms are very similar to that of humans in many respects, but side effects, such as nephrotoxicity or hepatotoxicity, which have not been observed in animal experiments on rodents occur repeatedly in humans. Therefore, the data generated from animals could not always be extrapolated to humans. For example, troglitazone showed severe hepatotoxic effects in man that had not been observed in regulatory animals [14], which could be due to adverse effects in drug-induced liver injury caused by species-specific susceptibilities [15]. The reasons for the species differences also include physiological parameters in which mice and humans differ, such as body weight and organ-specific excretionn processes in the kidney and the liver. Drugs excreted via the liver encounter different physiological parameters, such as species differences in biliary excretion. The bile flow in rats and mice is 90 and 100 mL/day/kg, respectively, whereas the bile flow in humans is 5 mL/day/kg [16]. Anatomically, humans and mice can store the bile in the gallbladder, whereas rats do not have a gallbladder and therefore continuously excrete the bile into the intestine. The biliary excretion of endogenous as well as exogenous compounds, such as drugs, is dependent on the activity of SLC and ABC transporters. Membrane transporters play a pivotal role in the absorption, distribution, metabolism, and elimination (ADME) of drugs. Therefore, it is crucial to compare the data generated from rodents with humans in in vitro assays to evaluate the impact of the transporter to DDI for humans during the potential use in therapy. Dresser et al. demonstrated species-dependent differences in the interaction of OCT1 with n-tetraalkylammonium derivatives [6,17].

The aim of this project was to figure out as to what extent species differences play a role in the transport function of OCT1. For that, we carried out interaction studies of chemical substances with hOCT1, rOct1, and mOct1 under the same conditions. As the first part of this project, we compared the affinity of the known substrate 1-methyl-4-phenylpyridinium (MPP) and the inhibition data of the known inhibitor decynium22 toward hOCT1 with the data of the orthologous mouse and rat Oct1. While in the second part, we correlated the hOCT1 interaction data of several drugs and also of pesticides with the data of mouse and rat Oct1. In this context, the involvement of the SLC transporter OCT1 in the interaction with pesticides ought to be examined to compare a broad spectrum of chemical entities that humans are exposed to. The interaction of a vast number of drugs with OCTs is intensively investigated. In contrast, the interaction of pesticides with SLC transporters, and particularly with OCTs, is barley examined, despite the increasing interest from regulatory authorities and producers of pesticides. In this project, we elucidated the impact of pesticides in the inhibition of OCT1, since these compounds could be involved in pesticide–drug interactions.

Hundreds of pesticides are used worldwide in agricultural holdings and large agricultural industries. To avoid or minimize the exposure of employees and consumers to pesticides, there are internationally harmonized definitions of the Maximum Residue Level (MRL) of pesticides in foodstuffs as well as the tolerable daily intake for humans as Acceptable Daily Intake (ADI). These parameters help to control the potential chronic toxicity by continued intake of foodstuffs contaminated with pesticides. The ADI is obtained by feeding rats certain amounts of pesticides through their food for a very long time. If the rats tolerate this chemical without any health consequences, the daily allowable dose (ADI) is achieved in mg of active substance per kg of body weight per day. For safety reasons, the permitted daily dose for humans should be only 1% of the permitted daily dose for rats. Nevertheless, the pharmacokinetics or ADME processes of several pesticides in humans and the involvement of membrane transporters in the liver and kidney, which are crucial for the absorption, elimination, and DDI, are not well understood. Therefore, the additional intention of this work was to expound the interaction of human OCT1 with pesticides and to correlate with the mouse and rat Oct1 interaction. Important parameters suh as ADI are generated by the exposure of animals to these chemical entities to prevent the potential pesticide toxicity to humans. Hence, it is very important to compare the interaction of the membrane transporter with pesticides across different species, particularly with rodents.

2. Results

2.1. Functional Characterization of Human, Mouse, and Rat OCT1

To compare the fundamental functional characteristics of human, mouse, and rat OCT1 under comparable conditions in stable transfected HEK293 cells, initial hOCT1-, mOct1-, and rOct2-mediated time-dependent uptake experiments were performed. Using MPP as substrate, the uptake into OCT1-HEK cells was measured over a period of 0.5 to 20 min, as shown in Figure 1. The MPP uptake facilitated by hOCT1, mOct1, and rOct1 increased linear up to 3 min and was saturated at 10 min for all species. Initial 1 min uptake of hOCT1-HEK, mOct1-HEK and rOct-HEK cells was 20.3-, 15.6-, and 14.3-fold higher than the uptake of the control cells; therefore, further MPP uptake experiments were terminated for all OCT1 transporters at 1 min.

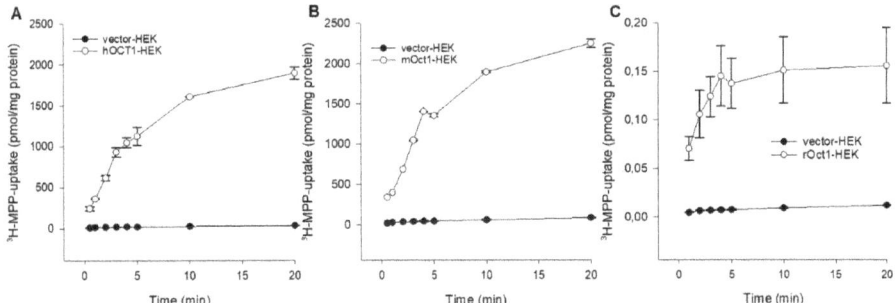

Figure 1. Time dependent uptake of 3H-MPP in (**A**) hOCT1-, (**B**) mOct1-, and (**C**) rOct1-HEK293 cells. Human, mouse, and rat organic cation transporter 1 (OCT1) transfected HEK293 cells were incubated for increasing time points at 37 °C in the presence of labeled 3H-1-methyl-4-phenylpyridinium (MPP) (2 nM), in case of hOCT1 and mOct1 the concentration was filled up to 10 µM with unlabeled MPP. Each data point represents the mean of two or three independent experiments ± average deviation. Experiments were carried out in triplicates.

To determine and compare the affinity of hOCT1, mOct1, and rOct1 in the same expression system and under the same experimental conditions, concentration-dependent MPP uptake was conducted. In transporter-transfected and vector-transfected HEK293 cells, we measured the uptake of MPP in a transport buffer containing 2 nM [^{3}H]-labeled MPP in the presence of increasing concentrations of non-labeled MPP. The K_m value of hOCT1, mOct1, and rOct1 were determined to be 73 ± 7 µM, 36 ± 13 µM, and 57 ± 5 µM, as shown in Figure 2A–C, respectively. The substrate turnover calculated as the V_{max} value of mOct1 (1423 ± 124 pmol/mg/min) and rOct1 (2740 ± 63 pmol/mg/min) was inconsiderably (<2.5-fold difference) lower than the V_{max} value of hOCT1 (3498 ± 103 pmol/mg/min) for MPP.

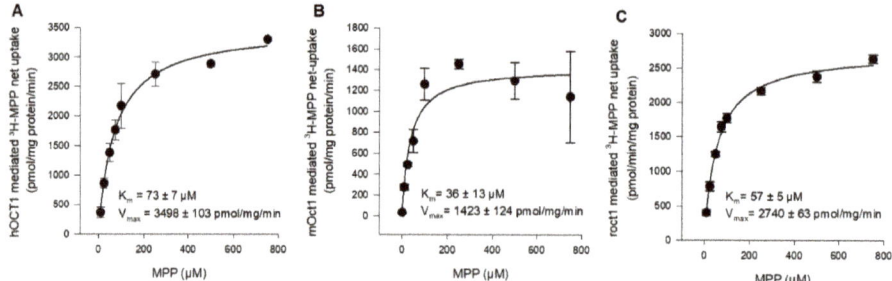

Figure 2. Kinetics of (**A**) hOCT1-, (**B**) mOct1-, and (**C**) rOct1-mediated 3H-MPP transport. Human, mouse, and rat OCT1-transfected HEK293 cells were incubated for 1 min at 37 °C in the presence of labeled (2 nM) and increasing concentrations of non-labeled MPP. Net uptake was fitted to the Michaelis–Menten equation to obtain the affinity constant K_m and maximum transport velocity V_{max} by non-linear regression analysis using Sigma Plot 13.0 software. Each data point represents the mean of two independent experiments ± average deviation. Experiments were carried out in triplicates.

Decynium22 is a well-known, high-affinity inhibitor of OCT1, OCT2, and OCT3 [2,17,18]. To our knowledge, there are no systematical studies under the same conditions to evaluate the concentration-dependent inhibition of hOCT1, mOct1, and rOct1 by decynium22. For further functional characterization and comparison of the three species, the inhibitory potential of the increasing decynium22 concentrations on OCT1-mediated uptake of MPP was measured, and the IC_{50} value of decynium22 for hOCT1, mOct1, and rOct1 was calculated to be 12.1 ± 0.8 µM, 5.3 ± 0.4 µM, and 10.5 ± 0.4 µM (Figure 3).

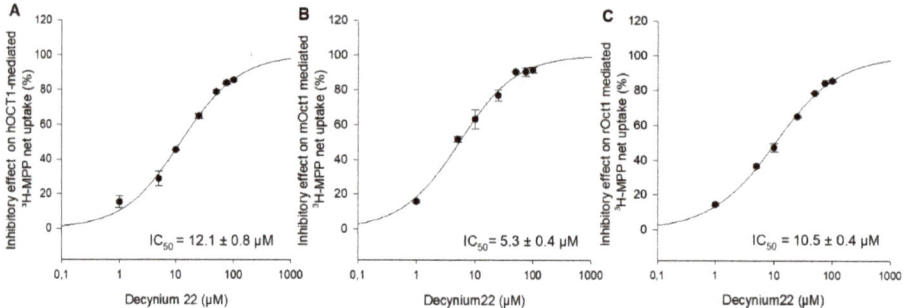

Figure 3. Inhibitory effects of decynium22 on (**A**) hOCT1-, (**B**) mOct1-, and (**C**) rOct1-mediated ³H-MPP transport in stable transfected HEK293 cells. Uptake of MPP at Km value was measured in the presence of increasing concentrations of decynium22 (1–100 µM). Each data point represents the mean inhibitory effect (%) calculated from the net-uptake of two independent experiments ± average deviation. Each experiment was carried out in triplicates. IC_{50} values were calculated by sigmoidal 3Hill analysis using Sigma Plot 13.0 software.

2.2. Comparison of the Interaction of hOCT1, mOct1, and rOct1 with Drugs and Pesticides

After the basic functional validation, a comparison of hOCT1, mOct1, and rOct1 interaction with fifteen drugs from different classes of compounds used for specific therapeutic targets as well as nine pesticides frequently applied in agricultural industries were evaluated.

Inhibition assays towards human OCT1, mouse Oct1, and rat Oct1 were conducted to compare the species-dependent interaction of ketoconazole, clonidine, verapamil, quinine, elacridar, quinidine, procainamide, ritonavir, ranitidine, zosuquidar, metformin, amiodarone, cimetidine, cyclosporine

A, and reserpine. The OCT1-facilitated MPP uptake was inhibited in the presence of 10 or 100 µM of each drug. Ketoconazole, clonidine, verapamil, quinine, elacridar, quinidine, and procainamide inhibited the transport activity of hOCT1, mOct1, and rOct1 at 100 µM by more than 50%. The seven above-mentioned drugs showed high, comparable, and species-independent inhibitory effects on hOCT1, mOct1, and rOct1, as depicted in Table 1. Slight differences at a very low level were observed, for example, for ritonavir and zosuquidar. Ritonavir demonstrated at 100 µM a reduction in rOct1- and hOCT1-mediated MPP uptake to 78% and 61%. In contrast, ritonavir stimulated at 100 µM the mOct1 transport activity by up to 16%. Zosuquidar revealed the low inhibition of the hOCT1-facilitated transport of MPP and no inhibition of rOct1 but a slight (23%) stimulation of the MPP uptake by mOct1. However, neither of the drugs showed clear interaction differences between human, mouse, and rat OCT1 transport activity.

Table 1. Inhibitory effects of various cationic drugs to human, mouse and rat OCT1-mediated ^{3}H-MPP uptake.

Drugs (15)	Type of Drug	Charge at pH 7.4	hOCT1		mOct1		rOct1	
			10 µM	100 µM	10 µM	100 µM	10 µM	100 µM
Ketoconazole *	antifungal	82% uncharged 18% cation	47	83	46	74	43	75
Clonidine	hypertension	100% cation	73	83	72	82	62	80
Verapamil *	class IV antiarrhythmic agent	100% cation	39	82	29	64	29	64
Quinine *	anti malaria	100% cation	20	59	−7	50	−1	44
Elacridar	tumor drug resistance	100% cation	31	57	61	76	53	70
Quinidine *	class I antiarrhythmic agent	100% cation	13	53	−5	46	19	37
Procainamide *	class I antiarrhythmic agent	100% cation	10	43	−5	58	21	58
Ritonavir *	antiretroviral HIV	100% cation	17	39	8	−16	17	22
Ranitidine *	H2 histamine receptor antagonist	100% cation	10	38	−12	12	11	45
Zosuquidar	antineoplastic drug	37% uncharged 63% cation	2	20	−4	−23	0	4
Metformin *	type 2 diabetes	100% cation	11	13	12	9	−19	−4
Amiodarone *	class III antiarrhythmic agent	100% cation	9	10	−29	9	−25	1
Cimetidine *	H2 histamine receptor antagonist	75% uncharged 25% cation	8	9	−25	21	19	20
CyclosporinA *	immunsuppressant	100% cation	10	7	−27	6	−15	8
Reserpine	hypertension	70% uncharged 30% cation	7	6	−12	2	−17	12

* Asterisks show the compounds which are already published to interact with hOCT1 but not with all rodent Oct1 [8,19,20].

The following pesticides were examined to elucidate their inhibitory potential on the OCT-mediated MPP uptake: imazalil, propamocarb, azoxystrobin, prochloraz, atrazin, amitraz, glyphosate, imidacloprid, and paraquat. The highest inhibition of OCTs was observed with imazalil, propamocarb, and azoxystrobin. They reduced the transporter-mediated uptake of MPP in the presence of 100 µM by 50% or more. The other pesticides showed no or only slight inhibitory effects. Some pesticides showed stimulation of OCT1-mediated MPP uptake, as summarized in Table 2. None of the pesticides demonstrated a clear differential species-dependent interaction within human, mouse, and rat OCT1 transport activity.

Table 2. Inhibitory effects of various pesticides to human, mouse and rat OCT1 mediated 3H-MPP uptake.

Pesticides (n = 9)	Type of Pesticide	Charge at pH 7.4	Inhibitory Effects (%)					
			hOCT1		mOct1		rOct1	
			10 µM	100 µM	10 µM	100 µM	10 µM	100 µM
Imazalil	fungicide	81% uncharged 19% cation	56	84	84	97	68	92
Propamocarb	fungicide	100% uncharged	9	49	29	63	24	57
Azoxystrobin	fungicide	100% uncharged	17	44	−2	49	0	42
Prochloraz	fungicide	100% cation	14	42	29	28	25	33
Atrazin	herbicide	100% uncharged	−8	15	−1	1	−65	−33
Amitraz	insecticide	100% cation	8	12	−23	21	−30	10
Glyphosat	herbicide	73% anion 27% ± charge	1	7	−9	22	−52	−19
Imidacloprid	insecticide	100% ± charge	4	1	23	−9	−5	−36
Paraquat *	herbicide	100% cation	0	−1	17	−9	1	−35

* The asterisk shows the compound which is already published to interact with hOCT1 but not with all rodent Oct1 [21].

Correlation analyses were carried out to visualize the interaction studies performed with drugs and pesticides toward hOCT1-, mOct1-, and rOct1-transfected HEK293 cells. The inhibitory effect of fifteen drugs and nine pesticides at both concentrations was plotted to evaluate interaction outcome of two transporters of different species. The Figure 4A–C present the functional correlation of hOCT1 versus mOct1, hOCT1 versus rOct1, and mOct1 versus rOct1. The correlation coefficient R^2 of all three plots was higher than 0.7, representing a good functional correlation of OCT1 within the species.

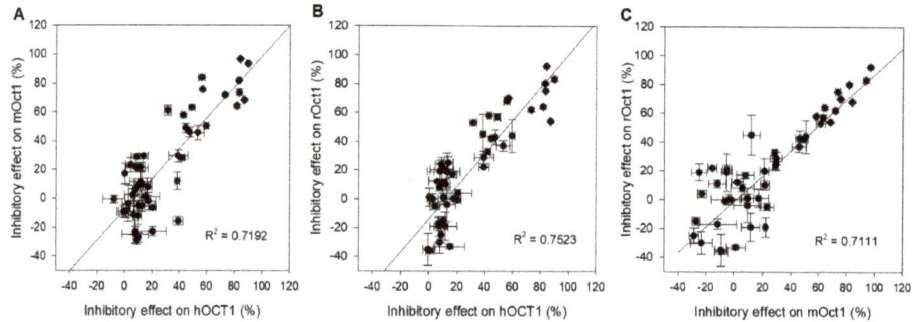

Figure 4. Scatter plot analysis correlating inhibitory effects of (**A**) hOCT1 and mOct1, (**B**) hOCT1 and rOct1, and (**C**) mOct1 and rOct1. The correlation coefficient R^2 value for all three combinations is higher than 0.7, indicating a good correlation between species. Data points represent mean and standard deviation of one individual experiment. Mean values in detail are presented in Tables 1 and 2.

Furthermore, to compare the drug and pesticide interaction of human OCT1 with other members of organic cation transporters belonging to the SLC22A and SLC47A (hOCT2 and hMATE1) families, additional inhibition studies with drugs and pesticides were performed. The hOCT2-mediated MPP as well as hMATE1-mediated metformin uptake was inhibited at 10 and 100 µM of fourteen cationic drugs and nine mainly cationic pesticides. The inhibition studies were measured in stable transfected HEK293 cells at comparable conditions. As shown in Table 3, decynium22 revealed transporter-dependent high inhibition down to 3% to 10% of metformin or MPP uptake by hMATE1, hOCT1, and hOCT2. The highest inhibition of hOCT1, hMATE1, and hOCT2 at 100 µM of pesticides was achieved with imazalil to 16%, 17%, and 39% remaining transporter activity.

Table 3. Inhibitory effects of various cationic drugs to hOCT1- and hOCT2-mediated ^{3}H-MPP uptake and MATE1-mediated ^{14}C-metformin uptake.

Drugs (14)	hOCT1		Inhibitory Effects (%) hOCT2		hMATE1	
	10 µM	100 µM	10 µM	100 µM	10 µM	100 µM
Decynium22 *	87	90	42	90	76	97
Clonidine	73	83	69	80	24	60
Ketoconazol *	47	83	33	64	87	98
Verapamil *	39	82	35	43	44	82
Elacridar	31	57	−5	14	42	71
Quinidine *	13	53	0	24	11	24
Procainamide *	10	43	22	38	22	30
Ritonavir *	17	39	15	24	69	91
Ranitidine *	10	38	9	30	19	76
Zosuquidar	2	20	−19	14	23	65
Metformin *	11	13	10	6	5	36
Amiodarone *	9	10	9	19	1	12
CyclosporinA	10	7	−26	−27	18	6
Reserpine	7	6	3	8	72	83

* Asterisks show the compounds which are already published to interact with hOCT1 but not with all rodent Oct1 [8,19,20].

The correlation analyses of the drug and pesticide interaction with hOCT1 versus hOCT2, as plotted in Figure 5A, shows with a correlation coefficient R^2 of 0.67 a good correlation for the selected compounds. Yet, for a few compounds (e.g., elacridar), there is no clear correlation between hOCT1 and hOCT2 (see Table 3).

Human OCT1 and MATE1 show for a few compounds inhibitory effects at the same level, e.g., imazalil at a very high level (83%), and amitraz at a very low level (12%) (see Table 4). However, the inhibitory effects of a large number of the compounds do not reveal a functional correlation of hOCT1 and hMATE1, as presented in Figure 5B. The calculated functional correlation coefficient R^2 was 0.45, which is remarkably lower than the coefficient between the OCT1 species or between hOCT1 and hOCT2.

Table 4. Inhibitory effects of various pesticides to hOCT1- and hOCT2-mediated ^{3}H-MPP uptake and MATE1-mediated ^{14}C-metformin uptake.

Pesticides (9)	OCT1		Inhibitory Effects (%) OCT2		MATE1	
	10 µM	100 µM	10 µM	100 µM	10 µM	100 µM
Imazalil	56	84	39	61	33	83
Propamocarb	9	49	24	54	22	25
Azoxystrobin	17	44	33	38	27	68
Prochloraz	14	42	32	33	7	70
Atrazin	−8	15	1	10	18	32
Amitraz	8	12	9	27	−11	12
Glyphosat	1	7	12	2	−1	14
Imidacloprid	4	1	−3	19	−8	29
Paraquat *	0	−1	−6	−4	3	4

* The asterisk shows the compound which is already published to interact with hOCT1 but not with all rodent Oct1 [21].

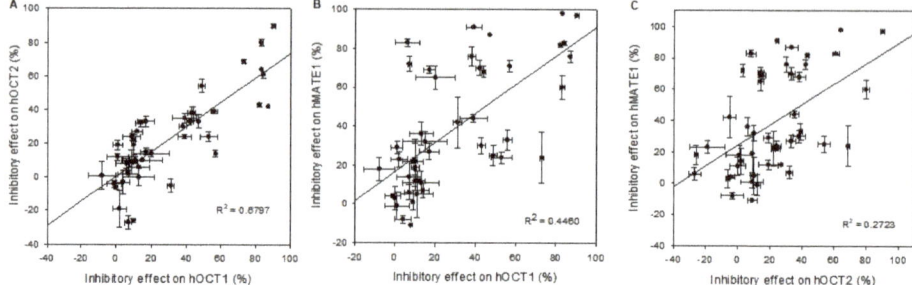

Figure 5. Scatter plot analysis correlating inhibitory effects of (**A**) hOCT1 vs. hOCT2, (**B**) hOCT1 vs. hMATE1, (**C**) and hOCT2 vs. hMATE1. The correlation coefficient R^2 value for the combination hOCT1 vs. hOCT2 is near 0.7, indicating a good correlation between cation transporters, while the combination hOCT1 vs. hMATE1 shows only an R^2 value of 0.45 and for hOCT2 vs. hMATE1 R^2 = 0.27. Data points represent mean and standard deviation of one individual experiment. Mean values are presented in detail in Tables 3 and 4.

3. Discussion

Laboratory animals are indispensable tools in the initial preclinical drug development and evaluation of the pharmacokinetics of new molecular entities (NMEs). In vivo, they deliver pivotal data in terms of toxicity and achievement of the therapeutic target as well as ADME. The parameters received from animal experiments reflect the systemic performance of the compound after treatment. Additional in vitro experiments are crucial to address specific interactions of NME with metabolizing enzymes, target proteins, permeability of the plasma membrane as well as transporter proteins, which mediate the intake or the release of the compounds for the cells. Therefore, the potential species differences should also be considered in the in vitro experimental setups.

The objective of this study was to compare the drug and pesticide interaction with human and rodent organic cation transporter 1 (OCT1; SLC22A1). There are several studies demonstrating the interaction of drugs with human, mouse and rat OCT1. Nevertheless, the direct comparison of the data is difficult, since most of the results are generated with different expression systems, substrates, and experimental conditions. Consequently, in our study, functional characterization and validation of the stable in HEK293 cell transfected human, mouse, and rat OCT1 was carried out, starting with the time-dependent MPP uptake, where all three transporters were saturated after 10 min and the linear uptake extended to 3 min. In the first time-dependent functional evaluation of rOct1 and hOCT1 by injecting cRNA in *Xenopus laevis* oocytes, a linear uptake of ^{14}C-TEA of 90 min and 120 min ^{3}H-MPP uptake was observed [1]. The substantial difference on the linearity of the uptake in X. laevis oocytes and HEK293 cells could be the expression of the OCTs in the plasma membrane, which is not comparable. In several studies, the group of Mladen Tzvetkov demonstrated the linear uptake of several compounds in OCT1-expressing HEK293 cells within 2 min [9,11,22]. The affinity of the OCT1 transporter different species for specific small molecules could differ within the same expression system, as demonstrated by Dresser et al. They compared the interaction and affinity of n-tetraalkylammonium derivates with human, mouse, rat, and rabbit OCT1 expressed in X. laevis oocytes and showed 4-fold higher affinity of mOct1 to TBA than the hOCT1 [17]. Therefore, it was very important to determine the affinity of the three transporters to MPP (K_m values) under the same conditions. In our study, the K_m values of human and rodent OCT1 were in a comparable range. Nevertheless, the affinities for mOct1 and rOct1 were slightly higher than the affinity for hOCT1. However, these differences were not significant according to Student's t-test ($p > 0.05$).

This indicates also a study of Gründemann and colleagues [23], where the K_m value of hOCT1-HEK293 cells was determined to be 32 µM, which is 2.2-fold lower than was observed in our study, even though the experimental conditions were comparable except for the fact that the HBSS buffer used in this study contained bicarbonate. K_m values of 10 µM and 5.6 µM were determined for mOct1 and rOct1 expressed *X. laevis* oocytes [24,25]. For further validation of hOCT1-, mOct1-, and rOct1-expressing HEK293 cells, the concentration-dependent inhibitory potential of the well-known OCT inhibitor [6] decynium22 was determined and the K_m values were calculated. Similarly, the IC_{50} values of decynium22 for hOCT1 and rOct1 were almost the same and mOct1 exhibited 2-fold higher affinity for decynium22 than the human and rat OCT1. In another study, decynium22 inhibited the MPP uptake in isolated rat hepatocytes as well as in hOCT1-expressing *X. laevis* oocytes, with IC_{50} values of 1.4 and 4.7 µM, respectively [2,26]. The difference on the substrate and inhibitor selectivity as well as affinity with in the orthologues OCT1 transporter could be the specific amino acid variation within the amino acid sequence. As very well discussed by Wright and Dantzler [27] and demonstrated by mutation analysis and the replacement of aspartate 475 to glutamate (D475E) in rOct1 amino acid sequence, the affinity for methylnicotinamide, tetraethylammonium (TEA), and choline increased by 4-, 8- and 15-fold, respectively. In contrast, the affinity of the mutant D475E rOct1 for MPP remained unchanged in comparison to the wild-type rOct1 [28]. Several studies demonstrated numerous hOCT1 polymorphisms as well as a worldwide genetic variability of hOCT1, indicating specific polymorphisms M420del could lead to loss-of-function. For example, 9% of the Caucasian population possesses OCT1 without functional activity [29]. Nevertheless, several SNP's that prompt a specific amino acid exchange in hOCT1 revealed alternated affinity as well as substrate or inhibitor selectivity [9,11,22].

To elucidate the interaction of drugs and pesticides with human, mouse, and rat OCT1, we performed the inhibition of OCT1-mediated uptake of MPP with two concentrations (10 and 100 µM) for each of the 15 drugs and nine pesticides. Seven drugs showed an inhibitory potential with a reduction of the uptake rate to more than 50%. The highest inhibition for hOCT1 was observed at 100 µM for ketoconazole > clonidine > verapamil > quinine > elacridar > quinidine > procainamide. Other drugs revealed very low inhibitory effects on hOCT1 activity. Nevertheless, most of the inhibitor drugs showed comparable inhibition between hOCT1, mOct1, and rOct1, with only slight variation. The results achieved in this study at 10 µM drug inhibitory potential to hOCT1 in % reflect the published IC_{50} values of 2.6–7.4 µM for ketoconazole, 0.6–23 µM for clonidine, 1–13 µM for verapamil, 3.5–96 µM for quinine, 5–340 µM for quinidine, 15–74 µM for procainamide, and 5–34 µM for ritonavir [8]. Elacridar inhibited the OCT1-mediated MPP uptake down to 69% and 39% remaining transport activity at 10 and 100 µM. In this study, we demonstrate, for the first time, the interaction/inhibition of hOCT1, mOct1, and rOct1 by elacridar (also known as GF 120918), an inhibitor of several ABC-efflux transporters.

Pesticides are, unfortunately, a part of our nutrition. Therefore, the responsible agencies worldwide try to protect the consumers by setting the Maximum Residue Level (MRL). However, the MRL is often exceeded accidentally or intentionally [30,31]. Consumers are continually exposed to pesticides, primarily through residues in foodstuff [32] and by close neighborhood to farms intensively treated with pesticides, which leads to an intake of pesticides through inhalation as well as through the skin by contaminated air. Food safety reports 2014 of the German federal office of consumer protection and food safety as well as the commission of the European community for monitoring of pesticide residues in plant products confirmed that pesticide residues were found to different extent in several foods (vegetables). Glyphosate is the most used pesticide worldwide and 4000 exposures were reported by the US poison center each year. Almost 10% of these cases were intentional (suicide) ingestions [33]. Thousands of accidental and intentional deaths by ingestion of paraquat are also observed. A plasma concentration of 734 µg/mL was determined in a patient who intentionally ingested glyphosate. The half-life of glyphosate is 3.1 h [33].

Glyphosate was found in human urine samples possibly as a result of dietary intake or from occupational use [34]. A urinary excretion study from farm families exposed to glyphosate demonstrated a maximum concentration of 233 µg/mL [35]. Similarly, paraquat, imazalil, azoxystrobin, atrazine, amitraz as well as imidacloprid were excreted and identified in urine [36–41]. Prochloraz was not detected in urine but several of its metabolites were, e.g., 2,4,6-trichlorophenoxyacetic acid, which was detected mainly as a glucuronide conjugate [42]. The kidney actively secretes numerous pesticides. Therefore, several transporter proteins expressed in proximal tubule cells could be involved in the active secretion of pesticides. The transport of paraquat by hOCT2-expressing HEK cells was reported recently [21]. The interaction of azoxystrobin, propamocarb, and several other pesticides inhibit the efflux activity of rabbit Abcg2 at the MRL level [43]. However, the MRL in foodstuff show enormous concentration differences. For example, propamocarb MRL in cereals is 0.1 mg/kg while in vegetables, it is 500-fold higher (50 mg/kg). Therefore, we used relatively high concentrations (10 and 100 µM) of the nine pesticides, which are mainly positively charged at the physiological pH, to elucidate their inhibitory potential on human, mouse, and rat OCT1. The choice of the high concentrations of the pesticides for the inhibition of OCT1-mediated MPP uptake enabled us to directly compare the inhibitory potential of each pesticide to OCT1 activity. The highest species-independent inhibition of OCT1 was observed for imazalil, followed by propamocarb > azoxystrobin > prochloraz. The hOCT1-, mOct1-, and rOct1-mediated MPP uptake was decreased between 3% and 75%. The inhibition of OCT1 and OCT2 as well the stimulation of MATE2K by propamocarb was reported by Guéniche et al. (2020), but the study also confirmed that propamocarb is not a substrate of the cation transporter [44]. To our knowledge, up to now, there is no data that showed the excretion of propamocarb in urine. Therefore, OCTs as well as MATE2K are most probably not involved in the renal secretion of propamocarb. Nevertheless, the detection of imazalil, azoxystrobin, and prochloraz metabolites in urine might be an active elimination facilitated by the OCTs as well as by MATEs.

Atrazin, amitraz, glyphosat, imidacloprid, and paraquat showed at 100 µM either a marginal inhibitory effect or a stimulation of OCT1 activity. Several tested compounds, particularly ritonavir, amiodarone, glyphosate and atrazine, demonstrated a stimulatory effect between 16% and 65%. Drug-induced cis-stimulation of the reference substrate uptake was observed previously for various influx as well as for efflux transporters and numerous compounds. Hagos et al. demonstrated 24% to 86% stimulation of OAT3 (SLC22A8) as well as OAT4 (SLC22A11)-mediated estrone sulfate uptake by melphalan, respectively [45]. Irinotecan caused 93% stimulation of estrone sulfate uptake by OATP1B1 (SLCO1B1), as reported by Marada et al. (2015) [46]. The mechanism behind these phenomena is still not clear. One possible explanation is the binding of the compound to a specific site of the transporter which generates a higher turnover for the substrate. The consequence is a higher accumulation of the reference substrate in the cells even at relatively low concentrations. This modulation of the transporter is most probably caused by allosteric effects or cooperativity of specific sites within the transporter.

Chen et al. (2007) reported results comparable to our studies concerning the interaction of paraquat with OCT1 but, in contrast, they demonstrated the transport of paraquat by OCT2, while we did not observe a significant interaction for paraquat with hOCT2. Since these pesticides did not interact significantly with OCTs as well as with MATEs, the renal secretion mediated by the cationic transporter that were examined in this study and are located in the kidney could be excluded. Most of these pesticides interact with several efflux transporters. Therefore, it would need further studies to understand the role of SLC transporters in the renal secretion mechanism of the pesticides. In this study, we evaluated the inhibitory potential of drugs and pesticides to hOCT1-, mOCT1- and rOct1-mediated uptake of MPP. Based on our data, we cannot deny that some of the drugs and pesticides that showed an inhibitory potential are also substrates of the OCTs. For a differentiation between inhibitor and substrate there are several options for further studies: If the substance to be examined is available radioactively or fluorescently labeled, a direct measurement of the accumulation in the HEK cells is possible, but the ultimate method to determine the OCT1-mediated uptake of non-labeled drugs and pesticides is by the HPLC tandem LC–MS/MS method. For a precise understanding of the interaction of the above-mentioned drugs and pesticides, further OCT1-mediated substrate uptake by LS–MS/MS analysis are needed.

In conclusion, the present study elucidated, for 26 structurally different and, at pH 7.4, mainly positively charged compounds, a good functional correlation between human, mouse, and rat OCT1. Additionally, we found substantial inhibitory potential for three of the selected pesticides with

OCT1, which was not species dependent. Nevertheless, potential species differences within OCT1 could not be excluded for other drugs and pesticides that were not considered in this study. Hence, for clinically relevant new molecular entities, it is recommended to perform functional in vivo as well as in vitro comparisons of the transport in humans and rodents.

4. Materials and Methods

4.1. Material

^{3}H-MPP (1-Methyl-4-phenylpyridinium iodide) and ^{14}C-metformin were purchased from American Radiolabeled Chemicals Saint louis; Missouri, USA. All non labelled chemicals were obtained from Sigma-Aldrich, Darmstadt, Germany. For transfection, the following cDNAs were used: hOCT1 (GeneBank: accession number: NM_003057.2), mOct1 (NM_009202.5), rOct1 (NM_012697.1), hMATE1 (NM_018242.2), and hOCT2 (NM_003058.3). The hOCT1 cloned has the genotype Ser14, Arg61, Cys88, Phe160, Gly401,Met408, Met420 and Gly465, which corresponds to the OCT1*1B allele according to the nomenclature suggested by Seitz et al. [29].

4.2. Transfection and Cell Culture

The respective cDNA of the cation transporters has been cloned into the expression vector pcDNA5/FRT. Human embryonic kidney (HEK-293-Flp-In) cells (Invitrogen, Darmstadt, Germany) were transfected using Lipofectamine 2000 (Invitrogen, Darmstadt, Germany) according to the manufacturer's protocol. Twenty-four hours after transfection, 175 µg/mL hygromycin B was added to the medium to select stable clones. After two to three weeks, single colonies were picked and expanded. The growth medium for stably transfected HEK-293 cells was Dulbecco's modified Eagle's medium (DMEM, high glucose) supplemented with 10% fetal bovine serum (Biochrom, Berlin, Geramny), 1% penicillin (10.000 Units/mL)/streptomycin (10 mg/mL). Cell lines were grown in a humidified atmosphere containing 5% CO_2 at 37 °C.

4.3. Transporter Mediated Uptake of Radiolabeled Substrates

For uptake assays, 2×10^5 cells in 0.5 mL growth medium per well were seeded into 24-well plates, coated with poly-D-lysine and cultured for 3 days. Then, growth medium was aspirated and each well was rinsed three times with 0.5 mL incubation buffer (HBSS buffer supplemented with 20 mM HEPES, pH 7.4) and incubated at least 20 min at 37 °C as described previously [47]. For hMATE1, it was necessary to generate an intracellular acidification; therefore, the cells were pre-incubated for at least 30 min in a 30 mM NH_4Cl containing incubation buffer at pH 7.4 and 37 °C.

The incubation buffer was removed and 200 µL incubation buffer containing radiolabeled and non-radiolabeled substances was added to each well and incubated at 37 °C for 1 min. After incubation, the uptake was terminated by aspirating the reaction mixture and washing the cells three times with 0.4 mL ice-cold PBS buffer. Cells were solubilized with 0.6 mL of 1N NaOH overnight. [^{3}H] or [^{14}C] content was measured after addition of 2.5 mL scintillation solvent (Roti®eco plus, Carl Roth, Karlsruhe, Germany) in a Beckmann LS6000 scintillation counter.

To determine the affinity (K_m) of MPP as a substrate of organic cation transporter, saturation experiments at initial rate period were performed as determined in time dependency experiments (data not shown). Organic cation transporter transfected HEK and empty vector-HEK cells were incubated for 1 min with 2 nM [^{3}H] MPP and increasing concentrations of non-labeled MPP: 1, 10, 25, 50, 100, 250, 500, and 750 µM. Experiments were conducted on at least two separate days. On each day, all experiments were performed as triplicates.

4.4. Inhibition Experiments

Inhibition experiments for IC_{50} determination were performed for 1 min with the known inhibitor of organic cation transporter, decynium22, at the respective calculated K_m-values of MPP (containing

2nM ^{3}H MPP). The MPP uptake was cis-inhibited by following concentrations of decynium22: 1, 5, 10, 25, 50, 75, and 100 µM. Experiments were conducted on at least 2 separate days. On each day, all experiments were performed as triplicates.

For screening experiments, cis-inhibition was carried out in duplicate by measuring the uptake of the labeled probe substrate in the absence and presence of 10 µM or 100 µM of the respective pesticide or drug. Transporter- and vector transfected HEK293 cells were incubated for 1 min with 2 nM ^{3}H-MPP or 1 µM ^{14}C-metformin. Inhibitory effects in percent were calculated from net-uptake.

4.5. Determination of Protein Concentration

The cellular protein amount was determined using a method described by Bradford [48]. On each experimental day, six wells per cell line of an additional 24-well plate were analyzed in parallel to the transport experiments. Cell monolayers in 24-well plates were washed three times with 0.5 mL incubation buffer and afterwards stored at −20 °C. For protein determination, the plates were thawed and each well was incubated for lyses 30–60 min in 100 µL 1× lyses buffer (Promega, Manheim, Germany). Cell lysate was filled up with ddH$_2$O to 1 mL per well and mixed thoroughly. The protein determination was performed in 96-well plates (flat bottom; Sarstedt, Nümbrecht, Germany) in duplicate. BSA was used as standard for a calibration curve ranging from 50 to 300 µg/mL. A total of 20 µL of BSA standards or 20 µL sample (1:1 diluted in ddH$_2$O) were mixed with 200 µL 1x Bradford reagent (Carl Roth) per well. After 10–20 min of incubation at room temperature, absorption was measured at 595 nm (Microplate Reader, Wallac Victor2 Perkin Elmer, Rodgau-Jügesheim, Germany). A standard curve was plotted from absorbance of 0–300 µg of BSA and the concentration of each test sample was determined using the standard curve.

4.6. Data Analysis

For the K_m calculation of MPP, the transporter-mediated uptake (pmol/mg protein/min) was plotted against MPP concentrations. The K_m and V_{max} values were obtained using SigmaPlot 13 by fitting the Michaelis–Menten equation V = V_{max}*[S]/(K_m + [S]), where V refers to the rate of substrate transport, V_{max} refers to the maximum rate of substrate transport, [S] refers to the concentration of substrate, and Km is defined as the concentration of substrate at the half-maximal transport rate. The inhibitory effect I (%) was calculated according to the formula I(%) = 100 − ($V_{\text{with inhibitor}}$*100/$V_{\text{w/o inhibitor}}$), and, for the IC$_{50}$ calculation of the inhibitor, the inhibitory effect I (%) was plotted against inhibitor concentrations and fitted using a 3-parameter Hill equation with I_{max} set to 100 using SigmaPlot 13.

Author Contributions: Conceptualization, S.F., A.K. and Y.H.; validation, S.F. and A.K.; investigation, S.F. and A.K. resources, writing—original draft preparation, Y.H.; writing—review Y.H., S.F. and A.K. and editing, Y.H.; project administration, A.K.; funding acquisition, Y.H., S.F. and A.K. All authors have read and agreed to the published version of the manuscript.

Funding: German Federal Ministry of Education and Research (BMBF).

Acknowledgments: For excellent technical support Anja Herdlitschke, Rovena Halpape and Andrea Mareike Cordes. Muhammad Rafehi for proofreading.

Conflicts of Interest: The authors declare no conflict of interest.

References

1. Gründemann, D.; Gorboulev, V.; Gambaryan, S.; Veyhl, M.; Koepsell, H. Drug excretion mediated by a new prototype of polyspecific transporter. *Nature* **1994**, *372*, 549–552. [CrossRef] [PubMed]
2. Zhang, L.; Dresser, M.J.; Gray, A.T.; Yost, S.C.; Terashita, S.; Giacomini, K.M. Cloning and functional expression of a human liver organic cation transporter. *Mol. Pharmacol.* **1997**, *51*, 913–921. [CrossRef] [PubMed]
3. Koepsell, H.; Schmitt, B.M.; Gorboulev, V. Organic cation transporters. *Rev. Physiol. Biochem. Pharmacol.* **2003**, *150*, 36–90. [CrossRef] [PubMed]

4. Gorboulev, V.; Ulzheimer, J.C.; Akhoundova, A.; Ulzheimer-Teuber, I.; Karbach, U.; Quester, S.; Baumann, C.; Lang, F.; Busch, A.E.; Koepsell, H. Cloning and characterization of two human polyspecific organic cation transporters. *DNA Cell Biol.* **1997**, *16*, 871–881. [CrossRef] [PubMed]
5. Nies, A.T.; Koepsell, H.; Winter, S.; Burk, O.; Klein, K.; Kerb, R.; Zanger, U.M.; Keppler, D.; Schwab, M.; Schaeffeler, E. Expression of organic cation transporters OCT1 (SLC22A1) and OCT3 (SLC22A3) is affected by genetic factors and cholestasis in human liver. *Hepatol.* **2009**, *50*, 1227–1240. [CrossRef] [PubMed]
6. Koepsell, H.; Lips, K.; Volk, C. Polyspecific organic cation transporters: Structure, function, physiological roles, and biopharmaceutical implications. *Pharm.Res.* **2007**, *24*, 1227–1251. [CrossRef] [PubMed]
7. Han, T.K.; Everett, R.S.; Proctor, W.R.; Ng, C.M.; Costales, C.L.; Brouwer, K.L.R.; Thakker, D.R. Organic cation transporter 1 (OCT1/mOct1) is localized in the apical membrane of Caco-2 cell monolayers and enterocytes. *Mol. Pharmacol.* **2013**, *84*, 182–189. [CrossRef]
8. Koepsell, H. Organic Cation Transporters in Health and Disease. *Pharmacol. Rev.* **2020**, *72*, 253–319. [CrossRef]
9. Tzvetkov, M.V.; dos Santos Pereira, J.N.; Meineke, I.; Saadatmand, A.R.; Stingl, J.C.; Brockmöller, J. Morphine is a substrate of the organic cation transporter OCT1 and polymorphisms in OCT1 gene affect morphine pharmacokinetics after codeine administration. *Biochem. Pharmacol.* **2013**, *86*, 666–678. [CrossRef]
10. Koepsell, H. The SLC22 family with transporters of organic cations, anions and zwitterions. *Mol. Asp. Med.* **2013**, *34*, 413–435. [CrossRef]
11. Matthaei, J.; Kuron, D.; Faltraco, F.; Knoch, T.; Dos Santos Pereira, J.N.; Abu Abed, M.; Prukop, T.; Brockmöller, J.; Tzvetkov, M.V. OCT1 mediates hepatic uptake of sumatriptan and loss-of-function OCT1 polymorphisms affect sumatriptan pharmacokinetics. *Clin. Pharmacol. Ther.* **2016**, *99*, 633–641. [CrossRef] [PubMed]
12. Tu, M.; Sun, S.; Wang, K.; Peng, X.; Wang, R.; Li, L.; Zeng, S.; Zhou, H.; Jiang, H. Organic cation transporter 1 mediates the uptake of monocrotaline and plays an important role in its hepatotoxicity. *Toxicology* **2013**, *311*, 225–230. [CrossRef] [PubMed]
13. Giacomini, K.M.; Huang, S.M.; Tweedie, D.J.; Benet, L.Z.; Brouwer, K.L.; Chu, X.; Dahlin, A.; Evers, R.; Fischer, V.; Hillgren, K.M.; et al. Membrane transporters in drug development. *Nat. Rev. Drug Discov.* **2010**, *9*, 215–236. [PubMed]
14. Lauer, B.; Tuschl, G.; Kling, M.; Mueller, S.O. Species-specific toxicity of diclofenac and troglitazone in primary human and rat hepatocytes. *Chem. Biol. Interact.* **2009**, *179*, 17–24. [CrossRef]
15. Tuschl, G.; Lauer, B.; Mueller, S.O. Primary hepatocytes as a model to analyze species-specific toxicity and drug metabolism. *Expert Opin. Drug Metab. Toxicol.* **2008**, *4*, 855–870. [CrossRef]
16. Lai, Y. Identification of interspecies difference in hepatobiliary transporters to improve extrapolation of human biliary secretion. *Expert Opin. Drug Metab. Toxicol.* **2009**, *5*, 1175–1187. [CrossRef]
17. Dresser, M.J.; Gray, A.T.; Giacomini, K.M. Kinetic and selectivity differences between rodent, rabbit, and human organic cation transporters (OCT1). *J. Pharmacol. Exp. Ther.* **2000**, *292*, 1146–1152.
18. Okuda, M.; Urakami, Y.; Saito, H.; Inui, K. Molecular mechanisms of organic cation transport in OCT2-expressing Xenopus oocytes. *Biochim. Biophys. Acta* **1999**, *1417*, 224–231. [CrossRef]
19. Vermeer, L.M.M.; Isringhausen, C.D.; Ogilvie, B.W.; Buckley, D.B. Evaluation of Ketoconazole and Its Alternative Clinical CYP3A4/5 Inhibitors as Inhibitors of Drug Transporters: The In Vitro Effects of Ketoconazole, Ritonavir, Clarithromycin, and Itraconazole on 13 Clinically-Relevant Drug Transporters. *Drug Metab. Dispos.* **2016**, *44*, 453–459. [CrossRef]
20. Panfen, E.; Chen, W.; Zhang, Y.; Sinz, M.; Marathe, P.; Gan, J.; Shen, H. Enhanced and Persistent Inhibition of Organic Cation Transporter 1 Activity by Preincubation of Cyclosporine A. *Drug Metab. Dispos.* **2019**, *47*, 1352–1360. [CrossRef]
21. Chen, Y.; Zhang, S.; Sorani, M.; Giacomini, K.M. Transport of paraquat by human organic cation transporters and multidrug and toxic compound extrusion family. *J. Pharmacol. Exp. Ther.* **2007**, *322*, 695–700. [CrossRef]
22. Meyer, M.J.; Seitz, T.; Brockmöller, J.; Tzvetkov, M.V. Effects of genetic polymorphisms on the OCT1 and OCT2-mediated uptake of ranitidine. *PLoS ONE* **2017**, *12*. [CrossRef] [PubMed]
23. Gründemann, D.; Hahne, C.; Berkels, R.; Schömig, E. Agmatine is efficiently transported by non-neuronal monoamine transporters extraneuronal monoamine transporter (EMT) and organic cation transporter 2 (OCT2). *J. Pharmacol. Exp. Ther.* **2003**, *304*, 810–817. [CrossRef] [PubMed]

24. Kakehi, M.; Koyabu, N.; Nakamura, T.; Uchiumi, T.; Kuwano, M.; Ohtani, H.; Sawada, Y. Functional characterization of mouse cation transporter mOCT2 compared with mOCT1. *Biochem. Biophys. Res. Commun.* **2002**, *296*, 644–650. [CrossRef]
25. Gorboulev, V.; Shatskaya, N.; Volk, C.; Koepsell, H. Subtype-specific affinity for corticosterone of rat organic cation transporters rOCT1 and rOCT2 depends on three amino acids within the substrate binding region. *Mol. Pharmacol.* **2005**, *67*, 1612–1619. [CrossRef]
26. Martel, F.; Martins, M.J.; Azevedo, I. Inward transport of 3H-MPP+ in freshly isolated rat hepatocytes: Evidence for interaction with catecholamines. *Naunyn Schmiedebergs Arch. Pharmacol.* **1996**, *354*, 305–311. [CrossRef]
27. Wright, S.H.; Dantzler, W.H. Molecular and cellular physiology of renal organic cation and anion transport. *Physiol. Rev.* **2004**, *84*, 987–1049. [CrossRef]
28. Gorboulev, V.; Volk, C.; Arndt, P.; Akhoundova, A.; Koepsell, H. Selectivity of the polyspecific cation transporter rOCT1 is changed by mutation of aspartate 475 to glutamate. *Mol. Pharmacol.* **1999**, *56*, 1254–1261. [CrossRef]
29. Seitz, T.; Stalmann, R.; Dalila, N.; Chen, J.; Pojar, S.; Dos Santos Pereira, J.N.; Krätzner, R.; Brockmöller, J.; Tzvetkov, M.V. Global genetic analyses reveal strong inter-ethnic variability in the loss of activity of the organic cation transporter OCT1. *Genome Med.* **2015**, *7*. [CrossRef]
30. Tsiplakou, E.; Anagnostopoulos, C.J.; Liapis, K.; Haroutounian, S.A.; Zervas, G. Pesticides residues in milks and feedstuff of farm animals drawn from Greece. *Chemosphere* **2010**, *80*, 504–512. [CrossRef]
31. Pirsaheb, M.; Limoee, M.; Namdari, F.; Khamutian, R. Organochlorine pesticides residue in breast milk: A systematic review. *Med. J. Islam. Repub. Iran.* **2015**, *29*, 228. [PubMed]
32. Hamilton, D.; Ambrus, A.; Dieterle, R.; Felsot, A.; Harris, C.; Petersen, B.; Racke, K.; Wong, S.-S.; Gonzalez, R.; Tanaka, K.; et al. Pesticide residues in food–acute dietary exposure. *Pest Manag. Sci.* **2004**, *60*, 311–339. [CrossRef] [PubMed]
33. Roberts, D.M.; Buckley, N.A.; Mohamed, F.; Eddleston, M.; Goldstein, D.A.; Mehrsheikh, A.; Bleeke, M.S.; Dawson, A.H. A prospective observational study of the clinical toxicology of glyphosate-containing herbicides in adults with acute self-poisoning. *Clin. Toxicol. (Phila.)* **2010**, *48*, 129–136. [CrossRef] [PubMed]
34. Niemann, L.; Sieke, C.; Pfeil, R.; Solecki, R. A critical review of glyphosate findings in human urine samples and comparison with the exposure of operators and consumers. *J. Verbr. Lebensm.* **2015**, *10*, 3–12. [CrossRef]
35. Acquavella, J.F.; Alexander, B.H.; Mandel, J.S.; Gustin, C.; Baker, B.; Chapman, P.; Bleeke, M. Glyphosate biomonitoring for farmers and their families: Results from the Farm Family Exposure Study. *Environ. Health Perspect.* **2004**, *112*, 321–326. [CrossRef] [PubMed]
36. Chan, B.S.; Lazzaro, V.A.; Seale, J.P.; Duggin, G.G. The renal excretory mechanisms and the role of organic cations in modulating the renal handling of paraquat. *Pharmacol. Ther.* **1998**, *79*, 193–203. [CrossRef]
37. Faniband, M.H.; Littorin, M.; Ekman, E.; Jönsson, B.A.G.; Lindh, C.H. LC-MS-MS Analysis of Urinary Biomarkers of Imazalil Following Experimental Exposures. *J. Anal. Toxicol.* **2015**, *39*, 691–697. [CrossRef]
38. Jamin, E.L.; Bonvallot, N.; Tremblay-Franco, M.; Cravedi, J.-P.; Chevrier, C.; Cordier, S.; Debrauwer, L. Untargeted profiling of pesticide metabolites by LC-HRMS: An exposomics tool for human exposure evaluation. *Anal. Bioanal. Chem.* **2014**, *406*, 1149–1161. [CrossRef]
39. Kuklenyik, Z.; Panuwet, P.; Jayatilaka, N.K.; Pirkle, J.L.; Calafat, A.M. Two-dimensional high performance liquid chromatography separation and tandem mass spectrometry detection of atrazine and its metabolic and hydrolysis products in urine. *J. Chromatogr. B Analyt. Technol. Biomed. Life Sci.* **2012**, *901*, 1–8. [CrossRef]
40. Gao, X.; Tan, Y.; Guo, H. Simultaneous determination of amitraz, chlordimeform, formetanate and their main metabolites in human urine by high performance liquid chromatography-tandem mass spectrometry. *J. Chromatogr. B Analyt. Technol. Biomed. Life Sci.* **2017**, *1052*, 27–33. [CrossRef]
41. Tao, Y.; Dong, F.; Xu, J.; Phung, D.; Liu, Q.; Li, R.; Liu, X.; Wu, X.; He, M.; Zheng, Y. Characteristics of neonicotinoid imidacloprid in urine following exposure of humans to orchards in China. *Environ. Int.* **2019**, *132*, 105079. [CrossRef] [PubMed]
42. Needham, D.; Challis, I.R. The metabolism and excretion of prochloraz, an imidazole-based fungicide, in the rat. *Xenobiotica* **1991**, *21*, 1473–1482. [CrossRef] [PubMed]
43. Halwachs, S.; Schäfer, I.; Kneuer, C.; Seibel, P.; Honscha, W. Assessment of ABCG2-mediated transport of pesticides across the rabbit placenta barrier using a novel MDCKII in vitro model. *Toxicol. Appl. Pharmacol.* **2016**, *305*, 66–74. [CrossRef] [PubMed]

44. Guéniche, N.; Bruyere, A.; Ringeval, M.; Jouan, E.; Huguet, A.; Hégarat, L.L.; Fardel, O. Differential interactions of carbamate pesticides with drug transporters. *Xenobiotica* **2020**, 1–13. [CrossRef]
45. Hagos, Y.; Hundertmark, P.; Shnitsar, V.; Marada, V.V.; Wulf, G.; Burckhardt, G. Renal human organic anion transporter 3 increases the susceptibility of lymphoma cells to bendamustine uptake. *Am. J. Physiol. Renal. Physiol.* **2015**, *308*, F330–F338. [CrossRef]
46. Marada, V.V.; Florl, S.; Kuhne, A.; Burckhardt, G.; Hagos, Y. Interaction of human organic anion transporter polypeptides 1B1 and 1B3 with antineoplastic compounds. *Eur. J. Med. Chem.* **2015**, *92*, 723–731. [CrossRef]
47. Hagos, Y.; Stein, D.; Ugele, B.; Burckhardt, G.; Bahn, A. Human Renal Organic Anion Transporter 4 Operates as an Asymmetric Urate Transporter. *J. Am. Soc. Nephrol.* **2007**, *18*, 430–439. [CrossRef]
48. Bradford, M.M. A rapid and sensitive method for the quantitation of microgram quantities of protein utilizing the principle of protein-dye binding. *Anal. Biochem.* **1976**, *72*, 248–254. [CrossRef]

© 2020 by the authors. Licensee MDPI, Basel, Switzerland. This article is an open access article distributed under the terms and conditions of the Creative Commons Attribution (CC BY) license (http://creativecommons.org/licenses/by/4.0/).

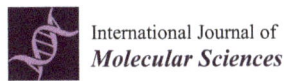

Article

Tofacitinib and Baricitinib Are Taken up by Different Uptake Mechanisms Determining the Efficacy of Both Drugs in RA

Jan Amrhein [1], Susanne Drynda [2], Lukas Schlatt [3], Uwe Karst [3], Christoph H. Lohmann [2], Giuliano Ciarimboli [1] and Jessica Bertrand [2,*]

1. Experimental Nephrology, Department of Internal Medicine D, University Hospital Münster, 48149 Münster, Germany; jan.amrhein@web.de (J.A.); gciari@uni-muenster.de (G.C.)
2. Department of Orthopedic Surgery, Otto-von-Guericke University, 39120 Magdeburg, Germany; susanne.drynda@med.ovgu.de (S.D.); christoph.lohmann@med.ovgu.de (C.H.L.)
3. Institute of Inorganic and Analytical Chemistry, University of Münster, 48149 Münster, Germany; lukas.schlatt@uni-muenster.de (L.S.); uk@uni-muenster.de (U.K.)
* Correspondence: jessica.bertrand@med.ovgu.de; Tel.: +49-391-67-15804

Received: 27 August 2020; Accepted: 9 September 2020; Published: 10 September 2020

Abstract: Background: Rheumatoid arthritis (RA) is a systemic autoimmune disease in which synovial fibroblasts (SF) play a key role. Baricitinib and Tofacitinib both act intracellularly, blocking the ATP-binding side of JAK proteins and thereby the downstream signalling pathway via STAT-3. Therefore, we investigated the role of organic cation transporters (OCTs) in Baricitinib and Tofacitinib cellular transport. Methods: OCT expression was analysed in SF isolated from RA and osteoarthritis (OA) patients, as well as peripheral blood mononuclear cells. The interaction of Baricitinib and Tofacitinib with OCTs was investigated using quenching experiments. The intracellular accumulation of both drugs was quantified using LC/MS. Target inhibition for both drugs was tested using Western blot for phosphorylated JAK1 and STAT3 upon stimulation with IL-6. Results: MATE-1 expression increased in OASF compared to RASF. The other OCTs were not differentially expressed. The transport of Baricitinib was not OCT dependent. Tofacitinib; however, was exported from RASF in a MATE-1 dependent way. Tofacitinib and Baricitinib showed comparable inhibition of downstream signalling pathways. Conclusion: We observed different cellular uptake strategies for Baricitinib and Tofacitinib. Tofacitinib was exported out of healthy cells due to the increased expression of MATE1. This might make Tofacitinib the favourable drug.

Keywords: RA; Tofacitinib; Baricitinib; organic cation transporter; MATE1

1. Introduction

Rheumatoid arthritis (RA) is a systemic autoimmune disease that predominantly affects synovial joints, causing progressive polyarthritis, joint destruction and disability [1]. Synovial fibroblasts (SF) are key players in the development of RA [2]. In healthy synovial joints the synovium is formed of a few fibroblast layers, which mainly regulate the production of synovial fluid [3]. Fibroblasts also play a role in the inert immune system, carrying Toll-like receptors and being able to secrete cytokines [4,5]. In RA, fibroblasts evolve a tumour-like phenotype which transforms them to Rheumatoid Arthritis synovial fibroblasts (RASF) [6]. RASF acquire an aggressive phenotype with increased proliferation, loss of cell–cell contacts and joint invasiveness, where they secrete proinflammatory cytokines and interact with other immune and stroma cells to perpetuate the inflammatory reaction [2].

Cytokine signalling is a crucial driver of inflammation processes in RA. Besides tumour necrosis factor alpha (TNF-α), Interleukin-6 (IL-6) mediates major inflammatory signalling pathways in RA [7].

Among other cytokines, it predominantly affects the JAK/STAT signalling. Janus kinases (JAKs) are non-receptor protein tyrosine kinases that consist of JAK1, JAK2, JAK3 and TYK2. IL-6 binds to the IL-6Rα/gp130 complex that is linked to JAKs [8]. Upon binding of IL-6 to the receptor complex JAKs get phosphorylated by each other [9]. The cytosolic signal transducer and activator of transcription proteins (STATs) are able to bind to phosphorylated residues of the JAKs and get phosphorylated as well. They dimerize, translocate into the cell nucleus and act as transcription factors for the production of further proinflammatory cytokines, as well as cell differentiation and cell proliferation inducing factors [8].

Baricitinib and Tofacitinib are both relative new drugs, so called tyrosine kinase inhibitors (TKIs), approved and recommended by the European League Against Rheumatism (EULAR) for the treatment of RA [10,11]. These TKIs both act intracellularly, where they block the ATP-binding side of JAK proteins and thereby the downstream signalling pathway via STAT proteins. The binding of JAK inhibitors reduces cell differentiation, proliferation and production of proinflammatory cytokines [12,13]. Patients, that show an inadequate response to the disease-modifying drugs methotrexate (MTX) and/or biologics, may receive Tofacitinib or Baricitinib. Therefore, it is important to determine the optimal treatment options for these patients with regard to efficacy and safety of Tofacitinib and Baricitinib. To date, it is not known why different TKIs exert different effects in patients with the same disease. Differences in the uptake mechanism could explain these differences.

Around 40% of all orally administered drugs show cationic characteristics, and therefore need specific transport systems to penetrate nonpolar cell membranes to reach their intracellular target [14]. Previous studies showed that other TKIs like Imatinib and Saracatinib were dependent on polyspecific (meaning that they can accept structurally different substances as substrate) organic cation transporters (OCTs) to reach their intracellular target [15–17]. OCTs are part of the solute carrier (SLC) family [18]. This family includes the human organic cation transporters (hOCT1, hOCT2, hOCT3), the novel organic cation transporters (hOCTN1, hOCTN2), and the multidrug and toxin extrusion proteins (hMATE1, hMATE2k). Many of these OCTs share the same substrates, but every transporter has an individual substrate/inhibitor interaction profile. Whereas hMATE1, hMATE2k and hOCTN1 mediate a H+/organic cation (OC) antiport, hOCT1, hOCT2 and hOCT3 transport along the electrochemical gradient of their substrates. OCTs are widely expressed in different cells and are essential for the secretion of organic cations (OCs) in the liver and kidney [19]. Even though they transport mainly endogenous and exogenous OCs, interactions with zwitterions and anions have been reported [20,21].

As Tofacitinib and Baricitinib are established drugs for the treatment of RA, we investigated the uptake pathways of these drugs under RA relevant conditions focussing on their interaction with different OCTs and on their therapeutic efficiency in RASF.

2. Results

2.1. Tofacitinib Could Be a Target for OCT Mediated Cellular Uptake

Predictions on the pKa of Baricitinib and Tofacitinib, using the online tool Chemicalize of ChemAxon, showed that Baricitinib is not charged in neutral pH solutions (red box Figure 1B), whereas Tofacitinib is partially positively charged (red box, Figure 1A). Adjusting the pH to more acidic values, like in RA synovial fluid, supposes an increase of positively charged species of the two drugs. However, Baricitinib would largely stay uncharged, whereas Tofacitinib gets more positively charged making it a potential substrate for organic cation transporters. Therefore, we investigated the expression pattern of OCTs in OASF and RASF (Figure 1C). We observed no difference in the expression of *hOCT1* and *hOCT3* between RA and OA synovial fibroblasts. *hOCT2* was not detectable. *hOCTN2* was also only weakly expressed and no difference was seen between RASF and OASF. RASF, however, expressed significantly more *hOCTN1* ($F_{(9, 44)} = 12.06$, 95% CI: 0.4480 to 1.157, $p < 0.0001$). *MATE-1* was lower expressed in RASFs compared to OASF ($F_{(9, 44)} = 12.06$, 95% CI: -0.6278 to -0.01494, $p = 0.0358$). This effect is even more pronounced in PBMCs from RA and OA patients (supplementary Figure S1). As both TKIs influence the IL-6 dependent pathways, we stimulated RASF with IL-6 and investigated the changes in the OCT expression pattern (Figure 1D). We observed an increase of *hMATE-1* expression, levelling out the differences between RASF and OASF. The other analysed OCTs were not changed in their expression.

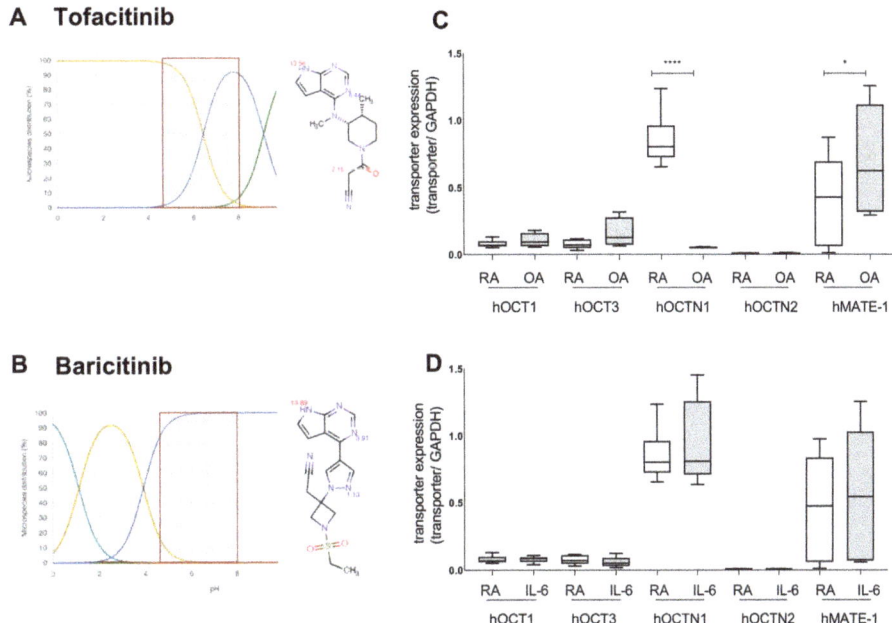

Figure 1. Tofacitinib could be a target for OCT mediated cellular uptake. (**A**,**B**) pKA prediction for Tofacitinib (**A**) and Baricitinib (**B**). The yellow curves indicate the presence of cationic form, the blue curves indicate the neutral form and the green curves of the anionic form of the substances at the given pH-values. The red boxes indicate the physiological pH-range. (**C**) Quantitative RT-PCR for the expression pattern of OCTs, and *hMATE-1* from OASF and RASF. GAPDH was used as housekeeping gene for normalization. (**D**) Quantitative RT-PCR investigating the expression pattern of OCTs, and *hMATE-1* in RASF after stimulation with 10 ng/mL IL-6 for 24 h. *GAPDH* was used as housekeeping gene for normalization. Statistical analyses were performed using an ordinary one-way ANOVA and Sidak correction for multiple testing. *: $p < 0.05$; ****: $p < 0.0001$

2.2. Baricitinib Uptake Is Not Transporter Dependent

First, we investigated a potential interaction of Baricitinib with different OCTs using the ASP+ quenching method as a readout. We observed no significant interaction with any of the expressed OCTs in a physiological range of Baricitinib concentration (Figure 2A,B). To investigate a potential transporter dependent accumulation of Baricitinib in SF, we used OASF and RASF for LC/MS determination of intracellular Baricitinib concentrations. We observed no change in Baricitinib concentration neither depending on the temperature, nor depending on the disease (RASF vs OASF). We observed a higher intracellular Baricitinib concentration using 1 µM (Figure 2C), compared to the approximate serum concentration of 0.15 µM Baricitinib (Figure 2D). However, no temperature-dependent change in Baricitinib concentration was detected, indicating that the uncharged Baricitinib might be able to penetrate the cell membrane without active transport.

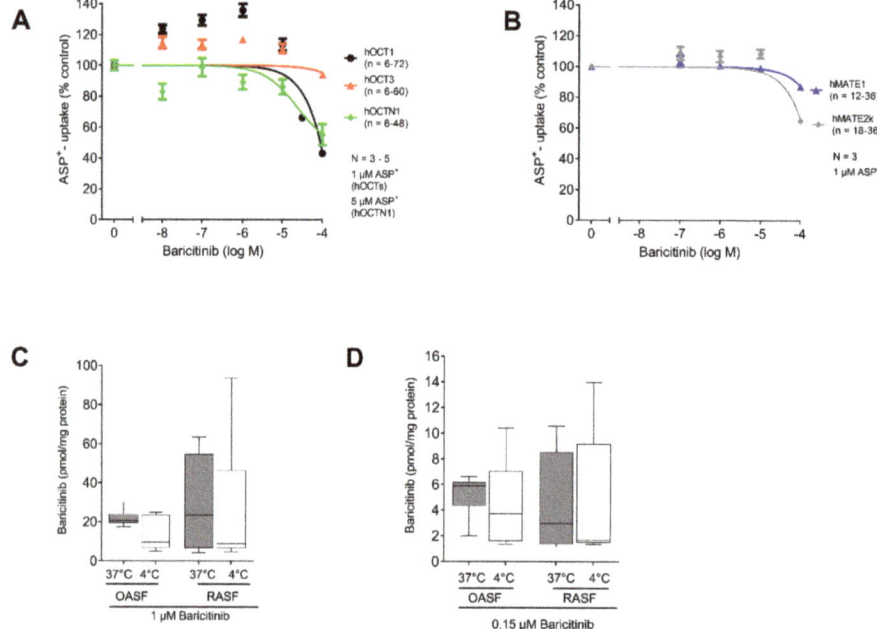

Figure 2. Baricitinib uptake is not transporter dependent. (**A**) ASP$^+$ determined apparent affinity of Baricitinib to hOCT1, hOCT3 and hOCTN1. No significant interaction was observed (n = 3–5). (**B**) ASP$^+$ determined affinity of hMATE1 and hMATE2k after intracellular acidification (n = 3). No significant interaction was observed. Data in (**A**,**B**) are presented as mean ± SEM and fitted using a non-linear fit. (**C**) LC/MS measurement of temperature dependent Baricitinib (1 µM) uptake in RASF and OASF (F (1.332, 10.21) = 1.570; p = 0.2470; n = 3). (**D**) LC/MS measurement of temperature dependent Baricitinib uptake (0.15 µM) in RASF and OASF (F (2.071, 16.56) = 0.44, p = 0.6578, n = 3). Statistical analyses were performed using a RM ANOVA. No post-hoc testing was performed, as the ANOVA was not significant. Data in (**C**,**D**) are presented as box plot with whiskers indicating the min and max values, as well as the median.

2.3. MATE-1 Mediates Tofacitinib Transport

To test the affinity of Tofacitinib to different OCTs, we again performed the ASP$^+$ quenching assay. We observed no interaction of Tofacitinib with the OCTs (Figure 3A). Next, we investigated the interaction with MATE transporters using previous acidification. Interestingly, we found concentration-dependent inhibition of ASP$^+$ uptake by Tofacitinib in hMATE1 transfected HEK cells with an IC50 of 19.8 µM (Figure 3B). To validate this finding, we used hMATE1-transfected HEK cells and observed a significant decrease in Tofacitinib intracellular accumulation at 37 °C (F (1.805, 12.63) = 20.71, 95% CI: −39.45 to −23.47, p < 0.0001). This suggests a transporter mediated export of Tofacitinib via hMATE1 (Figure 3C). When investigating 1 µM Tofacitinib concentration in OASF at 37 °C and 4 °C, we again observed significantly lower Tofacitinib concentrations at 37 °C compared to 4 °C (1 µM) (F (2.123, 12.74) = 10.15, 95% CI: −3.405 to −0.9026, p = 0.0045) (Figure 3D). This effect was not as pronounced in RASF, which might be explained by the lower hMATE1 expression in RASF compared to OASF (F (2.123, 12.74) = 10.15, 95% CI: −2.549 to 0.6115, p = 0.225). Using the approximate serum concentration of Tofacitinib for therapeutic use, we found the same pattern again, indicating that this effect is also present at low Tofacitinib concentrations (OASF: F (1.969, 15.75) = 6.925, 95% CI: −2.118 to −0.3189, p = 0.012) (Figure 3E).

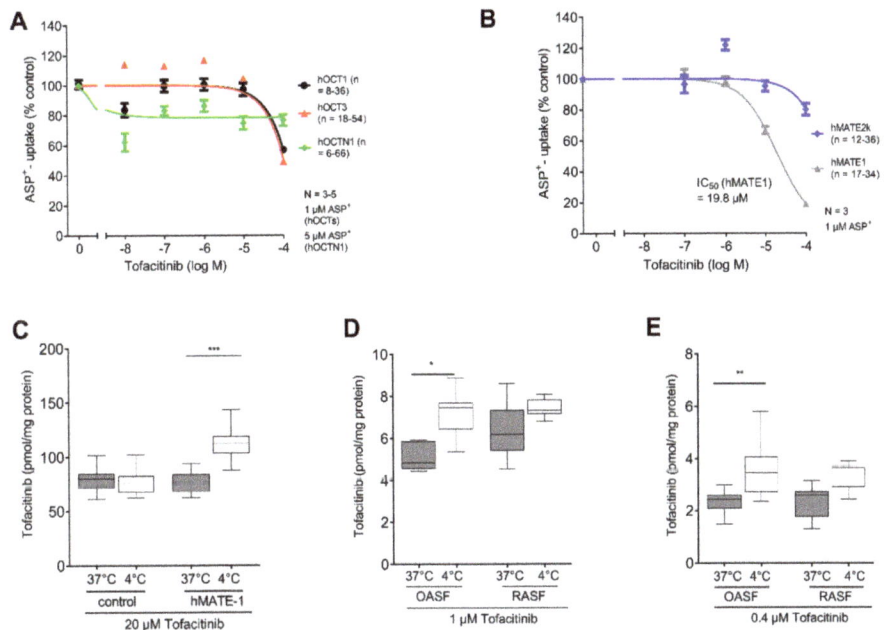

Figure 3. MATE-1 mediates Tofacitinib transport. (**A**) ASP$^+$ determined apparent affinity of Tofacitinib to hOCT1, hOCT3 and hOCTN1. No significant interaction was observed (n = 3–5). (**B**) ASP$^+$ determined apparent affinity of hMATE1 and hMATE2k after intracellular acidification (n = 3). MATE-1 shows an apparent affinity IC50 = 19.8 µM to MATE-1. Data in (**A**,**B**) are presented as mean ± SEM and fitted using a non-linear fit. (**C**) LC/MS determined intracellular Tofacitinib concentration of HEK cells (control) and HEK cells overexpressing MATE-1 at 37 °C and 4 °C (n = 3). (**D**) LC/MS measurement of temperature dependent Baricitinib (1 µM) uptake in RASF and OASF (n = 3). (**E**) LC/MS measurement of temperature dependent Baricitinib uptake (0.4 µM) in RASF and OASF (n = 3). Statistical analyses were performed using a RM ANOVA and Sidak correction for multiple testing. Data in (**C**,**D**) are presented as box plot with whiskers indicating the min and max values, as well as the median. *: $p < 0.05$; **: $p < 0.01$; ***: $p < 0.005$

2.4. Tofacitinib and Baricitinib Showed Comparable Inhibition of IL-6-Induced STAT3-Phosphorylation

As it was shown that Baricitinib and Tofacitinib are taken up by fibroblasts via different uptake mechanisms, we analysed the inhibition of JAK1 phosphorylation as well as the downstream target STAT3. Using 10 ng/mL IL-6 we activated the Jak1-STAT3 signalling pathway. We observed an increased time-dependent phosphorylation of Jak1 in RASF using IL-6 (untreated vs. 30 Min IL-6; 95% CI: −0.24 to −0.04; p = 0.02). Baricitinib did not influence phosphorylation JAK1 during the tested time course (Figure 4A). Tofacitinib, in contrast, time dependently inhibited the phosphorylation of JAk1 (Figure 4A). However, due to the very low amounts of pJak1 detectable, these results did not reach statistical significance. OASF were less responsive towards IL-6 stimulation. They showed only a weak phosphorylation of Jak1 (untreated vs. 30 min IL–6 95% CI: −0.1 to 0.002; p = 0.05), and no difference was observed using Baricitinib or Tofacitinib to inhibit the IL-6 induced phosphorylation (Figure 4B). Next, we investigated the phosphorylation of STAT3. As expected, 10 ng/mL IL-6 resulted in an increased time dependent phosphorylation of STAT3 in RASF (Time effect: $F(1.67, 33.37)$ = 8.62; p = 0.002). Using either Baricitinib or Tofacitinib, this phosphorylation was inhibited, indicating an efficient inhibition of IL-6 induced signalling using both TKIs (Treatment effect: $F(2, 24)$ = 11.27; p = 0.0004). No significant difference was observed between both drugs (Figure 4C). We also investigated the efficacy of IL-6 blockade in OASF. There was less phosphorylation of STAT3 in unstimulated OASF, and these fibroblasts were also less responsive compared to RASF (Figure 4D). The treatment with either Tofacitinib or Baricitinib completely abolished the IL-6 induced phosphorylation of STAT3 (Treatment effect: F (1.179, 9.432) = 16.35; p = 0.002). Again, no difference was observed between both TKIs.

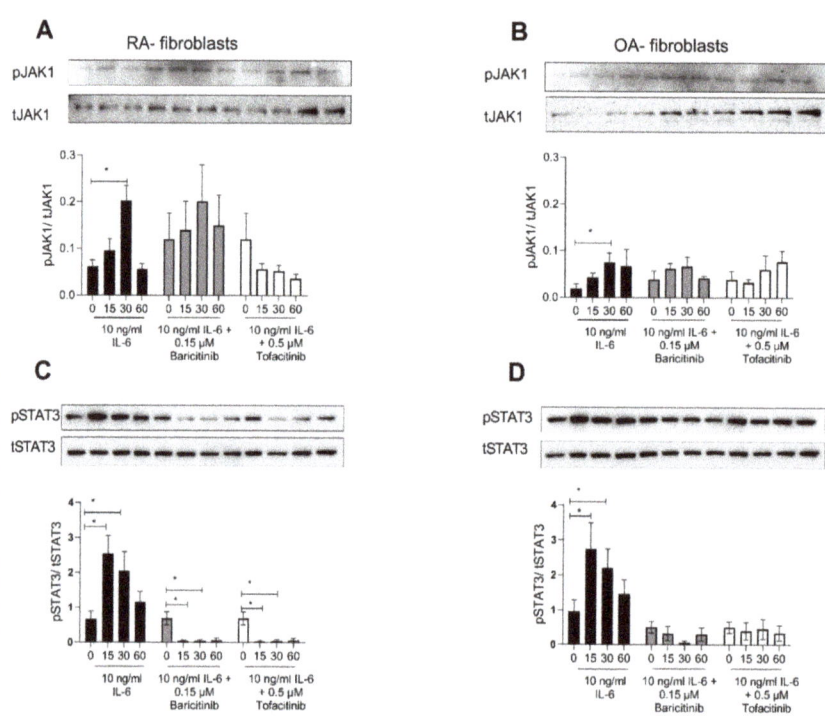

Figure 4. Tofacitinib and Baricitinib showed comparable inhibition of IL-6 induced STAT3-phosphorylation. (**A**) Western blot for pJAK1 compared to total Jak1 in RASF stimulated for 0, 15, 30 or 60 min with 10 ng/mL Il-6. Cells were also treated with 0.15 µM Baricitinib or 0.5 µM Tofacitinib. Quantification of at least 5 independent experiments are given in the graph underneath the blot. (**B**) Western blot for pJAK1 compared to total Jak1 in OASF stimulated with 10 ng/mL Il-6 and treated with 0.15 µM Baricitinib or 0.5 µM Tofacitinib. Quantification is given in the graph underneath the blot. (**C**) Western blot for pSTAT3 compared to total STAT3 in RASF stimulated for 0,15, 30 or 60 min with 10 ng/mL Il-6. Cells were also treated with 0.15 µM Baricitinib or 0.5 µM Tofacitinib. Quantification of at least five independent experiments is given in the graph underneath the blot. (**D**) Western blot for pSTAT3 compared to total STAT3 in OASF stimulated with 10 ng/mL Il-6 and treated with 0.15 µM Baricitinib or 0.5 µM Tofacitinib. Quantification is given in the graph underneath the blot. A two-way RM-ANOVA was performed for statistical testing. Data are presented as mean values with SEM. A p-value $p \leq 0.05$ was considered to show statistical significance and is indicated by *.

3. Discussion

Both tested TKIs, Tofacitinib and Baricitinib, are approved as therapeutic drugs for the treatment of RA. Tofacitinib predominantly inhibits JAK1 and JAK3, and to a lesser degree JAK2 [13]. Baricitinib mainly inhibits JAK2, and acts only to a minor degree on the phosphorylation of JAK1 and JAK3 [12].

Tofacitinib was the first JAK inhibitor approved by the FDA in 2012 and subsequently by the EMA in 2017 for use in patients with moderate-to-severe RA at a dose of 5 mg twice daily. Tofacitinib in combination with MTX is indicated for the treatment of moderate to severe active RA in adult patients who have responded inadequately to, or who are intolerant to, one or more disease-modifying antirheumatic drugs. Tofacitinib can be given as monotherapy in the case of intolerance to MTX, or when treatment with MTX is inappropriate. Baricitinib 2 mg once daily (as monotherapy or combination therapy) was approved for RA patients with inadequate response to one or more tumour necrosis factor antagonist therapies in the US and for csDMARD-IR in Canada, while Baricitinib 2 mg and 4 mg (as monotherapy or combination therapy) were approved for RA patients with csDMARD-IR in Europe.

Variances in the clinical performance of both JAK inhibitors have been observed [22]. However, the reason for these differences are unknown given that they both TKIs target Janus Kinases resulting in a reduced STAT3 phosphorylation. However, each TKI has a different inhibitory profile against the different JAK isotypes [23,24]. This study aims to give an explanation for this observation by evaluating the intracellular uptake of both TKI into their targeted cells. A possible target in RA are synovial fibroblasts as they play an important role in the pathogenesis by contributing to joint destruction and producing cytokines [3]. RASF express several organic ion transporters which are capable of translocating TKIs, among them hOCTN1 and hMATE1, which have been previously reported to transport Saracatinib and Imatinib, respectively [14–17].

Baricitinib is not charged under physiological conditions, and therefore is no a target for organic cation transporters (Figure 1A). For this reason, we did not observe a transporter-mediated uptake in either the ASP^+ quenching tests (Figure 1C), nor the LC/MS detection of temperature dependent Baricitinib accumulation (Figure 2).

Investigating the role of organic cation transporters for the Tofacitinib accumulation in human RASF, we identified hMATE1 to predominantly mediate this transport (Figure 3C). Compared to OASF, hMATE1 expression is reduced in RASF (Figure 1C). We have previously shown that pro-inflammatory cytokines influence the MATE-1 expression [14]. RA is characterized by inflammatory processes that impact on various cellular activities [25]. Therefore, the influence of IL-6, which is also the main activator of JAK signalling, on OCT expression was analysed. IL-6 did not further impact on the expression of MATE-1 (Figure 1D).

Tofacitinib is charged under physiological pH-conditions (Figure 1B). Because transport of organic cations mediated by MATE-1 is pH dependent, we observed an export of Tofacitinib [21]. The synovial fluid in RA patients has been reported to exhibit an acidic pH, under these conditions MATE-1 is expected to mediate efflux of Tofacitinib [25,26]. To investigate the intracellular concentration of both TKIs we chose the maximum plasma concentration for Tofacitinib and Baricitinib for our experiment. The concentration for Baricitinib was described as 150 nM, and 400 nM for Tofacitinib [27,28]. As expected, we did not observe a temperature-dependent increase of Baricitinib in fibroblasts (Figure 2D). This indicates that, due to its neutral charge, Baricitinib can penetrate the cell membrane without active transport. However, our data do not exclude that other transporters might contribute to the transport of Baricitinib into the cells. Tofacitinib in contrast is actively transported into fibroblasts. We found that MATE1 is the responsible transporter (Figure 3C). Interestingly, we found that OASF show a temperature-dependent lowering of Tofacitinib concentrations, indicating an active export of the drug from the cells (Figure 3D,E). This correlates with the increased MATE1 expression in OASF, which is reduced under inflammatory conditions. For this reason, in RASF, Tofacitinib is not exported.

We investigated the potency of both TKIs in inhibiting IL-6-induced JAK1 phosphorylation. As expected, Baricitinib did not inhibit JAK1 phosphorylation in RASF (Figure 4A). OASF were less responsive to IL-6 treatment (Figure 4B,D). Investigating the downstream transcription factor for IL-6 signalling, we observed no difference between Baricitinib and Tofacitinib, indicating that both TKIs are efficiently inhibiting the inflammatory response (Figure 4C).

The results from this study indicate that Tofacitinib might be exported from healthy cells, thereby not inhibiting the JAK pathway. Under disease conditions; however, Tofacitinib stays in the diseased cells and effectively inhibits the disease pathway. We observed no difference in inhibition of IL-6-induced inflammatory signalling for Tofacitinib and Baricitinib.

4. Conclusions

Thus, the differences in cellular uptake strategies for Baricitinib and Tofacitinib might explain the differences in clinical performance. Knowing that Tofacitinib is transported from healthy cells due to the increased expression of MATE1 might make it the more favourable drug.

5. Materials and Methods

5.1. Cell Lines

HEK293 cells (CRL-1573; American Type Culture Collection, Rochville, MD, USA) stably transfected with hOCT1 and hOCT3 were a kind gift of Prof. Koepsell (University of Würzburg) and grown with 600 µg/mL geneticin. HEK293 cells stably transfected with a hMATE1 plasmid (a gift by Dr. Yonezawa, Kyoto University Hospital, Japan Biochem. Pharmacol. 74: 359–371, 2007) were selected with 500 µg/mL hygromycin B. HEK293 cells transfected with cDNAs of hOCTN1 subcloned into a doxycycline-inducible pEBTetD plasmid vector were generously provided by Prof. Gründemann (University of Cologne, Cologne, Germany) [15,16] and selected with 3 mg/L puromycin. 24 h before starting experiments, hOCTN1 expression was induced by 1 mg/L doxycycline.

All cells were grown under standard conditions in Dulbecco's modified eagle medium (DMEM)—low glucose, containing 3.7 g/L $NaHCO_3$, 1.0 g/L D-glucose, 10% foetal calf serum, 100 U/mL penicillin/streptomycin, 1 mM L-glutamine, gassed with 5% CO_2 at 37 °C.

5.2. Synovial Fibroblasts (SF) Culture and Isolation

SF were isolated from synovial tissue of rheumatoid arthritis (RA) ($n = 10$) and osteoarthritis (OA) ($n = 10$) patients undergoing joint replacement surgery. The Ethics Committee of the University of Magdeburg approved this study (IRR: 73/18), and all patients gave written consent prior to inclusion in the study. RA patients met the American College of Rheumatology criteria. Isolated fibroblasts were cultured under standard conditions for maximal eight passages. When indicated, RA synovial fibroblasts (RASF) were incubated with 10 ng/mL recombinant human IL-6 (R&D).

5.3. Peripheral Blood Mononuclear Cell (PBMC) Isolation and Cultivation

Human PBMCs were isolated from RA and OA patients. The Ethics Committee of the University of Magdeburg approved this study (IRR: 73/18) and all patients gave written consent prior to inclusion in the study. In brief, 10 mL blood samples were centrifuged at 400× g in a Megafuge (Thermofisher Scientific, Berlin, Germany) for 10 min at room temperature. The cell pellet was resuspended in PBS/0.1% BSA and centrifuged at 300× g at room temperature for 25 min without breaks using a Biocoll separating solution (Biochrom, Berlin, Germany). The generated lymphocyte ring was carefully taken off removed and washed two times twice with PBS/0.1% BSA. Cells were cultured in Roswell Park Memorial Institute medium (RPMI 1640, Sigma-Aldrich, Taufkirchen, Germany) supplemented with 2 mM L-glutamine, 10% foetal bovine serum, 1% penicillin/streptomycin solution at 37 °C with 5% CO_2.

5.4. Apparent Affinities of Baricitinib and Tofacitinib for OCTs with 4-(4-(Dimethylamino)styryl)-N-Methylpyridinium (ASP^+)

To investigate whether Baricitinib and Tofacitinib interact with OCTs (hOCT1, hOCT3, hOCTN1, hMATE1, hMATE2k), we used a dynamic cis-inhibition protocol of ASP^+ uptake, a known fluorescent substrate of all examined OCTs, with Baricitinib (10^{-8} to 10^{-4} M) and Tofacitinib (10^{-8} to 10^{-4} M), as described previously [14]. Briefly, HEK293 cells were seeded in 96-well plates and grown to 80–100% confluence. For experiments with hMATE-expressing cells, cellular pH was made acidic by 20 min preincubation with a modified ringer-like solution containing NH$_4$Cl (in mM: 30 NH$_4$Cl, 115 NaCl, pH 7.4). Baricitinib and Tofacitinib (Hycultech, Beutelsbach, Germany) were dissolved in DMSO in ringer-like solution (RLS = HCO$_3^-$ free Ringer-like solution containing (in mmol/L): NaCl 145, K$_2$HPO$_4$ 1.6, KH$_2$PO$_4$ 0.4, D-glucose 5, MgCl$_2$ 1, calcium gluconate 1.3 with pH adjusted to 7.4) to final concentrations in the range 10^{-4}–10^{-9} M. Fluorescence measurements were carried out with the TECAN®infinite F200 (Maennedorf, Switzerland). Transporter function was investigated measuring the slope of fluorescence emission (measured at 590 nm after excitation at 450 nm) increase in the first 60 s after ASP$^+$ addition. ASP$^+$ uptake without potential inhibitor was set to 100%.

5.5. Quantification of Baricitinib and Tofacitinib Uptake by Liquid Chromatography Mass Spectrometry (LC/MS)

HEK293 cells or RASF/OASF seeded into a six-well plate were grown to 80–100% confluence. Medium was removed and cells were incubated with Baricitinib and Tofacitinib in RLS at 37 °C or 4 °C for 10 min. After this incubation, cells were quickly washed with 1 mL ice-cold RLS, and then lysed with 300 µL 0.1% formic acid. Cell lysates were incubated for 15 min in an ultrasound bath at 4 °C and centrifuged at 4700× *g* for 5 min at 4 °C. 10 µL internal standard (IS) of Baricitinib (Baricitinib-D5, Illkirch Graffenstaden, France) and Tofacitinib (Tofacitinib 13C3, Clearsynth, Mumbai, India) were added to the cell lysates for quantification. Acetonitrile (VWR, Radnor, Pennsylvania,, USA) was added, mixed and centrifuged for 15 min with 16,200× *g* at 4 °C. 200 µL of the supernatant were diluted in distilled water to reach a final acetonitrile concentration of 12%. The samples were frozen at −80 °C.

Quantification of Baricitinib and Tofacitinib concentration was performed using a high power liquid chromatography device (HPLC) (AdvanceTM UHPLC, Bruker Daltonik, Bremen, Germany) linked to a triple quadrupole mass spectrometer (EVOQ® Elite triple quadrupole mass spectrometer, Bruker Daltonik, Bremen, Germany). A PAL HTC-xt autosampler (CTC Analytics AG, Zwingen, Switzerland) was used to inject 10 µl of the sample to the HPLC. Analytes were separated on an AccucoreTM C18 HPLC column (50 mm × 3 mm; 2.6 µm) (Thermo Scientific, Waltham, MA, USA). Amounts of 0.1% formic acid and acetonitrile were used as mobile phase A and B.

Flow rate was set to 1 mL/min. Baricitinib and Tofacitinib had a specific retention time in HPLC. Ionization of the substances was realized using electrospray ionization (ESI) in a positive ionization mode. Spray voltage was set to 3500 V, conus temperature to 350 °C, gas flow to 60 AU, sample and cone temperature to 350 °C. Exhaust gases were removed. First, Tofacitinib and Tofacitinib-IS, then Baricitinib and Baricitinib-IS were measured for 75 ms each. Full scan was applied to determine specific fission products of Baricitinib and Tofacitinib. Flow rate of the Cole-Parmer 74,900 single-syringe infusion pump (Vernon Hills, Illinois, USA) was set to 10 µL/min, spray voltage to 4000 V, gas flow to 10 AU, gas flow of the nebulizer to 10 AU and temperature to 25 °C. Quantification took place in multiple reaction mode (MRM) (Table 1). Each sample was measured three times and the mean was calculated thereof.

Quantification was attained comparing the content of Baricitinib and Tofacitinib in the sample to the added IS (Figure 5). The result was normalized to the protein content determined in Bradford assay. Analyses were performed using MS Workstation (Bruker Daltonik, Bremen, Germany), MS Data review Version 8.2 (Bruker Daltonik, Bremen, Germany), Origin Pro 2016 (OriginLab, Northampton, MA, USA), GraphPad Prism 5 (GraphPad Software, San Diego, CA, USA) and Excel 2016. Method optimization and validation resulted in detection limits of Baricitinib and Tofacitinib of 0.9 ng/mL and 1.0 ng/mL, and quantification limits of 3.0 ng/mL and 3.3 ng/mL, respectively.

Table 1. MRM transitions of Baricitinib, Tofacitinib, IS and collision energy. The grey-marked fragments had the highest measurement intensity and were used for quantification.

Analyte	Transition [m/z > m/z]	Collision Energy
Tofacitinib	313 > 149	28
	313 > 98	31
	313 > 173	37
Tofacitinib-13C3	316 > 149	28
	316 > 98	31
	316 > 173	37
Baricitinib	372 > 251	26
	372 > 186	31
	372 > 159	43
Baricitinib-d5	377 > 251	26
	377 > 186	31
	377 > 159	43

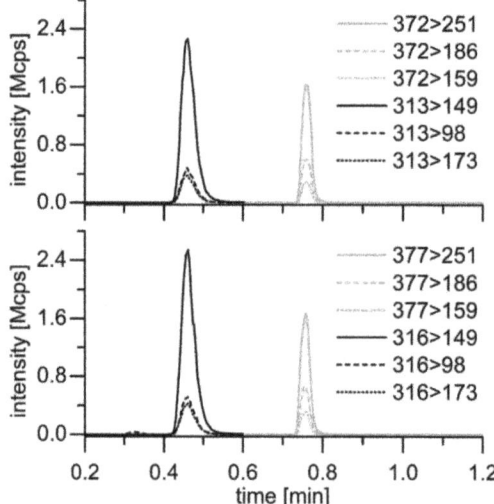

Figure 5. Transitions of Baricitinib and Tofacitinib (above) and IS (below). Tofacitinib is shown to the left in black, to the right Baricitinib in grey.

5.6. Quantitative Real-Time PCR (qRT-PCR)

RNA was isolated with the Qiagen RNeasy Midikit (Qiagen, Gilden, Germany) and Invitrogen Super Script III system was used for reverse transcription. qRT-PCR was performed using SYBR Green PCR Master Mix and the ABI PRISM 7900 Sequence Detection System (Applied Biosystems, Darmstadt, Germany) (primer pairs see supplementary Table S1). Gene expression is normalized to a semiquantitative standard curve and given in relation to the housekeeping gene GAPDH.

5.7. Western Blot Analysis

For each RASF/OASF sample, a total of 1×10^6 cells were seeded in a 25 cm^2 cell culture flask and the cells became adherent overnight. The cells were stimulated with 10 ng/mL IL-6 for 0, 15,

30 and 60 min with either Tofacitinib (1 µM, 0.4 µM) or Baricitinib (1 µM, 0.15 µM). Cells lysis was performed using NP-40- buffer and proteinase inhibitor cOmplete Ultra. Cell lysates were run on a 10% SDS-PAGE and transferred to a PVDF membrane. Blocking was performed in 5% BSA solution. Primary antibody against phospho-Jak1 (#74129), Jak-1 (#3344), phosphor-Stat3 (#9145), Stat-3 (#30835), GAPDH (#2118) diluted 1:1000 in 5% BSA were incubated over night at 4 °C. The secondary antibody was an HRP-conjugated anti-rabbit (#7074) 1:8000 in 5% BSA. All antibodies were bought from Cell Signaling (Danvers, MA, USA). Enhanced chemiluminescence (ECL) was used for Western blot detection, and quantification of bands was performed using ImageJ Software (U.S. National Institutes of Health, Bethesda, MD, USA, https://imagej.nih.gov/ij/, 1997-201).

5.8. Statistical Analysis

Data were analysed using GraphPad Prism, Version 5.0 (GraphPad Software, Inc., San Diego, CA, USA). To examine a statistical significance a two-way RM-ANOVA was performed. Sidak post-hoc multiple comparison test was performed to show intra individual significances. A *p*-value $p \leq 0.05$ was considered to show statistical significance. All experiments were repeated independently for at least three times.

Supplementary Materials: Supplementary materials can be found at http://www.mdpi.com/1422-0067/21/18/6632/s1. Figure S1: Expression of organic cation transporters in PBMCs of OA and RA patients. Table S1: Primer for qRT-PCR.

Author Contributions: J.A. performed the experiments, S.D. isolated RNA from PBMCs and provided the patient blood samples, L.S. and U.K. performed the LC/MS experiments, C.H.L. provided the tissue samples for fibroblast isolation, G.C. and J.B. discussed and interpreted the data, J.B. wrote the manuscript. All authors have read and agreed to the published version of the manuscript.

Funding: Susanne Drynda, Giuliano Ciarimboli and Jessica Bertrand received funding from Pfizer for the project leading to this manuscript. This research was funded by an unrestricted grant provided by Pfizer Pharma GmbH, Forschungsförderung 2017 (IIR #WI233723).

Acknowledgments: The authors acknowledge the excellent technical assistance of Carolin Schneider, Anja Schröder, Mandy Könnecke and Astrid Dirks. This project was supported by an unrestricted grant provided by Pfizer Pharma GmbH, Forschungsförderung 2017 (IIR #WI233723).

Conflicts of Interest: The authors declare no conflict of interest. The funders had no role in the design of the study; in the collection, analyses, or interpretation of data; in the writing of the manuscript, or in the decision to publish the results.

Abbreviations

ANOVA	Analysis of variance
ASP	4-(4-(dimethylamino)styryl)-*N*-methylpyridinium
AU	Arbitrary units
BSA	Bovine serum albumin
cDNA	complementary Deoxyribonucleic Acid
csDMARD-IR	conventional synthetic disease-modifying antirheumatic drug inadequate response
DMEM	Dulbecco's modified eagle medium
DMSO	Dimethyl sulfoxide
ECL	Enhanced chemiluminescence
EMA	European Medicines Agency
ESI	electrospray ionization
GAPDH	Glyceraldehyde 3-phosphate dehydrogenase
gp130	Glycoprotein 130
HEK 293 cells	Human embryonic kidney 293 cells
HPLC	High Performance Liquid Chromatography

IL-6	Interleukin-6
IL-6Ra	Interleukin 6 Receptor Alpha
IS	Internal standrad
JAK	Janus Kinase
LC/MS	Liquid chromatography/mass spectrometry
MATE	multidrug and toxin extrusion
MRM	multiple reaction mode
MTX	methotrexate
NP-40	Nonidet P-40
OA	osteoarthrits
OC	Organic cation
OCT	Organic cation transporter
OCTN	Novel organic cation transporter
PBMCs	peripheral blood mononuclear cell
pKa	Ionization Constant
RA	Rheumatoid arthritis
RLS	ringer-like solution
RM-ANOVA	Repeated Measures Analysis of variance
RNA	Ribonucleic acid
RT-PCR	Reverse transcription polymerase chain reaction
SF	Synovial fibroblasts
STAT	Signal transducer and activator of transcription
TKI	Tyrosine kinase inhibitor
TNF-alpha	tumour necrosis factor alpha
TYK	Tyrosine kinase

References

1. Smolen, J.S.; Aletaha, D.; McInnes, I.B. Rheumatoid arthritis. *Lancet* **2016**, *388*, 2023–2038. [CrossRef]
2. Huber, L.C.; Distler, O.; Tarner, I.; Gay, R.E.; Gay, S.; Pap, T. Synovial fibroblasts: Key players in rheumatoid arthritis. *Rheumatology* **2006**, *45*, 669–675. [CrossRef]
3. Ospelt, C. Synovial fibroblasts in 2017. *RMD Open* **2017**, *3*, e000471. [CrossRef] [PubMed]
4. Brentano, F.; Schorr, O.; Gay, R.E.; Gay, S.; Kyburz, D. RNA released from necrotic synovial fluid cells activates rheumatoid arthritis synovial fibroblasts via Toll-like receptor 3. *Arthritis Rheum.* **2005**, *52*, 2656–2665. [CrossRef] [PubMed]
5. Ospelt, C.; Brentano, F.; Rengel, Y.; Stanczyk, J.; Kolling, C.; Tak, P.P.; Gay, R.E.; Gay, S.; Kyburz, D. Overexpression of toll-like receptors 3 and 4 in synovial tissue from patients with early rheumatoid arthritis: Toll-like receptor expression in early and longstanding arthritis. *Arthritis Rheum.* **2008**, *58*, 3684–3692. [CrossRef] [PubMed]
6. Fassbender, H.G. Histomorphological basis of articular cartilage destruction in rheumatoid arthritis. *Coll. Relat. Res.* **1983**, *3*, 141–155. [CrossRef]
7. Wei, S.T.; Sun, Y.H.; Zong, S.H.; Xiang, Y.B. Serum Levels of IL-6 and TNF-alpha May Correlate with Activity and Severity of Rheumatoid Arthritis. *Med. Sci. Monit.* **2015**, *21*, 4030–4038. [CrossRef]
8. Malemud, C.J. The role of the JAK/STAT signal pathway in rheumatoid arthritis. *Ther. Adv. Musculoskelet. Dis.* **2018**, *10*, 117–127. [CrossRef]
9. Harrison, D.A. The Jak/STAT Pathway. *Cold Spring Harb. Perspect. Biol.* **2012**, *4*. [CrossRef]
10. Smolen, J.S.; Breedveld, F.C.; Burmester, G.R.; Bykerk, V.; Dougados, M.; Emery, P.; Kvien, T.K.; Navarro-Compan, M.V.; Oliver, S.; Schoels, M.; et al. Treating rheumatoid arthritis to target: 2014 update of the recommendations of an international task force. *Ann. Rheum. Dis.* **2016**, *75*, 3–15. [CrossRef]
11. Smolen, J.S.; Landewe, R.B.M.; Bijlsma, J.W.J.; Burmester, G.R.; Dougados, M.; Kerschbaumer, A.; McInnes, I.B.; Sepriano, A.; van Vollenhoven, R.F.; de Wit, M.; et al. EULAR recommendations for the management of rheumatoid arthritis with synthetic and biological disease-modifying antirheumatic drugs: 2019 update. *Ann. Rheum. Dis.* **2020**, *79*, 685–699. [CrossRef]

12. Al-Salama, Z.T.; Scott, L.J. Baricitinib: A Review in Rheumatoid Arthritis. *Drugs* **2018**, *78*, 761–772. [CrossRef] [PubMed]
13. Dhillon, S. Tofacitinib: A Review in Rheumatoid Arthritis. *Drugs* **2017**, *77*, 1987–2001. [CrossRef] [PubMed]
14. Schmidt-Lauber, C.; Harrach, S.; Pap, T.; Fischer, M.; Victor, M.; Heitzmann, M.; Hansen, U.; Fobker, M.; Brand, S.M.; Sindic, A.; et al. Transport mechanisms and their pathology-induced regulation govern tyrosine kinase inhibitor delivery in rheumatoid arthritis. *PLoS ONE* **2012**, *7*, e52247. [CrossRef] [PubMed]
15. Harrach, S.; Barz, V.; Pap, T.; Pavenstadt, H.; Schlatter, E.; Edemir, B.; Distler, J.; Ciarimboli, G.; Bertrand, J. Notch Signaling Activity Determines Uptake and Biological Effect of Imatinib in Systemic Sclerosis Dermal Fibroblasts. *J. Investig. Dermatol.* **2019**, *139*, 439–447. [CrossRef] [PubMed]
16. Harrach, S.; Edemir, B.; Schmidt-Lauber, C.; Pap, T.; Bertrand, J.; Ciarimboli, G. Importance of the novel organic cation transporter 1 for tyrosine kinase inhibition by saracatinib in rheumatoid arthritis synovial fibroblasts. *Sci. Rep.* **2017**, *7*, 1258. [CrossRef] [PubMed]
17. Harrach, S.; Schmidt-Lauber, C.; Pap, T.; Pavenstadt, H.; Schlatter, E.; Schmidt, E.; Berdel, W.E.; Schulze, U.; Edemir, B.; Jeromin, S.; et al. MATE1 regulates cellular uptake and sensitivity to imatinib in CML patients. *Blood Cancer J.* **2016**, *6*, e470. [CrossRef]
18. Hediger, M.A.; Romero, M.F.; Peng, J.B.; Rolfs, A.; Takanaga, H.; Bruford, E.A. The ABCs of solute carriers: Physiological, pathological and therapeutic implications of human membrane transport proteinsIntroduction. *Pflügers Arch.* **2004**, *447*, 465–468. [CrossRef]
19. Koepsell, H.; Endou, H. The SLC22 drug transporter family. *Pflugers Arch.* **2004**, *447*, 666–676. [CrossRef]
20. Takeda, M.; Khamdang, S.; Narikawa, S.; Kimura, H.; Kobayashi, Y.; Yamamoto, T.; Cha, S.H.; Sekine, T.; Endou, H. Human organic anion transporters and human organic cation transporters mediate renal antiviral transport. *J. Pharmacol. Exp. Ther.* **2002**, *300*, 918–924. [CrossRef]
21. Tanihara, Y.; Masuda, S.; Sato, T.; Katsura, T.; Ogawa, O.; Inui, K. Substrate specificity of MATE1 and MATE2-K, human multidrug and toxin extrusions/H(+)-organic cation antiporters. *Biochem. Pharmacol.* **2007**, *74*, 359–371. [CrossRef] [PubMed]
22. Westhovens, R. Clinical efficacy of new JAK inhibitors under development. Just more of the same? *Rheumatology* **2019**, *58*, i27–i33. [CrossRef] [PubMed]
23. O'Shea, J.J.; Kontzias, A.; Yamaoka, K.; Tanaka, Y.; Laurence, A. Janus kinase inhibitors in autoimmune diseases. *Ann. Rheum. Dis.* **2013**, *72*, 111–115. [CrossRef] [PubMed]
24. O'Shea, J.J.; Plenge, R. JAK and STAT signaling molecules in immunoregulation and immune-mediated disease. *Immunity* **2012**, *36*, 542–550. [CrossRef]
25. McInnes, I.B.; Schett, G. Cytokines in the pathogenesis of rheumatoid arthritis. *Nat. Rev. Immunol.* **2007**, *7*, 429–442. [CrossRef]
26. Farr, M.; Garvey, K.; Bold, A.M.; Kendall, M.J.; Bacon, P.A. Significance of the hydrogen ion concentration in synovial fluid in rheumatoid arthritis. *Clin. Exp. Rheumatol.* **1985**, *3*, 99–104.
27. Dowty, M.E.; Lin, J.; Ryder, T.F.; Wang, W.; Walker, G.S.; Vaz, A.; Chan, G.L.; Krishnaswami, S.; Prakash, C. The pharmacokinetics, metabolism, and clearance mechanisms of tofacitinib, a janus kinase inhibitor, in humans. *Drug Metab. Dispos.* **2014**, *42*, 759–773. [CrossRef]
28. Shi, J.G.; Chen, X.; Lee, F.; Emm, T.; Scherle, P.A.; Lo, Y.; Punwani, N.; Williams, W.V.; Yeleswaram, S. The pharmacokinetics, pharmacodynamics, and safety of baricitinib, an oral JAK 1/2 inhibitor, in healthy volunteers. *J. Clin. Pharmacol.* **2014**, *54*, 1354–1361. [CrossRef]

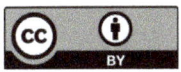

© 2020 by the authors. Licensee MDPI, Basel, Switzerland. This article is an open access article distributed under the terms and conditions of the Creative Commons Attribution (CC BY) license (http://creativecommons.org/licenses/by/4.0/).

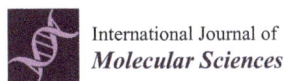

Article

Farnesoid X Receptor Activation Stimulates Organic Cations Transport in Human Renal Proximal Tubular Cells

Teerasak Wongwan [1], Varanuj Chatsudthipong [1] and Sunhapas Soodvilai [1,2,*]

1. Research Center of Transport Proteins for Medical Innovation, Department of Physiology, Mahidol University, Bangkok 10400, Thailand; teerasak.won@student.mahidol.ac.th (T.W.); varanuj.cha@mahidol.ac.th (V.C.)
2. Excellent Center for Drug Discovery, Mahidol University, Bangkok 10400, Thailand
* Correspondence: sunhapas.soo@mahidol.ac.th; Tel.: +66-2-2015610

Received: 13 July 2020; Accepted: 12 August 2020; Published: 24 August 2020

Abstract: Farnesoid X receptor (FXR) is a ligand-activated transcription factor highly expressed in the liver and kidneys. Activation of FXR decreases organic cation transporter (OCT) 1-mediated clearance of organic cation compounds in hepatocytes. The present study investigated FXR regulation of renal clearance of organic cations by OCT2 modulation and multidrug and toxin extrusion proteins (MATEs). The role of FXR in OCT2 and MATEs functions was investigated by monitoring the flux of ^3H–MPP$^+$, a substrate of OCT2 and MATEs. FXR agonists chenodeoxycholic acid (CDCA) and GW4064 stimulated OCT2-mediated ^3H–MPP$^+$ uptake in human renal proximal tubular cells (RPTEC/TERT1 cells) and OCT2-CHO-K1 cells. The stimulatory effect of CDCA (20 µM) was abolished by an FXR antagonist, Z-guggulsterone, indicating an FXR-dependent mechanism. CDCA increased OCT2 transport activity via an increased maximal transport rate of MPP$^+$. Additionally, 24 h CDCA treatment increased MATEs-mediated ^3H-MPP$^+$ uptake. Moreover, CDCA treatment increased the expression of OCT2, MATE1, and MATE2-K mRNA compared with that of the control. OCT2 protein expression was also increased following CDCA treatment. FXR activation stimulates renal OCT2- and MATE1/2-K-mediated cation transports in proximal tubules, demonstrating that FXR plays a role in the regulation of OCT2 and MATEs in renal proximal tubular cells.

Keywords: Nuclear receptor; renal excretion; kidney; drug transporters; bile acids

1. Introduction

The kidney is largely responsible for the elimination of metabolic waste products, therapeutic drugs, and xenobiotics, which contain organic cations (OCs) and anions (OAs) [1]. The secretion of OCs takes place in renal proximal tubules. This process requires the uptake of OCs from the blood into renal proximal tubular cells and subsequent elimination of these compounds into the tubular lumen across the luminal membrane. Three members of the organic cation transporters (OCTs), including OCT1, OCT2, and OCT3, are characterized [2]. Human OCT1 and OCT2 are highly expressed in liver and kidney, respectively, whereas OCT3 is ubiquitously expressed at a low level in multiple tissues [3]. OCs are transported into renal proximal tubular cells via the organic cation transporter (OCT) 2, a predominant OCT expressed in the basolateral membrane of human renal proximal tubular cells [4,5]. OCT2-mediated uptake of OCs is governed by an inside-negative membrane potential [4,6]. After uptake, OCs are then effluxed to the tubular lumen by several apical membrane transporters such as multidrug and toxin extrusion proteins (MATEs). Two MATE isoforms, MATE1 and MATE2-K, are expressed in renal proximal tubular cells [7,8]. Several endogenous compounds and therapeutic cationic drugs are eliminated via renal excretion that have been identified as substrates of both OCT2 and MATEs such as creatinine and metformin [5,9–13].

Altered expression or function of these transporters can affect organic cation drug renal secretion and subsequently alter their pharmacokinetics and efficacies [14,15]. Studies have reported nuclear receptor-mediated regulation of OCT2 and MATEs function. Specifically, the activation of pregnane X receptor (PXR) and androgen receptor increased OCT2 expression [16,17], whereas liver X receptor (LXR) activation decreased OCT2 expression and function [18]. In addition, kidney-specific multidrug and toxin extrusion proteins (MATE2K) expression was up-regulated upon the activation of Nrf2 pathway signaling [19]. Previous studies have shown that farnesoid X receptor (FXR), a ligand-activated transcriptional factor, is highly expressed in liver, kidney, intestine, and adrenal gland tissue [20]. FXR regulates several membrane transporters and channels, including the bile salt export pump (BSEP) [21], multidrug resistance-associated protein 2 (MRP2) [22], organic solute transporter OSTα/β [23,24], aquaporin 2(AQP2) [25], and MATE1 [26].

Previous studies showed that cholestasis resulted in a down-regu lation of OCT1 and impairment of hepatic-mediated OCT1 substrate uptake [27,28]. These processes might be controlled by the activation of FXR by bile acids, such as cholic acid and chenodeoxycholic acid (CDCA). These bile acids have been reported to act as endogenous ligands for FXR [29] and are increased in hepatic disease [30]. Down-regulation of OCT1 regarded as adaptive responses to cholestasis and may serve to diminish the hepatic accumulation of cationic substrate during liver injury [31]. Since OCT1 plays a role in the hepatic uptake-mediated biotransformation and the excretion of endogenous compounds and cationic drugs, decreases in OCT1 function may result in increased cationic plasma concentration. We hypothesize that other cation transporters expressed in the kidney, such as OCT2 and MATEs, may be critically important for cationic substrate elimination in hepatic disease. Here, we investigated the effect of FXR activation on renal OCT2 and MATEs function in renal proximal tubular cells.

2. Results

2.1. FXR Agonists Stimulate OCT2-Mediated ^{3}H-MPP$^+$ Uptake

To be certain that RPTEC/TERT1 cells are suitable cell model for investigating the role of FXR, we first tested whether the RPTEC/TERT1 cells express FXR by examination protein expression via Western blot analysis. As shown in Figure 1, we confirmed FXR protein expression in RPTEC/TERT1 cells. Relative to untreated cells, mRNA expression of a small heterodimer partner (SHP; a target gene of FRX activation [32,33]) was significantly increased following treatment with 20 µM CDCA for 24 h (Figure 1A,B). Next, we tested the effects of CDCA and GW4064, a potent synthetic agonists of FXR, on OCT2-mediated ^{3}H-MPP$^+$ uptake. As shown in Figure 1C, 24 h incubation with 20 µM CDCA and 5 µM GW4060 significantly stimulated OCT2-mediated ^{3}H-MPP$^+$ cellular uptake. While 20 µM CDCA stimulated uptake after 24 h, an extended incubation time did not lead to any further increase in OCT2-mediated ^{3}H-MPP$^+$ uptake (Figure 1D). In addition, we confirmed the effect of CDCA on OCT2-mediated ^{3}H-MPP$^+$ uptake in CHO-K1 cells expressing OCT2. Specifically, 24 h incubation with 20 and 30 µM CDCA significantly promoted ^{3}H-MPP$^+$ uptake in CHO-K1 cells (Figure 1E).

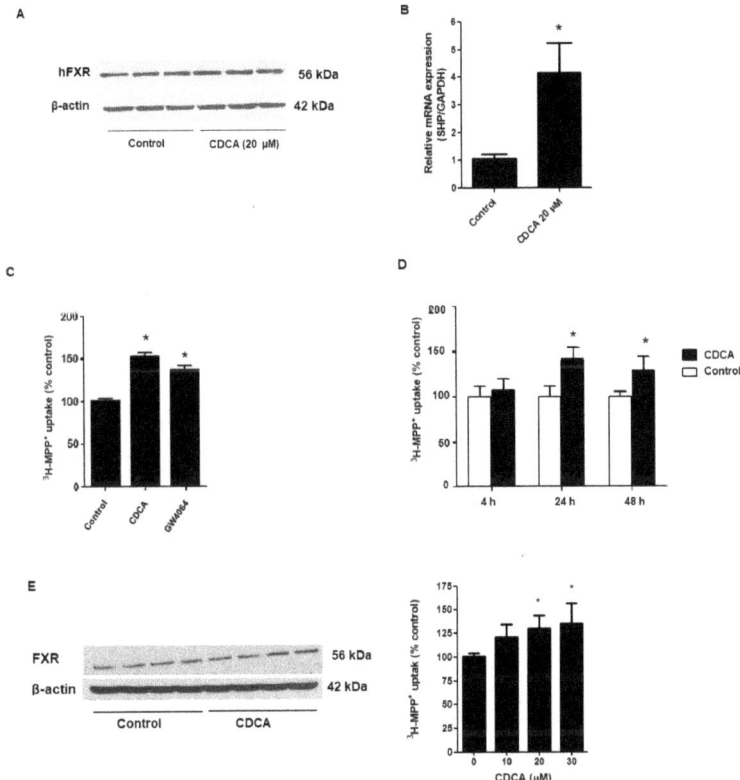

Figure 1. Effect of FXR agonists on OCT2-mediated ^{3}H–MPP$^+$ uptake. (**A**) protein expression of FXR and (**B**) mRNA expression of SHP in RPTEC/TERT1 cells following treating the cells with vehicle or 20 μM CDCA for 24 h; (**C**) effect of 20 μM CDCA and 5 μM GW4064 on ^{3}H-MPP$^+$ uptake; (**D**) Time-response effect of 20 μM CDCA; (**E**) FXR expression and ^{3}H-MPP$^+$ uptake in OCT2-CHO-K1 cells following incubation with 20 μM CDCA for 24 h. Data are expressed as a mean percentage of control (mean ± S.D.) from 3 independent experiments. *Significantly different from control ($p < 0.05$).

2.2. Stimulatory Effects of FXR Agonists Require FXR Activation

To determine whether the CDCA stimulation of ^{3}H-MPP$^+$ uptake is directly caused by FXR activation, we examined how FXR antagonists, Z-guggulsterone and DY268, affect CDCA-induced stimulation of ^{3}H-MPP$^+$ uptake. As shown in Figure 2, exposure to 10 μM Z-guggulsterone or DY268 had no significant effect on ^{3}H-MPP$^+$ uptake. CDCA-mediated uptake stimulation was attenuated by coincubation with Z-guggulsterone or DY268. These data indicate that CDCA uptake stimulation requires FXR activation.

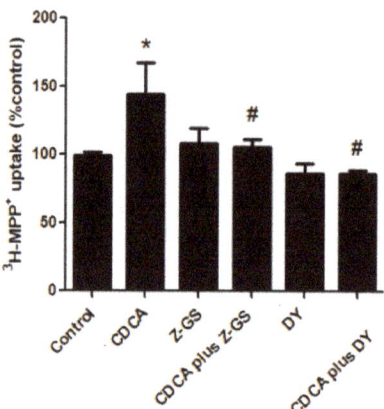

Figure 2. Effect of FXR activation on OCT2-mediated ^{3}H–MPP$^+$ uptake. RPTEC/TERT1 cells were treated with vehicle, 20 µM CDCA, FXR antagonists (10 µM Z-guggulsterone (Z-GS) or 10 µM DY268), and CDCA plus FXR antagonist for 24 h. The results are shown as mean ± S.D. of % control form 4 experiments. *Significantly different from control ($p < 0.05$) and # $p < 0.05$ compared with CDCA-treated cells.

2.3. Kinetic Study on FXR Activation on OCT2-mediated ^{3}H-MPP$^+$ Uptake

To investigate how FXR activation stimulates ^{3}H-MPP$^+$ uptake, we evaluated the kinetic parameters Kt and Jmax that reflect an affinity and functional membrane expression of OCT2, respectively. As shown in Figure 3, 24 h treatment with 20 µM CDCA in RPTEC/TERT1 cells significantly increased the Jmax from 6.48 ± 1.4 to 12.56 ± 3.1 pmol/min/cm^2 with no significant effect on Kt (22.83 ± 5.7 vs 19.75 ± 5.67 µM).

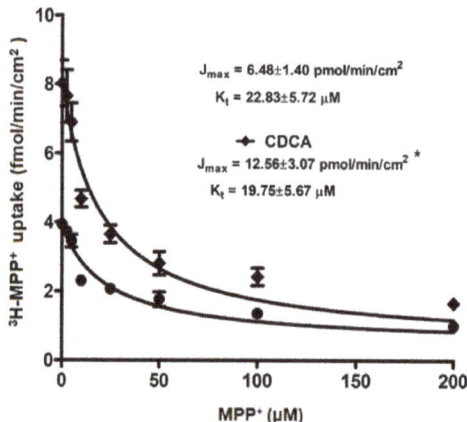

Figure 3. Kinetic study of OCT2-mediated ^{3}H-MPP$^+$ uptake in RPTEC/TERT1 cells. RPTEC/TERT1 cells were treated with vehicle or 20 µM CDCA for 24 h. ^{3}H-MPP$^+$ uptake was determined in the presence of unlabeled MPP$^+$ at 0–200 µM. The Jmax, and Kt values are reported as mean ± S.D. ($n = 3$). *Significantly different from control ($p < 0.05$).

2.4. FXR Activation Increases mRNA and Protein Expression of OCT2

To determine whether FXR activation affects OCT2 expression, RPTEC/TERT1 cells treated with vehicle or 20 µM CDCA for 24 h were probed for OCT2 mRNA and protein expression. Treatment of RPTEC/TERT1 cells with 20 µM CDCA significantly increased OCT2 mRNA expression compared with vehicle treatment. In addition, 20 µM CDCA treatment led to an increase in OCT2 protein expression as shown in Figure 4.

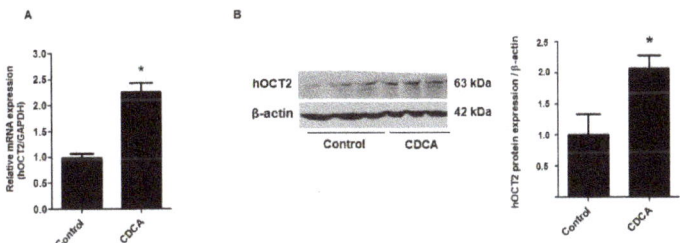

Figure 4. Effect of CDCA on expression of hOCT2. (**A**) mRNA expression of hOCT2 after treating with vehicle or 20 µM CDCA for 24 h. (**B**) Representative blots and the densitometry quantification of hOCT2 expression normalized by β-actin. The data are shown as mean ± S.D. from three independent experiments. * $p < 0.05$ compared with vehicle-treated group.

2.5. FXR Activation Increases Function and Expression of MATEs

Regulation of MATEs transport function by FXR activation was determined in RPTEC/TERT1 cells. These transporters function as organic cation/H$^+$ exchangers and are driven by a proton-gradient. Therefore, to test MATEs-mediated ^{3}H–MPP$^+$ uptake, we preincubated RPTEC/TERT1 cells with a K$^+$ based buffer containing ammonium chloride to generate intracellular acidification before transport measurement. Consequently, 20 µM CDCA treatment for 24 h significantly increased MATEs-mediated ^{3}H-MPP$^+$ compared with the vehicle-treated cells. CDCA stimulation was significantly inhibited by Z-guggulsterone and DY268 (Figure 5A). Next, we tested whether the observed correlation between FXR activation and MATEs transport function was a result of MATEs mRNA up-regulation. Using RPTEC/TERT1 cells, MATE1 and MATE2K mRNA expression were analyzed following treatment with 20 µM CDCA for 24 h. CDCA significantly increased both MATE1 and MATE2K mRNA expression (Figure 5B).

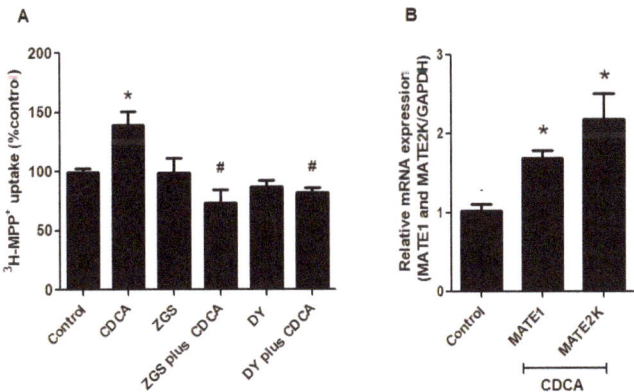

Figure 5. The effect of FXR activation on MATEs-mediated ^{3}H–MPP$^+$ uptake and MATEs expression in

RPTEC/TERT1 cells. (**A**) MATEs-mediated ^{3}H–MPP$^+$ uptake; treated with vehicle, 20 µM CDCA, FXR antagonists (10 µM Z-guggulsterone (Z-GS) or 10 µM DY268 (DY)), and CDCA plus FXR antagonists. (**B**) mRNA expression of MATE1 and MATE2K. The data are shown as mean ± S.D. ($n = 3$). * $p < 0.05$ compared with control and # $p < 0.05$ compared with CDCA-treated cells.

2.6. FXR Activation Stimulates Transepithelial Transport of ^{3}H-MPP$^+$

To determine the relationship between FXR activation and transcellular transport of OCs, we examined the effect of FXR activation on basolateral-apical transport of ^{3}H-MPP$^+$. As such, cell monolayers were incubated with vehicle control, 20 µM CDCA, 10 µM DY268, and 20 µM CDCA plus 10 µM DY268, and transepithelial transport of ^{3}H-MPP$^+$ was measured after 24 h. As shown in Figure 6, transcellular translocation of ^{3}H-MPP$^+$ from the basolateral to the apical chamber was significantly higher in the CDCA-treated cell monolayer compared with the vehicle-treated cells. Importantly, the stimulatory effect of CDCA was abolished by co-treatment with DY268.

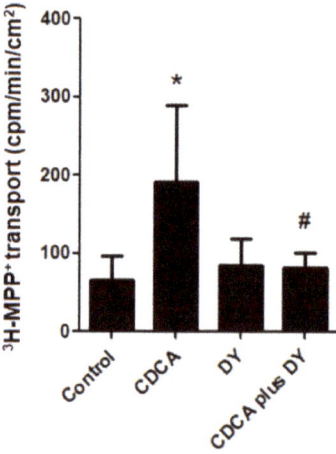

Figure 6. Effect of CDCA on transcellular transport of ^{3}H-MPP$^+$ in polarized cell monolayer. Polarized RPTEC/TERT1 cell monolayers were treated with vehicle, 20 µM CDCA, 10 µM DY268 (DY), and CDCA plus DY for 24 h. The values of basolateral to apical transport of ^{3}H-MPP$^+$ are expressed as mean ± S.D. of cpm/min/cm^2 form 3 experiments. Data from each experiment is obtained from 3 inserts. * $p < 0.05$ compared with vehicle-treated group and # $p < 0.05$ compared with CDCA-treated cells.

2.7. Pathological Concentration of Bile Acid Stimulates Renal OCT2 and MATEs

Previous studies have reported an increased concentration of unconjugated bile acids in liver diseases [30]. Therefore, we investigated the correlation between high unconjugated bile acid concentration and the stimulation of renal OCs transport. Cell monolayers were incubated with CDCA at 80 µM for 24 h followed by measurement of OCT2- and MATEs-mediated ^{3}H-MPP$^+$ transport. As shown in Figure 7, treatment a pathological concentration of CDCA significantly stimulated both OCT2- and MATEs-mediated ^{3}H-MPP$^+$ compared with vehicle-treated cells. The stimulatory effect of 80 µM CDCA on ^{3}H-MPP$^+$ uptake was correlated with an increase in mRNA expression of OCT2, MATE1, and MATE2K.

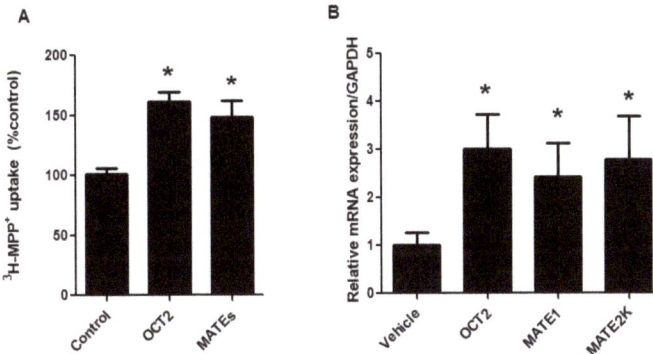

Figure 7. Effect of high concentration of CDCA on function and expression of OCT2 and MATEs. RPTEC/TERT1 cells were treated with vehicle or 80 µM CDCA for 24 h followed by measurements of (**A**) OCT2- and MATEs-mediated ^{3}H-MPP$^+$ uptake and (**B**) mRNA expression of OCT2, MATE1, and MATE2K. The data are expressed as mean ± S.D. from 3 independent experiments. * $p < 0.05$ compared with vehicle-treated group.

3. Discussion

Cationic transporters play a crucial role in the renal clearance of cationic endogenous and xenobiotic compounds [1,34]. Therefore, the altered expression and/or function of these transporters could affect the total profile excretion of these compounds. Previous reports showed that FXR activation regulates several hepatic transporters in different manners including down-regulation of OCT1 protein expression [27] or up-regulation of MATE1 protein expression [26]. The present study revealed that FXR activation regulates renal OCT2 and MATEs expression and function in the human proximal tubular cell line RPTEC/TERT1. Importantly, RPTEC/TERT1 cells express OCT2, MATE1, and MATE2K and represent an important in vitro model for studying renal transport [35]. Although the expression of FXR is present in the proximal tubular cells, we verified whether RPTEC/TERT1 cell line was suitable as a study model of FXR function. For this study, we initially confirmed that this cell line could be used for studying FXR activation by showing that FXR is expressed and activated by FXR agonist. Of note, we showed that FXR agonists increased OCT2-mediated ^{3}H-MPP$^+$ uptake in RPTEC/TERT1 cells. Importantly, the effect of CDCA on OCT2-mediated ^{3}H-MPP$^+$ uptake was not observed until after 24 h of incubation time; indicating that the FXR agonist has a slow mode of action on OCT2. Moreover, we showed that CDCA modulation of OCT2 is dependent upon FXR activation, as evidenced by our result showing that inhibition of FXR by pharmacological antagonists, guggulsterone and DY268 [36,37], attenuated the CDCA-mediated stimulation. Since RPTEC/TERT1 cells express both OCT2 and OCT3 [35], total ^{3}H-MPP$^+$ uptake into RPTEC/TERT1 cells could be mediated by either. However, we proved here that CDCA also stimulates OCT2 transport function in CHO-K1 cells expressing only OCT2. Taken together, these data imply that FXR activation by CDCA stimulates OCT2-mediated ^{3}H-MPP$^+$ uptake into RPTEC/TERT1 cells. However, we cannot rule out possible stimulatory effects of FXR activation on OCT3 in RPTEC/TERT1 cells. How FXR activation affects OCT3 should be further investigated in cells expressing OCT3 alone.

The stimulatory effect of FXR activation on OCT2 transport might via increase in either the functional number of transporters and/or transporter affinity with its substrate. Using kinetic data, we revealed that CDCA treatment increase in the Jmax of OCT2-mediated transport function. This result is indicative of an increase in the number of transporters at the membrane surface. FXR activation regulates several renal transporters and channel such as the organic solute transporters α and β (OSTα and OSTβ) and AQP2 by increase in mRNA and protein expressions [24,25], we investigated whether increased expression of OCT2 mediated the stimulatory effect of CDCA. We found that CDCA increased

OCT2 mRNA and protein expression in RPTEC/TERT1 cells. These results indicate that FXR activation increases ^{3}H-MPP$^+$ uptake into renal proximal tubular cells via the up-regulation of OCT2 mRNA and protein. Although previous studies have demonstrated that FXR modulates transporter and channel gene expression [24,25], we did not explore FXR direct binding and the up-regulation of OCT2 gene expression. FXR direct modulation of OCT2 expression needs to be determined in future studies.

Renal secretion of OCs requires both basolateral uptake and apical efflux. Therefore, we also investigated the correlation of FXR activation with the transporters expressed at apical membrane mediating secretion of OCs including MATE1 and MATE2K [8]. Our data demonstrated that CDCA stimulated the transport function of MATEs. Since FXR antagonists abolish this effect, we showed that the CDCA-mediated stimulation was controlled directly through FXR. The correlative relationship between FXR activation and OCT2/MATEs transport function was confirmed in basolateral to apical experiments. We demonstrated that FXR activation drove the flux of ^{3}H-MPP$^+$ from the basolateral chamber to the apical chamber. These results indicate that FXR activation stimulates OCT2/MATEs-mediated OC secretion in renal proximal tubular cells. Since RPTEC/TERT1 cells express both MATE1 and MATE2K, it is unclear what isoform FXR stimulated. Furthermore, we found that the stimulatory effect of FXR activation on ^{3}H-MPP$^+$ transport correlated well with the up-regulation of MATE1 and MATE2K mRNA. These results provide evidence that FXR activation stimulates OC secretion via up-regulation of both MATE1 and MATE2K.

There is increasing evidence that FXR is a critical regulatory factor in renal physiology and pathophysiology [38]. Previous studies have shown that pathological conditions related to hepatic injuries, such as ischemia/reperfusion and cholestasis, result in an up-regulation of the efflux transporter MATE1 and down-regulation of the uptake transporter OCT1 [27]. Dysregulation of these transporters can lead to the reduction of accumulated cationic compounds in hepatocytes [27]. Altered hepatic function could result in an increased plasma concentration of cations. Pathological conditions in the liver, such as acute hepatitis and obstructive jaundice, significantly increase the total serum concentrations of unconjugated bile acid including cholic acid, deoxycholic acid, and chenodeoxycholic acid (endogenous FXR agonists) up to 100 µM [29,30]. To model the consequences of pathologically high bile acid concentrations, we sought to correlate the modulation of bile acid concentration with renal OCT2, MATE1, and MATE2K expressions and functions. Our results revealed that high CDCA concentrations increase OCT2 and MATEs mRNA expression and modulate their function. These findings correlate with a previous study, which found that renal clearance of OCs in acute hepatic injury was increased due to high protein expression of OCT2 in the renal cortex [39]. Taken together, these data imply that renal FXR activation may be an adaptive response for the clearance of excess plasma OCs during hepatic clearance impairment.

4. Materials and Methods

4.1. Chemicals

N-methyl-^{3}H-4-phenylpyridinium acetate (^{3}H-MPP$^+$; 80 Ci/mmol) was purchased from American Radio Labeled Chemical Inc. (St. Louis, MO, USA). DY268 was purchased from Trocris (Thai Can Biotech, Bangkok, Thailand). Dulbecco's modified Eagle's medium (DMEM), Ham's F-12 nutrient mix (1:1), and TRIzol reagent, products of Invitrogen, were purchased from Gibthai (Bangkok, Thailand). iScrip cDNA Synthesis Kit and Luna Universal qPCR mastermix were obtained from Bio-Rad Thailand (Bangkok, Thailand), GW4064 (synthetic FXR agonist). Chenodeoxycholic acid (CDCA), Z-guggulsterone (FXR antagonist), tetrapentylammonium (TPeA), methyl-4-phenylpyridinium (MPP$^+$), and human OCT2 (HPA008567) antibody were purchased from Sigma-Aldrich (Bangkok, Thailand). Antibodies against FXR and β-actin were purchased from Merck Millipore (Bangkok, Thailand). Other chemicals used were of analytical grade from commercial sources.

4.2. Cell Cultures

RPTEC/TERT1 cells, an immortalized renal proximal tubular cell line expressing several drug transporters [35,40], was obtained from American Type Culture Collection (ATCC) and cultured in a mixture of DMEM and Ham's F-12 (1:1) supplemented with 10 ng/mL human epithelial growth factor, 5 µg/mL insulin, 5 µg/mL human transferrin, 5 ng/mL sodium selenite, 36 ng/mL hydrocortisone, 100 U/mL penicillin, and 100 µg/mL streptomycin. CHO-K1 cells expressing rbOCT2 were kindly gifted from Professor Stephen Wright, University of Arizona. These cells were maintained in Ham's F12 media supplemented with 10% FBS, 100 U/mL penicillin, and 100 µg/mL streptomycin, and 1% G418. All cells were cultured in a humidified incubator with 5% CO_2/95% air at 37 °C.

4.3. Measurement of OCT2 Transport Function

OCT2-mediated in ^{3}H-MPP$^+$ uptake in RPTEC/TERT1 cells was measured as previously described [18]. Briefly, RPTEC/TERT1 cell monolayers were washed twice with 1 mL of warm buffer pH 7.40 (NaCl 135 mM, KCl 5 mM, HEPES 13 mM, $CaCl_2.2H_2O$ 2.5 mM, $MgCl_2$ 1.2 mM, $MgSO_4.7H_2O$ 0.8 mM and D-glucose 28 mM) and incubated for further 15 min. The cell monolayers were incubated with buffer containing ^{3}H-MPP$^+$ for 5 min. The transport was stopped by three times washing with ice-cold buffer containing 100 µM unlabeled MPP$^+$. Cells were then lysed by adding 200 µL of 0.4 N NaOH in 10% SDS and left overnight. To neutralize the sample pH, 80 µL of 1 N HCl was added into each well. Accumulation of labeled MPP$^+$ was determined with a liquid scintillation and calculated as mole/min/cm^2 of the confluent monolayer surface.

4.4. Measurement of MATEs Transport Function

Measurement of MATEs-mediated ^{3}H-MPP$^+$ transport in RPTEC/TERT1 cells was performed as described by previous study [41]. Briefly, the cell monolayers were washed twice with 1 mL of warm K$^+$-based buffer (pH 7.4; KCl 130 mM, $MgSO_4.7H_2O$ 1.2 mM, $CaCl_2.2H_2O$ 1 mM, K_2HPO_4 2 mM, HEPES 20 mM, and D-glucose 5 mM) and were incubated for 15 min at 37 °C. To manipulate the intracellular acidification, the cell monolayers were further incubated with K$^+$-based buffer containing NH_4Cl 30 mM for 20 min at 37 °C [42,43]. Then, the cell monolayers were incubated with 200 µl of K$^+$ based-buffer (pH 8.0) containing ^{3}H-MPP$^+$ for 10 min. After incubation, the cell monolayers were washed three times with ice-cold buffer containing unlabeled MPP$^+$ 100 µM to stop transport activity. The cells were lysed by 0.4 N NaOH in 10% SDS and cellular accumulation of ^{3}H-MPP$^+$ was measured and calculated as fmol/min/cm^2 of the confluent monolayer surface.

4.5. Basolateral to Apical Transport of ^{3}H-MPP$^+$

RPTEC/TERT1 cells were cultured in in Transwell 12-well cultures (0.4 µm pore size; Corning Life Science, Corning, NY, USA) for 21 days. Basolateral and apical chambers were filled with 1 and 0.5 mL of media, respectively. Cell monolayer integrity was assessed using transepithelial electrical resistance (TEER). We selected the cell monolayers that achieved TEER values > 100 $\Omega \cdot cm^2$. On the day of experiment, the culture medium was withdrawn, and replaced with warm transport buffer and incubated with warm buffer for 30 min at 37 °C. Basolateral chamber was added with ^{3}H-MPP$^+$ for 30 min followed by sample collection (0.2 mL) from the apical chamber to determine ^{3}H-MPP$^+$ transepithelial transport. Transporter-mediated ^{3}H-MPP$^+$ transport was calculated by subtraction the total basolateral to apical transport of ^{3}H-MPP$^+$ with the transport of ^{3}H-MPP$^+$ in the presence of TPeA 100 µM, an inhibitor of OCTs.

4.6. Kinetic Analysis of OCT2-mediated ^{3}H-MPP$^+$ Uptake

The evaluation of OCT2 transport kinetics was performed as described previously [18]. RPTEC/TERT1 cell monolayers were incubated with transport buffer containing ^{3}H-MPP$^+$ 10 nM in the presence of various concentrations of unlabeled MPP$^+$. ^{3}H-MPP$^+$ uptake was calculated as mole/min/cm^2 of the confluent monolayer surface. This was followed by the calculation of kinetic parameters including a maximum transport rate of MPP$^+$ (Jmax) and the concentration of unlabeled MPP$^+$ that resulted in half-maximal transport (Kt) using the Michaelis–Menten equation of competitive interaction between labeled and unlabeled MPP$^+$ [44].

4.7. Real-Time PCR

Total RNA from RPTEC/TERT1 cells was extracted using TRIzol reagent (Invitrogen, Bangkok, Thailand). Synthesis of cDNA was performed using iScript cDNA Synthesis Kit (Bio-Rad, Bangkok, Thailand). A Luna Universal qPCR mastermix was then utilized for PCR amplification (Bio-Rad, Bangkok, Thailand). The primers used in this study are shown in Table 1.

Table 1. Primers (forward/reverse) for real-time PCR.

Target	Forward Primer (5'-3')	Reverse Primer (3'-5')
hOCT2	5-AGTCTGCCTGGTCAATGCT-3	5-AGGAATGGCGTGATGATGC-3
hMATE1	5-TGCTCCTGGGGGTCTTCTTA-3	5-GTGGGCCTGTGAATTGTGTG-3
hMATE2-K	5-TTGCACAGACCGTCTTCCTC-3	5-TGAGGAAGCTCCCGATCTCA-3
hSHP	5-GGCTTCAATGCTGTCTGGAGT-3	5-CTGGCACATCGGGGTTGAAGA-3
hGAPDH	5-CAAGCTCATTTCCTGGTATGAC-3	5-GTGTGGTGGGGGACTGAGTGTGG-3

The cycle threshold (CT) values were obtained from ABI Prism 7500 Sequence Detection System (Applied Biosystems (Thailand), Bangkok, Thailand), and the relative expression levels of mRNA were determined by the $2^{-\Delta\Delta Ct}$ method [45].

4.8. Western Blot Analysis

Proteins of RPTEC/TERT1 cells were separated by 10% SDS-polyacrylamide gel electrophoresis and subsequently transferred to a nitrocellulose membrane. Membranes were blocked with 5% non-fat dry milk for 2 h at room temperature and then blotted with primary antibodies for overnight at 4 °C. After that, the membranes were washed four times with Tris-buffered saline (TBST) for 10 min each. Subsequently, the membranes were incubated with horseradish peroxidase (HRP)-conjugated secondary antibody (Merck Millipore, Bangkok, Thailand) for 1 h. Proteins were detected and quantified by using an enhanced chemiluminescence (ECL) detection kit (Merck Millipore, Bangkok, Thailand) and the Gel and Graph Digitizing System (Uvitec, Cambridge, UK), respectively.

4.9. Statistical Analysis

Data are presented as mean and standard deviation (mean ± S.D.). Data of the kinetic study were analyzed by using unpaired student *t*-tests whereas other data were analyzed by using one-way analysis of variance (one-way ANOVA) tests with a post hoc Newman–Keuls test. The significant difference between each group of data was considered when $p < 0.05$.

5. Conclusions

We have demonstrated that FXR activation stimulates OC secretion in human renal proximal tubular cells. Moreover, the stimulatory effect of FXR on renal OC secretion may be mediated by the increase in OCT2/ MATEs-mediated OC transport. This effect is likely caused by enhanced OCT2 and MATE1/2K expression. Taken together, this study enhances our understanding of the role FXR may play in the regulation of renal OCT2- and MATEs-mediated renal OCs excretion.

Author Contributions: T.W. and S.S. conceived the studies and planned the experimental design. T.W. and S.S. performed the experiments analyzed the data. T.W., V.C., and S.S. interpreted the data. T.W. and S.S. wrote manuscript. V.C. and S.S. edited and proved the final manuscript. All authors have read and agreed to the published version of the manuscript.

Funding: This research project has been supported by the Thailand Research Funds and Mahidol University (grant no. RSA6280082 to S.S.) and the Royal Golden Jubilee (RGJ; grant no. PHD/0238/2553 to T.W.).

Acknowledgments: We would like to thank Professor Stephen Wright, University of Arizona for providing OCT2-CHO-K1 cells.

Conflicts of Interest: The authors declare no conflict of interest.

References

1. Wright, S.H. Role of organic cation transporters in the renal handling of therapeutic agents and xenobiotics. *Toxicol. Appl. Pharmacol.* **2005**, *204*, 309–319. [CrossRef] [PubMed]
2. Hosoyamada, M.; Sekine, T.; Kanai, Y.; Endou, H. Molecular cloning and functional expression of a multispecific organic anion transporter from human kidney. *Am. J. Physiol. Content* **1999**, *276*, F122–F128. [CrossRef] [PubMed]
3. Jonker, J.W.; Schinkel, A.H. Pharmacological and physiological functions of the polyspecific organic cation transporters: Oct1, 2, and 3 (SLC22A1-3). *J. Pharmacol. Exp. Ther.* **2003**, *308*, 2–9. [CrossRef] [PubMed]
4. Wright, S.H.; Dantzler, W.H. Molecular and cellular physiology of renal organic cation and anion transport. *Physiol. Rev.* **2004**, *84*, 987–1049. [CrossRef]
5. Yokoo, S.; Yonezawa, A.; Masuda, S.; Fukatsu, A.; Katsura, T.; Inui, K. Differential contribution of organic cation transporters, OCT2 and MATE1, in platinum agent-induced nephrotoxicity. *Biochem. Pharmacol.* **2007**, *74*, 477–487. [CrossRef]
6. Koepsell, H.; Lips, K.; Volk, C. Polyspecific organic cation transporters: Structure, function, physiological roles and biopharmaceutical implications. *Pharm. Res.* **2007**, *24*, 1227–1251. [CrossRef]
7. Terada, T.; Inui, K. Physiological and pharmacokinetic roles of H+/organic cation antiporters (MATE/SLC47A). *Biochem. Pharmacol.* **2008**, *75*, 1689–1696. [CrossRef]
8. Yonezawa, A.; Inui, K.-I. Importance of the multidrug and toxin extrusion MATE/SLC47A family to pharmacokinetics, pharmacodynamics/toxicodynamics and pharmacogenomics. *Br. J. Pharmacol.* **2011**, *164*, 1817–1825. [CrossRef]
9. Ciarimboli, G.; Deuster, D.; Knief, A.; Sperling, M.; Holtkamp, M.; Edemir, B.; Pavenstädt, H.; Lanvers-Kaminsky, C.; Zehnhoff-Dinnesen, A.A.; Schinkel, A.H.; et al. Organic cation transporter 2 mediates cisplatin-induced oto—and nephrotoxicity and is a target for protective interventions. *Am. J. Pathol.* **2010**, *176*, 1169–1180. [CrossRef]
10. Ciarimboli, G.; Lancaster, C.S.; Schlatter, E.; Franke, R.M.; Sprowl, J.A.; Pavenstädt, H.; Massmann, V.; Guckel, D.; Mathijssen, R.H.J.; Yang, W.; et al. Proximal tubular secretion of creatinine by organic cation transporter OCT2 in cancer patients. *Clin. Cancer Res.* **2012**, *18*, 1101–1108. [CrossRef]
11. Misaka, S.; Knop, J.; Singer, K.; Hoier, E.; Keiser, M.; Muller, F.; Glaeser, H.; Konig, J.; Fromm, M.F. The nonmetabolized beta-blocker nadolol is a substrate of Oct1, Oct2, Mate1, Mate2-k, and P-glycoprotein, but not of OATP1B1 and OATP1B3. *Mol. Pharm.* **2016**, *13*, 512–519. [CrossRef] [PubMed]
12. Nishizawa, K.; Yoda, N.; Morokado, F.; Komori, H.; Nakanishi, T.; Tamai, I. Changes of drug pharmacokinetics mediated by downregulation of kidney organic cation transporters Mate1 and Oct2 in a rat model of hyperuricemia. *PLoS ONE* **2019**, *14*, e0214862. [CrossRef] [PubMed]
13. Yonezawa, A.; Masuda, S.; Yokoo, S.; Katsura, T.; Inui, K. Cisplatin and oxaliplatin, but not carboplatin and nedaplatin, are substrates for human organic cation transporters (SLC22A1-3 and multidrug and toxin extrusion family). *J. Pharmacol. Exp. Ther.* **2006**, *319*, 879–886. [CrossRef] [PubMed]
14. Ivanyuk, A.; Livio, F.; Biollaz, J.; Buclin, T. Renal drug transporters and drug interactions. *Clin. Pharmacokinet.* **2017**, *56*, 825–892. [CrossRef]
15. Jonker, J.W.; Wagenaar, E.; van Eijl, S.; Schinkel, A.H. Deficiency in the organic cation transporters 1 and 2 (Oct1/Oct2 [Slc22a1/Slc22a2]) in mice abolishes renal secretion of organic cations. *Mol. Cell. Biol.* **2003**, *23*, 7902–7908. [CrossRef]
16. Shu, Y.; Bello, C.L.; Mangravite, L.M.; Feng, B.; Giacomini, K.M. Functional characteristics and steroid hormone-mediated regulation of an organic cation transporter in Madin-Darby canine kidney cells. *J. Pharmacol. Exp. Ther.* **2001**, *299*, 392–398.
17. Asaka, J.-I.; Terada, T.; Okuda, M.; Katsura, T.; Inui, K. Androgen receptor is responsible for rat organic cation transporter 2 gene regulation but not for rOCT1 and rOCT3. *Pharm. Res.* **2006**, *23*, 697–704. [CrossRef]

18. Wongwan, T.; Kittayaruksakul, S.; Asavapanumas, N.; Chatsudthipong, V.; Soodvilai, S. Activation of liver X receptor inhibits Oct2-mediated organic cation transport in renal proximal tubular cells. *Pflügers Archiv. Eur. J. Physiol.* **2017**, *469*, 1471–1481. [CrossRef]
19. Fukuda, Y.; Kaishima, M.; Ohnishi, T.; Tohyama, K.; Chisaki, I.; Nakayama, Y.; Ogasawara-Shimizu, M.; Kawamata, Y. Fluid shear stress stimulates MATE2-K expression via Nrf2 pathway activation. *Biochem. Biophys. Res. Commun.* **2017**, *484*, 358–364. [CrossRef]
20. Mencarelli, A.; Fiorucci, S. FXR an emerging therapeutic target for the treatment of atherosclerosis. *J. Cell. Mol. Med.* **2009**, *14*, 79–92. [CrossRef]
21. Ananthanarayanan, M.; Balasubramanian, N.; Makishima, M.; Mangelsdorf, D.J.; Suchy, F.J. Human bile salt export pump promoter is transactivated by the farnesoid X receptor/bile acid receptor. *J. Biol. Chem.* **2001**, *276*, 28857–28865. [CrossRef] [PubMed]
22. Kast, H.R.; Goodwin, B.; Tarr, P.T.; Jones, S.A.; Anisfeld, A.M.; Stoltz, C.M.; Tontonoz, P.; Kliewer, S.; Willson, T.M.; Edwards, P.A. Regulation of multidrug resistance-associated protein 2 (ABCC2) by the nuclear receptors pregnane X receptor, farnesoid X-activated receptor, and constitutive androstane receptor. *J. Biol. Chem.* **2001**, *277*, 2908–2915. [CrossRef] [PubMed]
23. Boyer, J.L.; Trauner, M.; Mennone, A.; Soroka, C.J.; Cai, S.-Y.; Tarek, M.; Zollner, G.; Lee, J.Y.; Ballatori, N. Upregulation of a basolateral FXR-dependent bile acid efflux transporter OSTalpha-OSTbeta in cholestasis in humans and rodents. *Am. J. Physiol. Gastrointest. Liver Physiol.* **2006**, *290*, G1124–G1130. [CrossRef] [PubMed]
24. Lee, H.; Zhang, Y.; Nelson, S.F.; Gonzales, F.J.; Edwards, P.A. FXR regulates organic solute transporters alpha and beta in the adrenal gland, kidney, and intestine. *J. Lipid Res.* **2006**, *47*, 201–214. [CrossRef]
25. Zhang, X.-Y.; Huang, S.; Gao, M.; Liu, J.; Jia, X.; Han, Q.; Zheng, S.; Miao, Y.; Li, S.; Weng, H.; et al. Farnesoid X receptor (FXR) gene deficiency impairs urine concentration in mice. *Proc. Natl. Acad. Sci. USA* **2014**, *111*, 2277–2282. [CrossRef]
26. Ferrigno, A.; Di Pasqua, L.G.; Berardo, C.; Siciliano, V.; Rizzo, V.; Adorini, L.; Richelmi, P.; Vairetti, M.P. The farnesoid X receptor agonist obeticholic acid upregulates biliary excretion of asymmetric dimethylarginine via MATE-1 during hepatic ischemia/reperfusion injury. *PLoS ONE* **2018**, *13*, e0191430. [CrossRef]
27. Denk, G.U.; Soroka, C.J.; Mennone, A.; Koepsell, H.; Beuers, U.; Boyer, J.L. Down-regulation of the organic cation transporter 1 of rat liver in obstructive cholestasis. *Hepatology* **2004**, *39*, 1382–1389. [CrossRef]
28. Nies, A.T.; Koepsell, H.; Winter, S.; Burk, O.; Klein, K.; Kerb, R.; Zanger, U.M.; Keppler, D.; Schwab, M.; Schaeffeler, E. Expression of organic cation transporters Oct1 (SLC22A1) and Oct3 (SLC22A3) is affected by genetic factors and cholestasis in human liver. *Hepatology* **2009**, *50*, 1227–1240. [CrossRef]
29. Fiorucci, S.; Biagioli, M.; Zampella, A.; Distrutti, E. Bile acids activated receptors regulate innate immunity. *Front. Immunol.* **2018**, *9*, 1853. [CrossRef]
30. Makino, I.; Nakagawa, S.; Mashimo, K. Conjugated and unconjugated serum bile acid levels n patients with hepatobiliary diseases. *Gastroenterology* **1969**, *56*, 1033–1039. [CrossRef]
31. Rizzo, G.; Renga, B.; Mencarelli, A.; Pellicciari, R.; Fiorucci, S. Role of FXR in regulating bile acid homeostasis and relevance for human diseases. *Curr. Drug Targets Immune Endocr. Metab. Disord.* **2005**, *5*, 289–303. [CrossRef] [PubMed]
32. Bae, E.H.; Choi, H.S.; Joo, S.Y.; Kim, I.J.; Kim, C.S.; Choi, J.S.; Ma, S.K.; Lee, J.; Kim, S.W. Farnesoid x receptor ligand prevents cisplatin-induced kidney injury by enhancing small heterodimer partner. *PLoS ONE* **2014**, *9*, e86553. [CrossRef] [PubMed]
33. Goodwin, B.; Jones, S.A.; Price, R.R.; Watson, M.A.; McKee, D.D.; Moore, L.B.; Galardi, C.; Wilson, J.G.; Lewis, M.C.; Roth, M.E.; et al. A regulatory cascade of the nuclear receptors FXR, SHP-1 and LRH-1 represses bile acid biosynthesis. *Mol. Cell* **2000**, *6*, 517–526. [CrossRef]
34. Nies, A.T.; Koepsell, H.; Damme, K.; Schwab, M. Organic cation transporters (Octs, Mates), in vitro and in vivo evidence for the importance in drug therapy. *Arrestins Pharmacol. Ther. Potential* **2010**, *201*, 105–167. [CrossRef]
35. Aschauer, L.; Carta, G.; Vogelsang, N.; Schlatter, E.; Jennings, P. Expression of xenobiotic transporters in the human renal proximal tubule cell line RPTEC/TERT1. *Toxicol. Vitr.* **2015**, *30*, 95–105. [CrossRef] [PubMed]
36. Cui, J.; Huang, L.; Zhao, A.; Lew, J.-L.; Yu, J.; Sahoo, S.; Meinke, P.T.; Royo, I.; Peláez, F.; Wright, S.D. Guggulsterone is a farnesoid X receptor antagonist in coactivator association assays but acts to enhance transcription of bile salt export pump. *J. Biol. Chem.* **2003**, *278*, 10214–10220. [CrossRef]

37. Yu, D.D.; Lin, W.; Forman, B.M.; Chen, T. Identification of trisubstituted-pyrazol carboxamide analogs as novel and potent antagonists of farnesoid x receptor. *Bioorganic Med. Chem.* **2014**, *22*, 2919–2938. [CrossRef]
38. Claudel, T.; Staels, B.; Kuipers, F. The farnesoid x receptor. *Arter. Thromb. Vasc. Biol.* **2005**, *25*, 2020–2030. [CrossRef]
39. Kurata, T.; Muraki, Y.; Mizutani, H.; Iwamoto, T.; Okuda, M. Elevated systemic elimination of cimetidine in rats with acute biliary obstruction: The role of renal organic cation transporter Oct2. *Drug Metab. Pharmacokinet.* **2010**, *25*, 328–334. [CrossRef]
40. Wieser, M.; Stadler, G.; Jennings, P.; Streubel, B.; Pfaller, W.; Ambros, P.F.; Riedl, C.; Katinger, H.; Grillari, J.; Grillari-Voglauer, R.; et al. hTERT alone immortalizes epithelial cells of renal proximal tubules without changing their functional characteristics. *Am. J. Physiol.* **2008**, *295*, F1365–F1375. [CrossRef]
41. Yasujima, T.; Ohta, K.-Y.; Inoue, K.; Ishimaru, M.; Yuasa, H. Evaluation of 4′,6-diamidino-2-phenylindole as a fluorescent probe substrate for rapid assays of the functionality of human multidrug and toxin extrusion proteins. *Drug Metab. Dispos.* **2010**, *38*, 715–721. [CrossRef] [PubMed]
42. Lang, K.; Wagner, C.; Haddad, G.; Burnekova, O.; Geibel, J. Intracellular pH activates 690 membrane-bound Na (+)/H (+) exchanger and vacuolar H (+)-ATPase in human embryonic kidney (HEK) 691 cells. *Cell. Physiol. Biochem.* **2003**, *13*, 257–262. [CrossRef] [PubMed]
43. Masuda, S.; Terada, T.; Yonezawa, A.; Tanihara, Y.; Kishimoto, K.; Katsura, T.; Ogawa, O.; Inui, K.-I. Identification and functional characterization of a new human kidney–specific H+/organic cation antiporter, kidney-specific multidrug and toxin extrusion 2. *J. Am. Soc. Nephrol.* **2006**, *17*, 2127–2135. [CrossRef]
44. Malo, C.; Berteloot, A. Analysis of kinetic data in transport studies: New insights from kinetic studies of Na+-d-glucose cotransport in human intestinal brush-border membrane vesicles using a fast sampling, rapid filtration apparatus. *J. Membr. Biol.* **1991**, *122*, 127–141. [CrossRef] [PubMed]
45. Livak, K.J.; Schmittgen, T.D. Analysis of relative gene expression data using real-time quantitative PCR and the 2−ΔΔCT method. *Methods* **2001**, *25*, 402–408. [CrossRef] [PubMed]

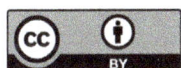

© 2020 by the authors. Licensee MDPI, Basel, Switzerland. This article is an open access article distributed under the terms and conditions of the Creative Commons Attribution (CC BY) license (http://creativecommons.org/licenses/by/4.0/).

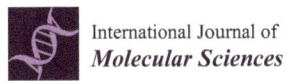

International Journal of
Molecular Sciences

Article

Rapid Regulation of Human Multidrug and Extrusion Transporters hMATE1 and hMATE2K

Marta Kantauskaitė [†], Anna Hucke [†], Moritz Reike, Sara Ahmed Eltayeb, Chuyan Xiao, Vivien Barz and Giuliano Ciarimboli *

Medicine Clinic D, Experimental Nephrology, University Hospital of Münster, 48149 Münster, Germany; marcikee@gmail.com (M.K.); anna_hucke@gmx.de (A.H.); moritz.reike@gmx.de (M.R.); Sara.Eltayeb@ukmuenster.de (S.A.E.); chuyanxiao_deutsch@163.com (C.X.); Vivien.Barz@ukmuenster.de (V.B.)
* Correspondence: gciari@uni-muenster.de; Tel.: +49-251-56981
† These authors equally contributed to the manuscript.

Received: 4 June 2020; Accepted: 20 July 2020; Published: 21 July 2020

Abstract: Vectorial transport of organic cations (OCs) in renal proximal tubules is mediated by sequential action of human OC transporter 2 (hOCT2) and human multidrug and toxic extrusion protein 1 and 2K (hMATE1 and hMATE2K), expressed in the basolateral (hOCT2) and luminal (hMATE1 and hMATE2K) plasma membranes, respectively. It is well known that hOCT2 activity is subjected to rapid regulation by several signaling pathways, suggesting that renal OC secretion may be acutely adapted to physiological requirements. Therefore, in this work, the acute regulation of hMATEs stably expressed in human embryonic kidney cells was characterized using the fluorescent substrate 4-(4-(dimethylamino)styryl)-N-methylpyridinium (ASP^+) as a marker. A specific regulation of ASP^+ transport by hMATE1 and hMATE2K measured in uptake and efflux configurations was observed. In the example of hMATE1 efflux reduction by inhibition of casein kinase II, it was also shown that this regulation is able to modify transcellular transport of ASP^+ in Madin–Darby canine kidney II cells expressing hOCT2 and hMATE1 on the basolateral and apical membrane domains, respectively. The activity of hMATEs can be rapidly regulated by some intracellular pathways, which sometimes are common to those found for hOCTs. Interference with these pathways may be important to regulate renal secretion of OCs.

Keywords: organic cations; transport; kidneys; regulation

---

1. Introduction

Kidneys are key players in the excretion of several substances of endogenous and exogenous origin. Besides by filtration in glomeruli, renal excretory function is sustained by secretion through the proximal tubules [1,2]. Tubular secretion is especially important for polar and charged molecules, which are subjected to a vectorial transport across proximal tubule cells by the orchestrated action of membrane transporters expressed either in the basolateral (facing blood) or apical (facing primary urine) membrane of the cells. In vectorial secretion processes, transporters expressed in the basolateral plasma membrane domain are responsible for the influx, whereas the ones expressed in the apical membrane domain are responsible for the efflux of substrates [3]. Tubular secretion is responsible for renal excretion of charged molecules, such as organic cations (OCs). Endogenous OCs are substances with important physiological function, such as serotonin and histamine, or are metabolism products, such as creatinine. A vast majority of exogenous OCs is represented by drugs such as metformin, verapamil, morphine, etc. [4,5].

The human organic cation transporter 2 (hOCT2) expressed in the basolateral membrane of proximal tubule cells mediates the first step of OC secretion, that is, the Na^+- and H^+-independent uptake of OCs [6,7] from the blood. The OC secretion into the urine is then accomplished by extrusion into the tubule lumen, a process that in humans is mediated mainly by human multidrug and toxin extrusion proteins 1 and 2K (hMATE1-2K) [8], pH-dependent transporters expressed in the apical membrane domain of proximal tubule cells [9–13]. This process is stimulated by the slightly acidic pH of primary urine. Substances that interact with hOCT2 can also interact with hMATEs [14–16], confirming that these transporters constitute a secretory axis for OCs in renal tubules. This transport vectorial system is involved also in the renal secretion of atypical substrates such as the chemotherapeutic drugs cisplatin and oxaliplatin. Since oxaliplatin is a better substrate of hMATE1 and hMATE2K than cisplatin, it is efficiently eliminated into the urine and causes less nephrotoxicity than cisplatin (Figure 1) [12,17,18].

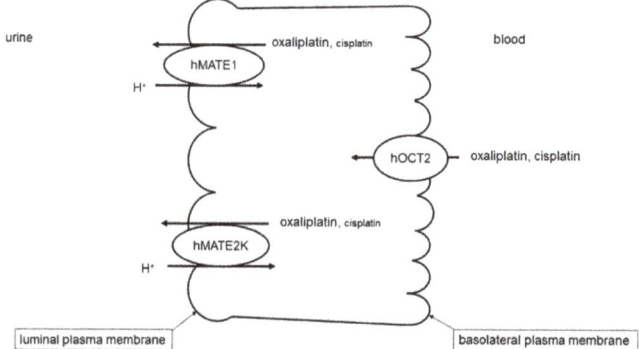

Figure 1. Renal secretion system for organic cations (OCs). In renal proximal tubule cells, the uptake of OCs from the blood is mediated by human organic cation transporter 2 (hOCT2) expressed on the basolateral domain of plasma membrane. The OC secretion from the cells into the urine is mediated by human multidrug and toxic extrusion protein 1 and 2K (hMATE1 and hMATE2K) expressed on the apical domain of plasma membrane. The slightly acidic pH of the urine favors secretion driven by hMATEs. In this example, oxaliplatin and cisplatin as substrates of the renal secretion system are shown. Lower affinity of cisplatin for hMATEs is indicated by the smaller font size.

It is well known that the activity of OCTs is subjected to specific acute regulation by several signaling pathways, which can elicit changes in transporter affinity or alter the number of transporters in the membrane [19]. However, information on regulation of MATEs is limited. The knowledge of specific regulation of transporters belonging to the same functional axis such as OCTs/MATEs is important, because such a regulation has the potential to modify the renal OC secretion, in this way changing body exposition to drugs and extent of nephrotoxicity. Therefore, in this work, the acute regulation of hMATEs has been comparatively investigated.

2. Results

Both human embryonic kidney (HEK) 293 cell lines transfected with either hMATE1 or hMATE2K were able to transport 4-(4-dimethylaminostyril)-N-methylpyridinium (ASP$^+$) in a concentration-dependent manner. Specific uptake was calculated by subtraction of unspecific uptake calculated in the presence of 1 mM cimetidine, a high affinity inhibitor of MATEs [20], from total ASP$^+$ uptake. Transport reached saturation both in hMATE- and hMATE2K-HEK cells, allowing calculation of the kinetic parameters V_{max} and K_m, which were, respectively, 4.5 ± 0.7 arbitrary fluorescence units (a.u.) and 14.2 ± 5.0 µM for hMATE1, and 15.3 ± 0.6 a.u. and 6.6 ± 1.0 µM for hMATE2K (Figure 2a, Table 1). The hMATE2K showed a slightly higher affinity for ASP$^+$ than hMATE1 in the uptake configuration. The V_{max} values cannot be directly compared, since they also depend on transfection efficiency, which can be different for hMATE1 and hMATE2K, on the gain used in the measurements, and on performance of the fluorimeter lamp. Additionally, in the efflux configuration (Figure 2b), hMATE2K seemed to have a slightly higher affinity for ASP$^+$ than hMATE1 (the K_m values calculated for efflux are not shown, since they cannot be exactly calculated because not all the intracellular ASP$^+$ is exchangeable; however the K_m ratio for the efflux mediated by hMATE1/hMATE2K was 1.5, suggesting a higher affinity of hMATE2K than hMATE1 for ASP$^+$ in the efflux configuration). Since not all the intracellular ASP$^+$ is exchangeable, these values must be considered as an approximation and cannot be directly compared to the K_m values measured in the uptake configuration.

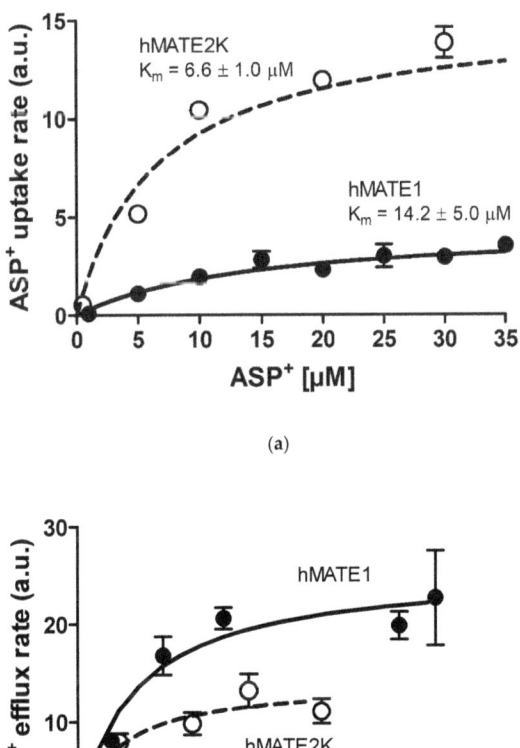

Figure 2. Saturation of 4-(4-dimethylaminostyril)-N-methylpyridinium (ASP$^+$) transport mediated by hMATE1 (closed symbols) and hMATE2K (open symbols) in both the uptake (**a**) and efflux conformation (**b**). (**a**) shows the specific ASP$^+$ uptake calculated subtracting unspecific (determined in the presence of 1 mM cimetidine) from total ASP$^+$ uptake (not shown). (**b**) shows the rate of ASP$^+$ efflux calculated as described in Materials and Methods. The calculated K_m values are indicated in the figure. The K_m values for efflux are not shown, since they can not be exactly calculated because not all the intracellular ASP$^+$ is exchangeable. Data are mean ± standard error of the mean (SEM) of three independent experiments, where each ASP$^+$ concentration was measured in at least six replicates per experiment. As explained in the text, the V_{max} values are not directly comparable, and for this reason are not shown.

Table 1. This table summarizes the affinities (K_m in µM) of hMATE1 and hMATE2K for ASP^+ measured in the uptake configuration.

Transport Direction	Transporter Affinity (K_m)	
	hMATE1	hMATE2K
Uptake	14.2 ± 5.0 µM	6.6 ± 1.0 µM

The rapid regulatory abilities of various cellular signal messengers on ASP^+ uptake by human MATE transporters are presented in Figure 3. Cells were incubated with each substance for 10 min, before measuring ASP^+ uptake. For activation of protein kinase A (PKA) and protein kinase C (PKC), we used 1 µM forskolin and 1 µM 1,2-dioctanoyl-sn-glycerol (DOG), respectively. For inhibition of phosphatidylinositol 3-kinase (PI3K), of Ca^{2+}/calmodulin (CaM), of $p56^{lck}$ tyrosine kinase ($p56^{lck}$), and of casein kinase II (CKII), we used 0.1 µM wortmannin, 5 µM calmidazolium, 5 µM aminogenistein, and 10 µM 4,5,6,7-tetrabromo-1H-benzimidazole (TBBz), respectively. The regulatory substances were used in a concentration range, which has been described to be specific for activation/inhibition of distinct signaling pathways and which was already used in HEK293 cells to study acute regulation of OCTs [19,21–27].

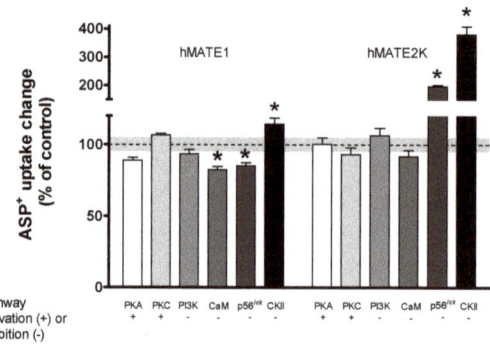

Figure 3. Acute regulation of ASP^+ uptake in hMATE1- and hMATE2K-HEK293 cells. HEK293 cells expressing hMATE1 or hMATE2K were incubated with a regulator of interest for 10 min before addition of 5 (hMATE1) or 2 (hMATE2K) µM ASP^+, respectively. Protein kinase A (PKA) was stimulated by incubation with 1 µM forskolin, whereas protein kinase C (PKC) was stimulated with 1 µM 1,2-dioctanoyl-sn-glycerol (DOG). Phosphatidylinositol 3-kinase (PI3K) was inhibited by 0.1 µM wortmannin, Ca^{2+}/calmodulin (CaM) by 5 µM calmidazolium, $p56^{lck}$ by 5 µM aminogenistein, and casein kinase II (CKII) by 10 µM 4,5,6,7-tetrabromo-1H-benzimidazole (TBBz). The uptake of ASP^+ in control wells was set as 100%. All conditions were compared to the control. Each column represents the mean ± SEM with 20–36 replicates measured in at least three independent experiments. The dotted line represents the control value = 100%, with a grey shading representing the SEM variation range. The stars (*) show a statistically significant difference compared to control experiments ($p < 0.05$, unpaired t-test).

The uptake mediated by hMATE1 seemed to be only slightly downregulated by CaM and $p56^{lck}$ inhibition (to −18 ± 2% and −15 ± 2% of controls, respectively). Interestingly, inhibition of CKII stimulated ASP^+ uptake (+14 ± 4%). Uptake mediated by hMATE2K was strongly stimulated by $p56^{lck}$ and CKII inhibition (to +97 ± 5% and +281 ± 29% of controls, respectively). Other substances (forskolin, DOG, wortmannin) had no significant influence on hMATE-mediated ASP^+ uptake.

Because of the huge regulatory effects of $p56^{lck}$ and CKII inhibition on ASP^+ uptake by hMATE2K, we investigated whether this regulation was due to the activity of Na^+/H^+ exchanger 1 (NHE1), which is the main regulator of pH in HEK cells [28]. For this reason, ASP^+ uptake regulation was measured in hMATE2K-HEK cells under inhibition of NHE1 by 1 µM cariporide, a concentration known to specifically inhibit NHE1 [29] (Figure 4).

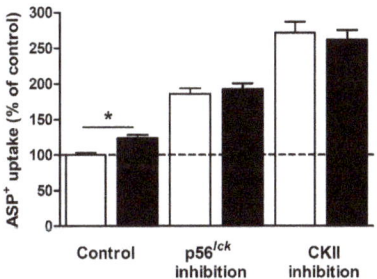

Figure 4. The effect of Na$^+$/H$^+$ exchanger 1 (NHE1) inhibition with 1 µM cariporide on regulation of ASP$^+$ uptake by hMATE2K. hMATE2K-HEK293 cells were incubated with a regulator of interest (p56^{lck} inhibition by 5 µM aminogenistein and CKII inhibition by 10 µM TBBz) alone (open bars) or in the presence of 1 µM cariporide (closed bars) for 10 min. After incubation, 2 µM ASP$^+$ solution was applied, and uptake through hMATE2K transporter was measured. Control condition indicates the uptake of ASP$^+$ without addition of regulator, which was set to 100%. Results in the presence or absence of cariporide were compared. Each column represents mean ± SEM of at least three independent experiments. The star (*) shows a statistically significant difference compared to experiments without cariporide ($p < 0.05$, unpaired t-test).

Ten minutes of incubation with 1 µM cariporide increased ASP$^+$ uptake by hMATE2K, probably because of efficient NHE1 inhibition and slight acidification of the cells, which stimulated ASP$^+$ uptake. Inhibition of NHE1 with cariporide did not change the stimulation of ASP$^+$ uptake by hMATE2K under p56^{lck} or CKII inhibition. To study the effects of pH on regulation of ASP$^+$ uptake by hMATE2K, we incubated the cells with NH$_4$Cl to make the cellular pH more acidic (Figure S4). This maneuver strongly increased the ASP$^+$ uptake by hMATE2K to 292 ± 14% (measured in at least three independent experiments) compared to control experiments, which were set to 100 ± 4% (not shown). Interestingly, under cell acidification, the stimulation of ASP$^+$ uptake by hMATE2K observed under p56^{lck} inhibition with aminogenistein disappeared, while the one produced by CKII inhibition with TBBz remained (Figure 5).

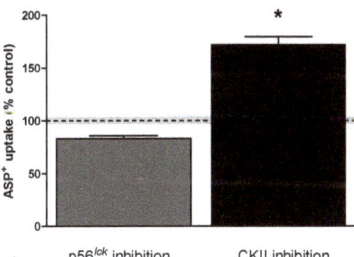

Figure 5. Acute regulation of ASP$^+$ uptake into hMATE2K-HEK cells after 30 mM NH$_4$Cl pre-treatment to acidify the cells, before 10 min incubation with the regulator of interest (5 µM aminogenistein for p56^{lck} inhibition or 10 µM TBBz for CKII inhibition). After this, incubation solution was replaced with 2 µM ASP$^+$, and uptake through hMATE2K was measured. The uptake of ASP$^+$ without addition of regulator was set to 100% (dashed line with grey shading representing the SEM variation range). Each column represents mean ± SEM of at least three independent experiments. The star (*) shows a statistically significant difference compared to control experiments without TBBz ($p < 0.05$, unpaired t-test).

Rapid Regulation of Efflux

We further investigated whether ASP$^+$ efflux mediated by hMATE1 or hMATE2K is also subjected to rapid regulation (Figures 6 and 7). Figure 6 shows an example of hMATE2K efflux regulation experiments performed under PKC activation with DOG compared to control experiments. Figure 7 shows the summary of the results on efflux mediated by hMATE1 and hMATE2K obtained under modulation of several signaling pathways.

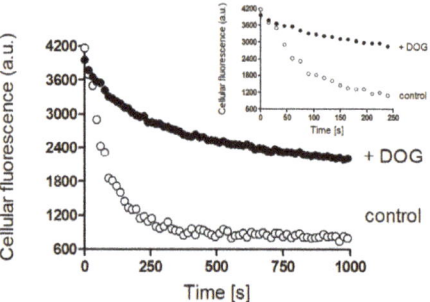

Figure 6. Example of acute regulation of ASP$^+$ efflux from hMATE2K-HEK293 cells under PKC activation with 1 µM DOG (closed circles). Prior to addition of DOG, hMATE2K cells were incubated with 25 µM ASP$^+$ for 30 min. After that, DOG was added for further 10 min. After this, incubation solution was removed, and cell monolayers were washed two times with ice-cold Ringer-like solution (pH 7.4). Each well was filled with Ringer-like solution and the decrease in fluorescence signal over time was measured. In control experiments, the efflux of ASP$^+$ without addition of regulator was measured (open circles). The experimental points of ASP$^+$ fluorescence decrease measured in the first 250 s are shown in the insert.

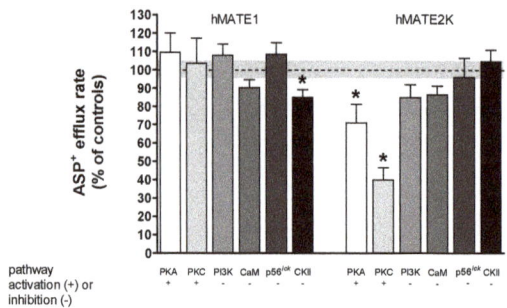

Figure 7. Acute regulation of ASP$^+$ efflux from hMATE1- and hMATE2K-HEK293 cells. Prior to the addition of regulator, hMATEs cells were incubated with 25 µM ASP$^+$ for 30 min. After that, regulator (PKA was stimulated by incubation with 1 µM forskolin, PKC with 1 µM DOG; PI3K was inhibited by 0.1 µM wortmannin, CaM by 5 µM calmidazolium, p56^{lck} by 5 µM aminogenistein, and CKII by 10 µM TBBz) was added for a further 10 min. After this, incubation solution was removed, and cell monolayers were washed two times with ice-cold Ringer-like solution (pH 7.4). Each well was filled with Ringer-like solution and the decrease in fluorescence signal was measured for 10 min. In control experiments, the efflux of ASP$^+$ without addition of regulator was set to 100%. All other conditions were compared with the control. Each column represents mean ± SEM from three different experiments. The dotted line represents the control value = 100%, with the grey shading representing the SEM variation range. The stars (*) show a statistically significant difference compared to control experiments ($p < 0.05$, unpaired t-test).

Since inhibition of CKII with TBBz seems to be able to regulate hMATE1 both in the uptake and in the efflux configuration, we tested whether this regulation can modulate the activity of the transport axis for OCs in Madin–Darby canine kidney (MDCK) II cells, a polarized cell system, where we expressed hOCT2 alone or together with hMATE1. The hMATE1 was transfected in MDCK II cells already stably expressing hOCT2-GFP. The cells were grown on filters (12 well Thin-cert, 1 μm transparent, Greiner Bio-One, Frickenhausen, Germany), allowing the separation of an apical and basolateral compartment. Expression of hOCT2 and hMATE1 was controlled by PCR and immunofluorescence analysis (Figures S7 and S8). The genetic manipulation of MDCK II cells resulted in the expression of hOCT2 and hMATE1 both at the mRNA and at the protein levels. Immunofluorescence labeling of hOCT2 and hMATE1 clearly showed that the two proteins were expressed in distinct cellular compartments, with hOCT2 mainly expressed in the basolateral and hMATE1 in the apical membrane domain. The cellular accumulation of ASP^+ was compared between hOCT2-MDCK and hOCT2-hMATE1-MDCK cells after addition of the fluorescent substrate to the basolateral compartment in order to mimic the physiological direction of transport in the kidneys (Figure 8). By addition of ASP^+ to the basolateral compartment, a higher intracellular ASP^+ accumulation was observed in hOCT2- compared with hOCT2-hMATE1-MDCK-cells, indicating that the presence of hMATE1 increased the ASP^+ efflux through the apical domain of the plasma membrane. Incubation with TBBz strongly increased the intracellular ASP^+ content in hOCT2-hMATE1- compared with hOCT2-MDCK-cells, probably due to an inhibition of ASP^+ efflux through the hMATE1, as observed in experiments with hMATE1-HEK293 cells (Figure 7).

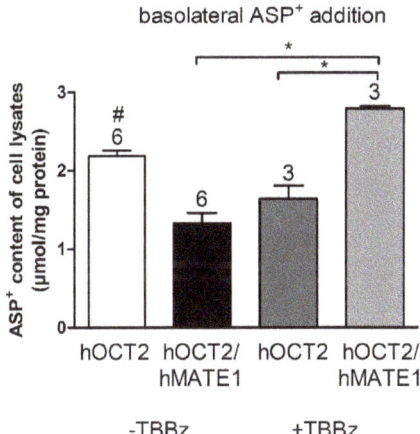

Figure 8. ASP^+ intracellular accumulation in Madin–Darby canine kidney (MDCK) II cells expressing hOCT2 or hOCT2 together with hMATE1. MDCK II cells expressing the transporters were grown on filters. Upon reaching confluence, we added ASP^+ (50 μM) to the basolateral compartment, and after 2 h incubation in the presence or absence of 10 μM TBBz, we lysed cells with 4% SDS, with fluorescence in cell lysates being quantified by comparison with cell lysates, where known ASP^+ concentrations were added. ASP^+ concentrations in cell lysates were normalized to protein content. Each column represents mean ± SEM from 3–6 different experiments. The stars (*) show a statistically significant difference between the groups and # represents a difference compared to all other groups ($p < 0.05$, ANOVA with Tukey's post-test).

3. Discussion

The kidneys deal with rapidly changing quantity of water and solutes, which derives from variable fluid and meal intake and metabolic activities. Transport systems are strongly involved in determining renal function consisting of secretion and reabsorption processes of water and solutes.

For this reason, a regulation of transporter activity to cope with different situations is conceivable. Indeed, the renal transport systems are targeted by several hormones, which can initiate a series of regulation pathways [19]. Focusing on renal secretion systems, this regulation has potential pharmacological and pathophysiological importance, since their inhibition may augment the bodily exposure to dangerous synthetic and natural xenobiotics, and their stimulation may be useful for prevention or treatment of pharmacological and occupational renal toxicity [30]. Posttranslational modifications such as phosphorylation/dephosphorylation, glycosylation, and ubiquitination processes are important modulators of protein function, structure, or localization [31]. For transporters, these modifications can alter their kinetic characteristics, such as K_m or V_{max} [32].

Considering the renal secretion axis of organic cations (OCs), it is well known that such posttranslational modifications can regulate the first step of secretion, that is, the uptake of OCs into the proximal tubule cells. This process is mainly mediated in humans by hOCT2. From experiments with hOCT2 and also with other orthologs and paralogs, it is well known that glycosylation and oligomerization are important for regulating the insertion of the transporter into the plasma membrane [33–36] and that multiple intracellular signaling pathways are involved in its rapid regulation [24,27]. Specifically, hOCT2 function was significantly reduced by inhibition of the Ca^{2+}/calmodulin complex and stimulation of PKC and of PKA [24]. However, there are only few investigations on the regulation of the final step of renal OC secretion, that is, the transport of OCs by hMATE1 and hMATE2K from proximal tubule cells into the urine. It is conceivable that pathways exist that can regulate renal secretion of organic cations acting both on hOCTs and hMATEs.

The present knowledge on MATE regulation is well summarized in [37]. Transcriptional regulation of MATE1 has been described, together with regulation of its function or mRNA expression under pathological situations such as ischemia/reperfusion injury and diabetes [37]. In inflamed or fibrotic fibroblasts, hMATE expression is downregulated by tumor necrosis factor (TNF)α, interleukin (IL)-16, IL-6, and platelet-derived growth factor (PDGF) [38,39], and stimulated by the Notch pathway [39]. In plasma membranes from human kidney cortex, the protein expression of hMATE was found to not be gender- or age-dependent, at least in renal samples from adults [40].

To increase the knowledge on hMATE regulation and find out whether there is a regulation of the OC secretory axis, we investigated in this work the hMATE rapid regulation, focusing on pathways that are known to modulate hOCT function.

Physiologically, hMATEs work as OC/H^+ exchangers, driven by the slight acidity of primary urine in proximal tubules. Working in vitro with HEK293 cells as an expression system for hMATEs, we can study the transport characteristics of the transporters, offering to the cells substrates from the extracellular site and investigating their uptake by hMATEs, which is driven by the negative membrane potential. This uptake can be stimulated by decreasing the intracellular pH. The HEK system can be also used to study the function of hMATEs as OC efflux transporters by loading the cells with substrates and measuring their efflux kinetics.

Using the fluorescent organic cation ASP^+ as a substrate, we showed that both ASP^+ uptake and efflux were pH-dependent (Figure S5) and that hMATE2K has a slightly higher affinity than hMATE1 for the substrate both in the efflux and in the uptake configuration. Performing efflux experiments over 30 min, we measured that up to 40% (41 ± 6%, $N = 4$, not shown) of ASP^+ is not exchangeable. For this reason, the K_m for ASP^+ in the efflux configuration cannot be exactly determined.

Rapid regulation of ASP^+ uptake was studied first. Here, hMATE1 activity was decreased by inhibition of the Ca^{2+}/calmodulin complex with calmidazolium and of $p56^{lck}$ tyrosine kinase with aminogenistein, while inhibition of CKII with TBBz stimulated hMATE1-mediated ASP^+ uptake, indicating that in HEK293 cells these pathways are endogenously active and regulate hMATE1 uptake. A search of putative calmodulin binding sites in hMATE1 using the calmodulin binding database of the Ikura Lab, Ontario Cancer Institute (http://calcium.uhnres.utoronto.ca/ctdb/ctdb/home.html), showed that it has a putative calmodulin binding sequence at position 533 (DGAKLSRK). Using the group-based prediction system GPS 5.0 [41], in the putative intracellular domains of hMATE1 amino acid sequence (Table S2), no direct p56^{lck} phosphorylation site could be identified, while a CKII potential phosphorylation site was detected at position S402 (Figure 9). ASP$^+$ uptake by hMATE2K was significantly stimulated by inhibition of p56^{lck} tyrosine kinase and of CKII. While CKII-induced regulation was stronger than that of the same type as was measured for hMATE1, the effect of p56^{lck} tyrosine kinase was opposite to what was observed for hMATE1. This strong stimulation of hMATE2K by inhibition of p56^{lck} tyrosine kinase and of CKII was not dependent on a changed activity of NHE1, since it was still present when the experiments were performed under NHE1 inhibition. However, the regulation by inhibition of p56^{lck} tyrosine kinase disappeared under cellular acidification, suggesting that it involves some interaction close to the H$^+$ binding site, probably in proximity of the N-terminus, where H$^+$-driven conformational changes of MATEs take place [42]. Indeed, a potential phosphorylation site for p56^{lck} was present in the putative second intracellular loop of hMATE2K at position Y104 (Figure 9). CKII has putative phosphorylation sites at S3, S508, and S519 (Figure 9).

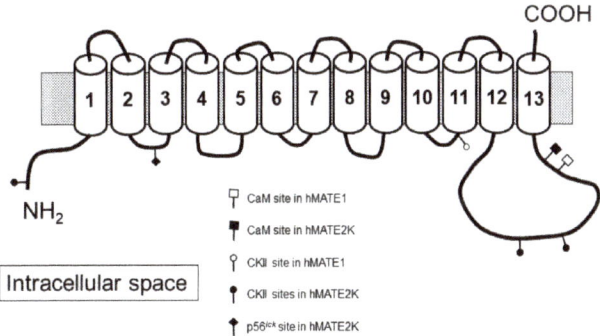

Figure 9. This figure shows a schematic secondary structure of hMATEs, as determined using the eukaryotic linear motif resource [43]. Both hMATE1 (NP_060712.2, NM_018242.3) and hMATE2K (NP_001093116.1, NM_001099646.2) are modelled as having 13 transmembrane domains (TMD), with intracellular amino- and extracellular carboxy-termini. Potential CaM, CKII, and p56^{lck} phosphorylation sites identified as explained in the Materials and Methods section are also shown. Several other potential phosphorylation sites for PKA (S23/S119/S249/S335/S336/T337/S538 in hMATE1; S469/S508/S534 in hMATE2K) and for PKC (T98/S101/T103/S335/S336/S538 in hMATE1; T325/T398/S469/S492/T496/S498/T505/T506/T530/S531/S534 in hMATE2K) were identified using GPS 5.0 [41], but for the sake of clarity, they are not indicated in the figure.

For what concerns regulation of ASP$^+$ efflux, inhibition of CKII caused a downregulation of efflux by hMATE1, in clear opposition to what observed for uptake, suggesting that incubation with TBBz stabilizes hMATE1 in an uptake configuration. In hMATE2K cells, this maneuver did not change the efflux of ASP$^+$, in strong contrast to what measured for ASP$^+$ uptake, also here suggesting that TBBz stabilizes the transporter rather than an uptake configuration. The other pathways did not change ASP$^+$ efflux, except for that concerning activation of PKA with forskolin and of PKC with DOG, which in hMATE2K cells significantly inhibited its function, suggesting that PKA and PKC inhibit the efflux by hMATE2K. A search of putative phosphorylation sites in hMATE2K showed that it has several potential PKA and PKC phosphorylation sites in intracellular domains (Table S2), suggesting that these sites may be the target of this regulation.

Can a regulation of the transporter axis change the renal secretion of substrates? This point was investigated in MDCK II cells, a polarized cell model, resembling the physiological polarization of renal tubules, where the hOCT2 alone or together with hMATE1 were expressed. Expression of hMATE1 reduced the cellular ASP$^+$ accumulation, probably by increasing its transport out of cells. Interestingly, inhibition of CKII resulted in a higher cellular ASP$^+$ content, confirming the results obtained with HEK293 cells, where incubation with TBBz reduced its efflux. For this reason, regulation of transporters involved in renal secretion of organic cations may be an approach to stimulate renal secretion or to decrease exposition of kidney cells to nephrotoxicants.

Comparing these results with the data from the literature, we found hOCT2 to be regulated by several different signaling pathways [24,27,44], while the activity of hMATEs both in the uptake and in the efflux configuration was found to be regulated only by few pathways (Table 2).

Table 2. Signaling pathways and their effects on hOCT2-, hMATE1-, and hMATE2K-mediated transport.

Signaling Pathway	hOCT2 Uptake	hMATE1 Uptake	hMATE1 Efflux	hMATE2K Uptake	hMATE2K Efflux
PKA	↓[24]	0	0	0	↓
PKC	↓[24]	0	0	0	↓
CKII	↑	↓	↑	↓	0
CaM	↑[24]	↑	0	0	0
p56^{lck}	↑[44]	↑	0	↓	0
PI3K	↓[24]	0	0	0	0

0 = no effect; ↑/↓ = the activity of the indicated kinase stimulates/inhibits the transporters. When no reference is indicated, the results refer to the present work.

4. Materials and Methods

Cell culture: Human embryonic kidney (HEK) 293 cells stably expressing hMATE1 or hMATE2K or the respective empty vector were used for the experiments. Generation of these cell lines has been already described elsewhere [45]. HEK293 cells were maintained at 37 °C, 5% CO$_2$, in 50 mL cell culture flasks (Greiner, Frickenhausen, Germany). Cell medium consisted of Dulbecco's minimal Eagle's medium (Biochrom, Berlin, Germany) supplemented with 10% fetal bovine serum, 1 g/L glucose, 2 mM glutamine, 3.7 g/L NaHCO$_3$, and 100 U/mL streptomycin/penicillin (Biochrom). Selection of cells transfected with hMATE1 or hMATE2K transporter was assured by the addition of hygromycin (200 or 175 mg/mL, respectively). Cell cultures were grown on 96-, 24-, or 12-well plates until 80–90% confluence was reached. Experiments were performed with cells from passages 40–65. A brief characterization of these cell lines is shown in the Figures S1–S3.

For some experiments, the MDCK II cell line was used, since it has a clear apical-basolateral polarity, well-defined cell junctions, and a rapid growth rate, and because it polarizes in cell culture [46]. MDCK II cells were transduced with hOCT2-GFP inserted into the vector pQCXIH (Clontech Laboratories, Takara Bio USA, Mountain View, CA, USA) by a retroviral transduction technique, as described in [47]. These cells were then transiently transfected with hMATE1 inserted into the pcDNA 3.1 vector [16] (a kind gift by Atushi Yonezawa, Kyoto University, Japan). Transfection was performed with Lipofectamine 2000 transfection reagent according to the manufacturer's instructions (Fisher Scientific, Schwerte, Germany).

Reagents: ASP$^+$ was purchased from Fischer Scientific. Wortmannin, calphostin C, calmidazolium, and aminogenistein were purchased from Calbiochem (Calbiochem, Merck Chemicals, Darmstadt, Germany). All other reagents were of the highest purity and were obtained from Sigma-Aldrich (Sigma-Aldrich, Merck Chemicals, Darmstadt, Germany).

Fluorescence measurements.: The fluorescent organic cation ASP$^+$ was used to monitor hMATE activity, as already performed in other works [45,48]. Measurements were performed using a microplate fluorescence reader with excitation at 465 nm and emission at 590 nm (Infinite F200, Tecan, Switzerland), as already described in detail [23].

Transport characteristics and acute regulation of hMATE1 and hMATE2K were studied using two different protocols. The first one aimed to test function and acute regulation of hMATEs in the uptake configuration, and the second one aimed to measure these parameters in an efflux configuration.

Before measurements, cell monolayers were washed with Ringer-like solution containing (in mM): NaCl 145, K_2HPO_4 1.6, KH_2PO_4 0.4, D-glucose 5, $MgCl_2$ 1, and calcium gluconate 1.3, with pH adjusted to 7.4 at 37 °C. For uptake kinetic experiments, OC transport was measured dynamically at 37 °C after addition of ASP^+ in a 1–35 µM concentration range as initial rate of fluorescence increase [23]. Slopes of fluorescence increase were linearly fitted and used as ASP^+ uptake measure. For measurements of transporter activity in the efflux configuration, we incubated cells for 10 min at 37 °C with ASP^+ in a 10–100 µM concentration range. After this incubation, cells were washed with ice-cold Ringer-like solution and the decrease of fluorescence was measured at 37 °C for 10 min. The slope of the initial fluorescence decrease was used as a measure of transporter efflux velocity. This part of the efflux seemed to be mediated mainly by hMATEs (Figure S3). To calibrate for cellular ASP^+ content at the beginning of efflux measurements, in unpaired experiments after incubation with ASP^+ and washing with ice-cold Ringer-like solution, we lysed cells with 4% sodium dodecyl sulfate (SDS) in 10 mM Tris-HCl (pH 7.4) and their fluorescence was compared with that measured in SDS cell lysates, where known ASP^+ concentrations were added, as explained in Figure S9. An example of the fluorescence decrease in efflux experiments is given in Figure 10. In both uptake and efflux experiments, we also evaluated pH dependence of ASP^+ transport by hMATEs (Figure S5).

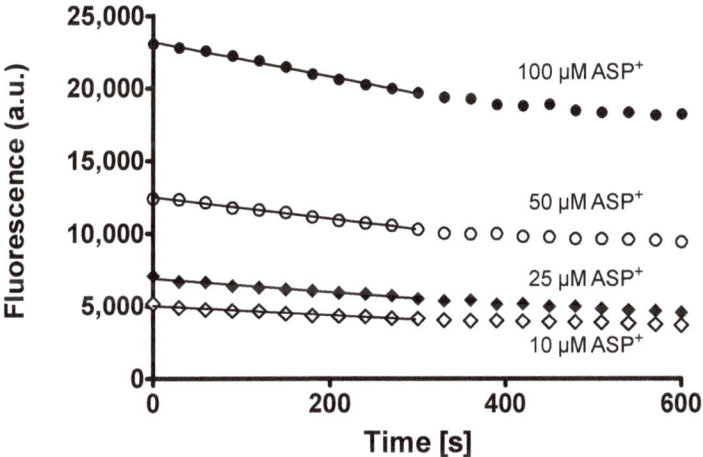

Figure 10. Example of efflux experiments performed after 10 min incubation of hMATE1-HEK cells with 10–100 µM ASP^+ at 37 °C. The decrease of cellular fluorescence upon time in seconds is shown for different ASP^+ concentrations used. The lines show the part of the fluorescence decrease used to calculate the slope of efflux velocity. Fluorescence is given as arbitrary units (a.u.).

In some experiments, the dependence of ASP^+ uptake by hMATEs on pH was investigated using intracellular acidification. To do this, cells were incubated with 30 mM NH_4Cl for 30 min and, before addition of ASP^+, the NH_4Cl solution was replaced by fresh Ringer-like solution (37 °C, pH 7.4). The course of pH changes induced by this procedure was investigated in unpaired experiments using 2′,7′-bis(2-carboxyethyl)-5(6)-carboxyfluorescein acetoxymethyl ester (BCECF-AM). BCECF-AM is a membrane permeable substance, which functions as pH-sensitive fluorescent dye [49,50]. Briefly, confluent hMATE-HEK cells were incubated in the dark with Ringer-like solution containing 5 µM BCECF-AM for 30 min. After incubation, the dye was removed, and the cells were incubated with Ringer-like solution with or without 30 mM NH_4Cl for 30 min. After this time, incubation solution was replaced by fresh Ringer-like buffer. All the solutions had a pH 7.4 at 37 °C. The pH changes were monitored with Tecan Infinite M200 (Tecan, Switzerland) by ratiometric measurements of BCECF fluorescence emission at 540 nm after excitation at the wavelengths of 440 nm (isosbestic point) and 490 nm (pH-dependent) (Figure S4).

Acute regulation of ASP^+ transport by hMATEs was studied in the uptake and in the efflux transporter configuration. Regulation of ASP^+ uptake was studied after 10 min incubation with known regulators of important signaling pathways, which are known to be active in HEK293 cells [19,21,23,24,26,27]. The concentrations of the potential regulators were chosen according to previous regulation studies of OCT function [19,21,23,24,26,27]. After pre-treatment with the potential regulator, ASP^+ was added to the cells and its uptake over time was monitored. In some experiments, cells were treated with NH_4Cl to induce an acidification and were then incubated 10 min with the regulator before replacing incubation solution with Ringer-like buffer and measuring ASP^+ uptake.

For regulation experiments of hMATE-mediated ASP^+ efflux, we loaded confluent hMATEs-HEK293 cells with 25 µM ASP^+ for 30 min. After that, regulator of interest or Ringer-like solution as a control was applied for 10 more minutes, still in the presence of ASP^+. Afterwards, incubation solution was removed, each well was washed with ice-cold Ringer-like solution, and the decrease in fluorescence was measured at 37 °C, as described above.

The effect of each regulator on ASP^+ uptake and efflux were compared with control conditions without potential regulator, which were set as 100%. In order to test the specificity of regulatory effects, we measured regulation by some effective substance also in the presence of 10 µM cariporide, an inhibitor of NHE1 [29].

Immunofluorescence analysis: MDCK-hOCT2-GFP cells transfected with hMATE1 and growing on filters for 7 days were fixed in 4% paraformaldehyde (PFA). After fixation, the cells were washed three times with Dulbecco's phosphate-buffered saline (PBS, Biochrom, Berlin, Germany) and permeabilized using 0.1% Triton X-100 for 5 min. After extensive washing with PBS, unspecific binding sites were blocked by overnight incubation at 4 °C with 10% bovine serum albumin (BSA, Sigma-Aldrich) in PBS. Cells were then incubated 60 min at room temperature with a rabbit anti-hMATE1 antibody (hMATE1 E13, sc-133390, Santa Cruz, Dallas, TX, USA) diluted 1:10 in 1% BSA in PBS. After three washing steps in PBS, the secondary antibody (anti-rabbit IgG Alexa Fluor 594, Cell Signaling, Frankfurt/Main, Germany) at a 1:1.000 dilution was incubated for 60 min followed by five more washing steps in PBS. The nuclei were blue-labeled with 2-(4-amidinophenyl)-1H-indole-6-carboxamidine (DAPI, Sigma-Aldrich). Finally, cells were covered with Fluoromount (Sigma-Aldrich), and fluorescence photographs were taken by epifluorescence microscopy (Observer Z1 with apotome, Zeiss, Göttingen, Germany). Negative control slides were included without addition of primary antibody (data not shown).

PCR analysis: For PCR analysis of MDCK II cells, total RNA from wild type (WT) cells or cells expressing hOCT2 alone or together with hMATE1 or only the empty vectors (EV) were isolated using the Qiagen RNeasy Midikit (Qiagen, Gilden, Germany) and reverse transcription was performed using the Superscript II system (Invitrogen, Carlsbad, CA), both according to the manufacturer's recommendations. Standard PCR was performed using specific primer pairs as listed in Table S1. The PCR products were separated using agarose gel electrophoresis.

Statistical analysis: Experimental data are presented as means ± SEM, with n referring to the number of totally measured replicates obtained in at least three independent experiments. Significant differences of regulatory substances were calculated using unpaired Student's t-test or ANOVA with Tukey's post-test for multiple comparisons. A p-value < 0.05 was considered statistically significant. Analyses were performed using GraphPad Prism, Version 5.3 (GraphPad Software, San Diego, CA, USA).

5. Conclusions

As found for other SLC transporter families, hMATEs, members of the renal secretion pathway of organic cations, can be acutely regulated. Although hMATEs are highly similar in their structure and substrate affinities, they do have some differences for what concerns responses to cellular messengers. Preliminary results suggest that such a regulation is effective in systems expressing uptake and extrusion transporters.

Supplementary Materials: Supplementary materials can be found at http://www.mdpi.com/1422-0067/21/14/5157/s1.

Author Contributions: Conceptualization, G.C.; methodology, G.C., A.H., M.K.; validation, C.X., S.A.E., V.B.; formal analysis, G.C.; investigation, A.H., M.K., M.R., C.X., S.A.E., V.B.; writing—original draft preparation, M.K.; writing—review and editing, G.C.; supervision, G.C.; project administration, G.C.; funding acquisition, G.C. All authors have read and agreed to the published version of the manuscript.

Funding: This research was funded by the Deutsche Forschungsgemeinschaft, grant number 107/11.1 to G.C.

Acknowledgments: We thank Astrid Dirks, Rita Schröter, and Ute Neugebauer for their excellent technical assistance. Furthermore, we thank Atsushi Yonezawa and Yohannes Hagos for hMATE1 plasmid and hMATE2K cell line donation, respectively, and Beatrice Snieder and Ulf Schulze for the hOCT2 viral transduction of MDCK II cells.

Conflicts of Interest: The authors declare no conflict of interest. The funders had no role in the design of the study; in the collection, analyses, or interpretation of data; in the writing of the manuscript; or in the decision to publish the results.

Abbreviations

ASP$^+$	4-(4-(dimethylamino)styryl)-N-methylpyridinium
a.u.	arbitrary units
BCECF-AM	2′,7′-bis(2-carboxyethyl)-5(6)-carboxyfluorescein acetoxymethyl ester
BSA	bovine serum albumin
CaM	calmodulin
CKII	casein-kinase II
DAPI	2-(4-amidinophenyl)-1H-indole-6-carboxamidine
DOG	1,2-dioctanoyl-sn-glycerol
HEK	human embryonic kidney
hMATE	human multidrug and toxins extrusion protein
hOCT	human organic cation transporter
IL	interleukin
MDCK	Madin–Darby canine kidney
NHE1	Na$^+$/H$^+$ exchanger 1
OCs	organic cations
PBS	phosphate-buffered saline
PDGF	platelet-derived growth factor
PFA	paraformaldehyde
PI3K	phosphatidylinositol 3-kinase
PKA	protein kinase A
PKC	protein kinase C
p56^{lck}	p56^{lck} tyrosine kinase
SDS	sodium dodecyl sulfate
SEM	standard error of the mean
TBBz	4,5,6,7-tetrabromo-1H-benzimidazole
TNF	tumor necrosis factor

References

1. Koepsell, H. Polyspecific organic cation transporters: Their functions and interactions with drugs. *Trends Pharmacol. Sci.* **2004**, *25*, 375–381. [CrossRef] [PubMed]
2. Wright, S.H. Role of organic cation transporters in the renal handling of therapeutic agents and xenobiotics. *Toxicol. Appl. Pharmacol.* **2005**, *204*, 309–319. [CrossRef]
3. Wright, S.H.; Dantzler, W.H. Molecular and cellular physiology of renal organic cation and anion transport. *Physiol. Rev.* **2004**, *84*, 987–1049. [CrossRef]

4. Wagner, D.J.; Hu, T.; Wang, J. Polyspecific organic cation transporters and their impact on drug intracellular levels and pharmacodynamics. *Pharmacol. Res.* **2016**, *111*, 237–246. [CrossRef]
5. Lai, R.E.; Jay, C.E.; Sweet, D.H. Organic solute carrier 22 (SLC22) family: Potential for interactions with food, herbal/dietary supplements, endogenous compounds, and drugs. *J. Food Drug Anal.* **2018**, *26*, S45–S60. [CrossRef]
6. Motohashi, H.; Sakurai, Y.; Saito, H.; Masuda, S.; Urakami, Y.; Goto, M.; Fukatsu, A.; Ogawa, O.; Inui, K.K. Gene expression levels and immunolocalization of organic ion transporters in the human kidney. *J. Am. Soc. Nephrol.* **2002**, *13*, 866–874.
7. Koepsell, H.; Lips, K.; Volk, C. Polyspecific organic cation transporters: Structure, function, physiological roles, and biopharmaceutical implications. *Pharm. Res.* **2007**, *24*, 1227–1251. [CrossRef]
8. Otsuka, M.; Matsumoto, T.; Morimoto, R.; Arioka, S.; Omote, H.; Moriyama, Y. A human transporter protein that mediates the final excretion step for toxic organic cations. *Proc. Natl. Acad. Sci. USA* **2005**, *102*, 17923–17928. [CrossRef] [PubMed]
9. Terada, T.; Inui, K. Physiological and pharmacokinetic roles of H^+/organic cation antiporters (MATE/SLC47A). *Biochem. Pharmacol.* **2008**, *75*, 1689–1696. [CrossRef]
10. Masuda, S.; Terada, T.; Yonezawa, A.; Tanihara, Y.; Kishimoto, K.; Katsura, T.; Ogawa, O.; Inui, K. Identification and functional characterization of a new human kidney-specific H^+/organic cation antiporter, kidney-specific multidrug and toxin extrusion 2. *J. Am. Soc. Nephrol.* **2006**, *17*, 2127–2135. [CrossRef] [PubMed]
11. Komatsu, T.; Hiasa, M.; Miyaji, T.; Kanamoto, T.; Matsumoto, T.; Otsuka, M.; Moriyama, Y.; Omote, H. Characterization of the human MATE2 proton-coupled polyspecific organic cation exporter. *Int. J. Biochem. Cell Biol.* **2011**, *43*, 913–918. [CrossRef]
12. Yonezawa, A.; Inui, K. Importance of the multidrug and toxin extrusion MATE/SLC47A family to pharmacokinetics, pharmacodynamics/toxicodynamics and pharmacogenomics. *Br. J. Pharmacol.* **2011**, *164*, 1817–1825. [CrossRef] [PubMed]
13. Zhang, X.; Wright, S.H. MATE1 has an external COOH terminus, consistent with a 13-helix topology. *Am. J. Physiol Renal Physiol.* **2009**, *297*, F263–F271. [CrossRef]
14. König, J.; Zolk, O.; Singer, K.; Hoffmann, C.; Fromm, M.F. Double-transfected MDCK cells expressing human OCT1/MATE1 or OCT2/MATE1: Determinants of uptake and transcellular translocation of organic cations. *Br. J. Pharmacol.* **2011**, *163*, 546–555. [CrossRef] [PubMed]
15. Inui, K.I.; Masuda, S.; Saito, H. Cellular and molecular aspects of drug transport in the kidney. *Kidney Int.* **2000**, *58*, 944–958. [CrossRef]
16. Sato, T.; Masuda, S.; Yonezawa, A.; Tanihara, Y.; Katsura, T.; Inui, K. Transcellular transport of organic cations in double-transfected MDCK cells expressing human organic cation transporters hOCT1/hMATE1 and hOCT2/hMATE1. *Biochem. Pharmacol.* **2008**, *76*, 894–903. [CrossRef]
17. Yonezawa, A.; Inui, K. Organic cation transporter OCT/SLC22A and H^+/organic cation antiporter MATE/SLC47A are key molecules for nephrotoxicity of platinum agents. *Biochem. Pharmacol.* **2011**, *81*, 563–568. [CrossRef] [PubMed]
18. Yokoo, S.; Yonezawa, A.; Masuda, S.; Fukatsu, A.; Katsura, T.; Inui, K. Differential contribution of organic cation transporters, OCT2 and MATE1, in platinum agent-induced nephrotoxicity. *Biochem. Pharmacol.* **2007**, *74*, 477–487. [CrossRef]
19. Ciarimboli, G.; Schlatter, E. Regulation of organic cation transport. *Pflügers Arch.* **2005**, *449*, 423–441. [CrossRef]
20. Matsushima, S.; Maeda, K.; Inoue, K.; Ohta, K.Y.; Yuasa, H.; Kondo, T.; Nakayama, H.; Horita, S.; Kusuhara, H.; Sugiyama, Y. The inhibition of human multidrug and toxin extrusion 1 is involved in the drug-drug interaction caused by cimetidine. *Drug Metab. Dispos.* **2009**, *37*, 555–559. [CrossRef]
21. Massmann, V.; Edemir, B.; Schlatter, E.; Al-Monajjed, R.; Harrach, S.; Klassen, P.; Holle, S.K.; Sindic, A.; Dobrivojevic, M.; Pavenstadt, H.; et al. The organic cation transporter 3 (OCT3) as molecular target of psychotropic drugs: Transport characteristics and acute regulation of cloned murine OCT3. *Pflügers Arch.* **2014**, *466*, 517–527. [CrossRef] [PubMed]
22. Schlatter, E.; Klassen, P.; Massmann, V.; Holle, S.K.; Guckel, D.; Edemir, B.; Pavenstädt, H.; Ciarimboli, G. Mouse organic cation transporter 1 determines properties and regulation of basolateral organic cation transport in renal proximal tubules. *Pflügers Arch.* **2014**, *466*, 1581–1589. [CrossRef] [PubMed]

23. Wilde, S.; Schlatter, E.; Koepsell, H.; Edemir, B.; Reuter, S.; Pavenstädt, H.; Neugebauer, U.; Schröter, R.; Brast, S.; Ciarimboli, G. Calmodulin-associated post-translational regulation of rat organic cation transporter 2 in the kidney is gender dependent. *Cell. Mol. Life Sci.* **2009**, *66*, 1729–1740. [CrossRef] [PubMed]
24. Biermann, J.; Lang, D.; Gorboulev, V.; Koepsell, H.; Sindic, A.; Schröter, R.; Zvirbliene, A.; Pavenstädt, H.; Schlatter, E.; Ciarimboli, G. Characterization of regulatory mechanisms and states of human organic cation transporter 2. *Am. J. Physiol. Cell Physiol.* **2006**, *290*, C1521–C1531. [CrossRef]
25. Ciarimboli, G.; Koepsell, H.; Iordanova, M.; Gorboulev, V.; Dürner, B.; Lang, D.; Edemir, B.; Schröter, R.; van Le, T.; Schlatter, E. Individual PKC-phosphorylation sites in organic cation transporter 1 determine substrate selectivity and transport regulation. *J. Am. Soc. Nephrol.* **2005**, *16*, 1562–1570. [CrossRef]
26. Ciarimboli, G.; Struwe, K.; Arndt, P.; Gorboulev, V.; Koepsell, H.; Schlatter, E.; Hirsch, J.R. Regulation of the human organic cation transporter hOCT1. *J. Cell Physiol.* **2004**, *201*, 420–428. [CrossRef]
27. Cetinkaya, I.; Ciarimboli, G.; Yalcinkaya, G.; Mehrens, T.; Velic, A.; Hirsch, J.R.; Gorboulev, V.; Koepsell, H.; Schlatter, E. Regulation of human organic cation transporter hOCT2 by PKA, PI3K, and calmodulin-dependent kinases. *Am. J. Physiol. Renal Physiol.* **2003**, *284*, F293–F302. [CrossRef]
28. Willoughby, D.; Masada, N.; Crossthwaite, A.J.; Ciruela, A.; Cooper, D.M. Localized Na^+/H^+ exchanger 1 expression protects Ca^{2+}-regulated adenylyl cyclases from changes in intracellular pH. *J. Biol. Chem.* **2005**, *280*, 30864–30872. [CrossRef]
29. Dhein, S.; Salameh, A. Na^+/H^+-exchange inhibition by cariporide (Hoe 642). A new principle in cardiovascular medicin. *Cardiovasc. Drug Rev.* **1999**, *17*, 134–146. [CrossRef]
30. Berkhin, E.B.; Humphreys, M.H. Regulation of renal tubular secretion of organic compounds. *Kidney Int* **2001**, *59*, 17–30. [CrossRef]
31. Czuba, L.C.; Hillgren, K.M.; Swaan, P.W. Post-translational modifications of transporters. *Pharmacol. Ther.* **2018**, *192*, 88–99. [CrossRef]
32. Xu, D.; You, G. Loops and layers of post-translational modifications of drug transporters. *Adv. Drug Deliv. Rev.* **2017**, *116*, 37–44. [CrossRef]
33. Keller, T.; Egenberger, B.; Gorboulev, V.; Bernhard, F.; Uzelac, Z.; Gorbunov, D.; Wirth, C.; Koppatz, S.; Dotsch, V.; Hunte, C.; et al. The large extracellular loop of organic cation transporter 1 influences substrate affinity and is pivotal for oligomerization. *J. Biol. Chem.* **2011**, *286*, 37874–37886. [CrossRef]
34. Pelis, R.M.; Suhre, W.M.; Wright, S.H. Functional influence of N-glycosylation in OCT2-mediated tetraethylammonium transport. *Am. J. Physiol. Renal. Physiol.* **2006**, *290*, F1118–F1126. [CrossRef] [PubMed]
35. Pelis, R.M.; Zhang, X.; Dangprapai, Y.; Wright, S.H. Cysteine accessibility in the hydrophilic cleft of the human organic cation transporter 2. *J. Biol. Chem.* **2006**, *281*, 35272–35280. [CrossRef] [PubMed]
36. Brast, S.; Grabner, A.; Sucic, S.; Sitte, H.H.; Hermann, E.; Pavenstädt, H.; Schlatter, E.; Ciarimboli, G. The cysteines of the extracellular loop are crucial for trafficking of human organic cation transporter 2 to the plasma membrane and are involved in oligomerization. *FASEB J.* **2012**, *26*, 976–986. [CrossRef] [PubMed]
37. Nies, A.T.; Damme, K.; Kruck, S.; Schaeffeler, E.; Schwab, M. Structure and function of multidrug and toxin extrusion proteins (MATEs) and their relevance to drug therapy and personalized medicine. *Arch. Toxicol.* **2016**, *90*, 1555–1584. [CrossRef] [PubMed]
38. Schmidt-Lauber, C.; Harrach, S.; Pap, T.; Fischer, M.; Victor, M.; Heitzmann, M.; Hansen, U.; Fobker, M.; Brand, S.M.; Sindic, A.; et al. Transport mechanisms and their pathology-induced regulation govern tyrosine kinase inhibitor delivery in rheumatoid arthritis. *PLoS ONE* **2012**, *7*, e52247. [CrossRef] [PubMed]
39. Harrach, S.; Barz, V.; Pap, T.; Pavenstädt, H.; Schlatter, E.; Edemir, B.; Distler, J.; Ciarimboli, G.; Bertrand, J. Notch signaling activity determines uptake and biological effect of Imatinib in systemic sclerosis dermal fibroblasts. *J. Investig. Dermatol.* **2019**, *139*, 439–447. [CrossRef] [PubMed]
40. Oswald, S.; Muller, J.; Neugebauer, U.; Schroter, R.; Herrmann, E.; Pavenstadt, H.; Ciarimboli, G. Protein abundance of clinically relevant drug transporters in the human kidneys. *Int. J. Mol. Sci.* **2019**, *20*, 5303. [CrossRef] [PubMed]
41. Xue, Y.; Ren, J.; Gao, X.; Jin, C.; Wen, L.; Yao, X. GPS 2.0, a tool to predict kinase-specific phosphorylation sites in hierarchy. *Mol. Cell Proteomics* **2008**, *7*, 1598–1608. [CrossRef]
42. Claxton, D.P.; Jagessar, K.L.; Steed, P.R.; Stein, R.A.; Mchaourab, H.S. Sodium and proton coupling in the conformational cycle of a MATE antiporter from *Vibrio cholerae*. *Proc. Natl. Acad. Sci. USA* **2018**, *115*, E6182–E6190. [CrossRef] [PubMed]

43. Gouw, M.; Michael, S.; Samano-Sanchez, H.; Kumar, M.; Zeke, A.; Lang, B.; Bely, B.; Chemes, L.B.; Davey, N.E.; Deng, Z.; et al. The eukaryotic linear motif resource—2018 update. *Nucleic. Acids Res.* **2018**, *46*, D428–D434. [CrossRef] [PubMed]
44. Frenzel, D.; Köppen, C.; Bauer, O.B.; Karst, U.; Schröter, R.; Tzvetkov, M.V.; Ciarimboli, G. Effects of single nucleotide polymorphism Ala270Ser (rs316019) on the function and regulation of hOCT2. *Biomolecules* **2019**, *9*, 578. [CrossRef]
45. Hucke, A.; Park, G.Y.; Bauer, O.B.; Beyer, G.; Köppen, C.; Zeeh, D.; Wehe, C.A.; Sperling, M.; Schröter, R.; Kantauskaite, M.; et al. Interaction of the new monofunctional anticancer agent Phenanthriplatin with transporters for organic cations. *Front. Chem.* **2018**, *6*, 180. [CrossRef] [PubMed]
46. Dukes, J.D.; Whitley, P.; Chalmers, A.D. The MDCK variety pack: Choosing the right strain. *BMC Cell Biol.* **2011**, *12*, 43. [CrossRef]
47. Schulze, U.; Vollenbröker, B.; Braun, D.A.; Le, T.V.; Granado, D.; Kremerskothen, J.; Fränzel, B.; Klosowski, R.; Barth, J.; Fufezan, C.; et al. The Vac14-interaction network is linked to regulators of the endolysosomal and autophagic pathway. *Mol. Cell Proteomics* **2014**, *13*, 1397–1411. [CrossRef] [PubMed]
48. Wittwer, M.B.; Zur, A.A.; Khuri, N.; Kido, Y.; Kosaka, A.; Zhang, X.; Morrissey, K.M.; Sali, A.; Huang, Y.; Giacomini, K.M. Discovery of potent, selective multidrug and toxin extrusion transporter 1 (MATE1, SLC47A1) inhibitors through prescription drug profiling and computational modeling. *J. Med. Chem.* **2013**, *56*, 781–795. [CrossRef] [PubMed]
49. Bright, G.R.; Fisher, G.W.; Rogowska, J.; Taylor, D.L. Fluorescence ratio imaging microscopy: Temporal and spatial measurements of cytoplasmic pH. *J. Cell Biol.* **1987**, *104*, 1019–1033. [CrossRef]
50. Grant, R.L.; Acosta, D. Ratiometric measurement of intracellular pH of cultured cells with BCECF in a fluorescence multi-well plate reader. *In Vitro Cell Dev. Biol. Anim.* **1997**, *33*, 256–260. [CrossRef]

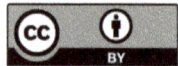

© 2020 by the authors. Licensee MDPI, Basel, Switzerland. This article is an open access article distributed under the terms and conditions of the Creative Commons Attribution (CC BY) license (http://creativecommons.org/licenses/by/4.0/).

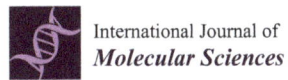

Communication

Identification of Prognostic Organic Cation and Anion Transporters in Different Cancer Entities by In Silico Analysis

Bayram Edemir

Department of Medicine, Hematology and Oncology, Martin Luther University Halle-Wittenberg, 06108 Halle (Saale), Germany; bayram.edemir@uk-halle.de; Tel.: +49-345-557-4890

Received: 5 June 2020; Accepted: 21 June 2020; Published: 24 June 2020

Abstract: The information derived from next generation sequencing technology allows the identification of deregulated genes, gene mutations, epigenetic modifications, and other genomic events that are associated with a given tumor entity. Its combination with clinical data allows the prediction of patients' survival with a specific gene expression pattern. Organic anion transporters and organic cation transporters are important proteins that transport a variety of substances across membranes. They are also able to transport drugs that are used for the treatment of cancer and could be used to improve treatment. In this study, we have made use of publicly available data to analyze if the expression of organic anion transporters or organic cation transporters have a prognostic value for a given tumor entity. The expression of most organic cation transporters is prognostic favorable. Within the organic anion transporters, the ratio between favorable and unfavorable organic anion transporters is nearly equal for most tumor entities and only in liver cancer is the number of unfavorable genes two times higher compared to favorable genes. Within the favorable genes, *UNC13B*, and *SFXN2* cover nine cancer types and in the same way, *SLC2A1*, *PLS3*, *SLC16A1*, and *SLC16A3* within the unfavorable set of genes and could serve as novel target structures.

Keywords: TCGA; human pathology atlas; gene ontology; organic cation transporter; organic anion transporter

---

1. Introduction

The organic cation and organic anion transporters belong to the superfamily of solute carrier (SLC) transporters and members are expressed in nearly all epithelia throughout the body [1]. The abbreviation of OAT, for organic anion transporter, is normally used for members of the SLC22 protein family. OAT1 for example is also known as SLC22A6 and OAT2 as SLC22A7. An overview about the nomenclature is given by Prof. Gerhard Burckhardt [2]. Members of the SLCO protein family are also called organic anion transporting polypeptides (OATP) [1]. In the same way, the abbreviation OCT, for organic cation transporter, is classically used for SLC22A1–SLC22A3 (OCT1–OCT3) [3]. Beside the SLC22A family, several other proteins are capable of the transport of organic anions and/or organic cations or are related with transport processes. Members of these protein families are expressed in nearly all epithelial cells. Physiologically, they are involved in the uptake and excretion of a broad range of substrates. For example, in liver and kidneys members of the organic anion transporter protein family are involved in the uptake of bile acid and the renal excretion of endogenous and xenobiotic compounds [2,4]. Further substrates include prostaglandins, steroid hormones, p-aminohippurate, monocarboxylates or acidic neurotransmitter metabolites, reviewed for example in [1,5,6].

Although involved in the transport of endogenous substrates, it has been shown for many members that they also transport xenobiotic-like drugs [6] and are thought to be involved in the intracellular accumulation of xenobiotic drugs [7]. Since they transport a wide range of substrates several studies have shown that members of the organic cation transporters and organic anion transporters are also capable to transport chemotherapeutics used for treatment of cancer, like platinum based chemotherapeutics, nucleoside analogs or kinase inhibitors [8]. Several studies focused on the identification of drugs that can be transported by a transport protein and its correlation to expression, treatment, and clinical outcome. It is important to know the expression pattern of members of the organic anion transporters and organic cation transporters in different tumor entities. The Cancer Genome Atlas (TCGA) provides next generation RNA-sequencing data for the most common tumor entities [9]. The data can be used to query the expression pattern of a gene of interest in different tumor samples. For many samples information also available includes clinical outcome, and the Human Pathology Atlas combined the gene expression level and generated a list of genes that are either favorable or unfavorable for clinical outcome of the patients [10]. So far, a systematic analysis of the prognostic value of organic anion transporters and organic cation transporters for the different tumor entities are missing. Here we made use of publicly available TCGA data to identify transporters that have either favorable or unfavorable prognostic value for the different tumor entities. We have also tried to identify common transporters that have a prognostic value in several tumor entities. The identified genes could serve as targets for the development of novel therapeutic drugs.

2. Results

The Human Pathology Atlas contains mRNA expression data from 17 different forms of human cancer. The expression data is derived from TCGA and correlation analyses based on mRNA expression levels in cancer tissue and the clinical outcome for patients have been performed to identify genes that are either favorable or unfavorable for overall survival of the patients. High expression of an unfavorable prognostic gene correlated with a poor patient survival outcome, and high expression of a favorable prognostic gene correlated with a longer patient survival. A prognostic gene for a given cancer was defined as a gene for which the expression level above or below the experimentally determined cutoff in an individual patient yields a significant ($p < 0.001$) difference in overall survival [10]. Figure S1 shows the number of identified genes for different tumor entities derived from the Human Pathology Atlas.

The range in total number of prognostic genes goes from 57 (testis cancer) up to 5964 in renal cancer. Interestingly, the number of unfavorable genes in liver cancer is nearly ten times higher as the number of favorable genes. Unfortunately, the lists derived from the Human Pathology Atlas do not discriminate between the different cancer subtypes, for example in renal cancer, between clear cell renal carcinoma, papillary renal cell carcinoma, and chromophobe renal cell carcinoma. We have used the list to identify genes related with organic anion transport and organic cation transport that are prognostic for patients' clinical outcome. To identify organic anion transport and organic cation transport related genes we used the Gene Ontology (GO) classification [11]. For the identification of organic cation transport, we used all genes that belong to the GO accession number GO:0015695 and for organic anion transport, all genes classified with the accession number GO:0015711. The list of genes were queried using the PANTHER classification system [12]. In total, 29 genes are classified as organic cation transport in the GO:0015695 and 453 as organic anion transport in the GO:0015711.

To get a more precise analysis we used the gene enrichment analysis to calculate if there is a positive (more than expected) or negative (less than expected) enrichment of a given GO for a given list of prognostic genes (Table 1) [12]. For the unfavorable list of genes, there is no significant enrichment of genes. However, there is a significant enrichment for favorable genes in the kidney (organic anion transport and organic cation transport), in lung and endometrial cancer (organic cation transport) and in liver cancer (organic anion transport).

Table 1. Enriched GO terms within the list of favorable genes. A significant raw p value (< 0.05) are highlighted in bold.

Tumor Entity	GO Biological Process	Fold Enrichment	Raw p-Value
Kidney	organic cation transport	2.57	**0.02**
	organic anion transport	1.58	**0.00007**
Lung	organic cation transport	9.43	**0.001**
	organic anion transport	1.06	0.8
Endometrial	organic cation transport	3.39	**0.03**
	organic anion transport	1.36	0.1
Liver	organic cation transport	2.65	0.3
	organic anion transport	3.57	**0.0000009**

The prognostic organic cation transport related genes for each tumor entity classified in the GO terms described above are shown in Table 2.

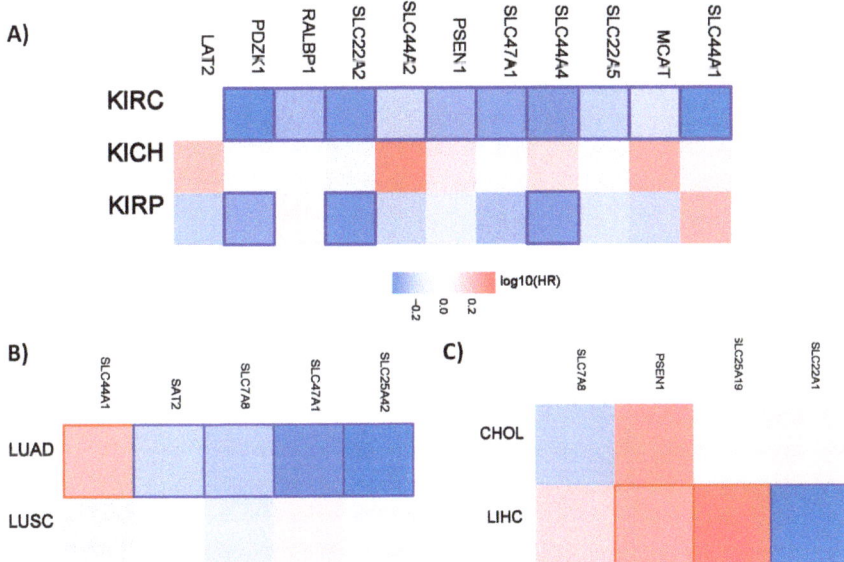

Figure 1. Hazard ratio of the organic cation transporter expression in different renal and lung cancer subtypes. The hazard ratio (HR) was calculated for (**A**) the different renal cancer (renal clear cell carcinoma (KIRC), renal papillary cell carcinoma (KIRP), and chromophobe renal cell carcinoma (KICH). (**B**) The hazard ratio for lung adenocarcinoma (LUAD) and lung squamous cell carcinoma (LUSC). (**C**) The hazard ratio for cholangiocarcinoma (CHOL) and liver hepatocellular carcinoma (LIHC). The red and blue color denote higher and lower risk, respectively. The rectangles with frames represent the statistically significant HR ($p < 0.05$).

Table 2. Prognostic organic cation transport related genes identified in different tumor entities. Genes present in two different tumor entities are highlighted in bold and genes present in three tumor entities are double underlined. Genes that are favorable for a given tumor entity but unfavorable for another tumor entity are underlined.

Tumor Entity	Unfavorable	Favorable
Breast Cancer	0	0
Cervical Cancer	SLC22A3	SLC25A42
Colorectal Cancer	0	0
Endometrial Cancer	SLC25A19	SAT2, SLC47A1, SLC22A5, MCAT
Glioma	0	0
Head and Neck Cancer	0	SLC44A4
Liver Cancer	SLC7A8, PSEN1, SLC25A19	SLC22A1
Lung Cancer	SLC44A1	SAT2, SLC7A8, SLC47A1, SLC25A42
Melanoma	0	0
Pancreatic Cancer	SLC44A2	SAT2, SLC22A5, SLC25A45, SLC25A29
Prostate cancer	0	0
Renal Cancer	LAT2	PDZK1, RALBP1, SLC22A2, SLC44A2, PSEN1, SLC47A1, SLC44A4, SLC22A5, MCAT, SLC44A1
Stomach cancer	0	MCAT
Testis cancer	LAT2	0
Thyroid cancer	0	0
Urothelial Cancer	SLC7A8, SLC22A3	SLC44A4, SLC25A29
Ovarian Cancer	0	RALBP1

The number of organic cation transport related genes with a favorable prognostic value is higher compared to unfavorable group. The expression of SAT2, SLC47A1, SLC22A5, and SLC44A4 are favorable in three different tumor entities. On the other hand, PSEN1, SLC7A8, SLC44A1, and SLC44A2 are unfavorable in some tumor entities (liver, lung, or pancreatic cancer) and in others (renal and lung cancer) they are favorable. The expression of ten organic cation transporters is favorable in renal cancer and only the expression of LAT2 is unfavorable. The Human Pathology Atlas does not discriminate between the different cancer subtypes. For example, renal cancer includes renal clear cell carcinoma (KIRC), renal papillary cell carcinoma (KIRP), and chromophobe renal cell carcinoma (KICH). We have used the GEPIA2 online tool to analyze the prognostic value of the organic cation transporters for the different tumor subtypes [13]. Figure 1 shows the results for the renal cancer and lung cancer subtypes.

Interestingly, all the favorable prognostic organic cation transporters in renal cancer are favorable for overall survival for patients with clear cell renal carcinoma. PDZK1, SLC22A2, and SLC44A4 have also a prognostic value for patients with renal papillary cell carcinoma. A similar pattern is also evident for the different lung and liver cancer subtypes. The organic cations only have a prognostic value for patients with lung adenocarcinoma but not for patients with lung squamous cell carcinoma. In the liver, the organic transporters only have a prognostic value for patients with liver hepatocellular carcinoma.

Since there are more genes classified as organic anion transporters, we used a column diagram to present the data. Figure S2 shows the number of organic anion transporters that have a prognostic value for the different tumor entities. The list with gene names is provided in the Table S1.

The number of genes more or less correlates with the total number of prognostic genes. In liver cancer the difference between favorable and unfavorable organic anion transporter organic anion transporter is smaller compared to total number.

Similar to the organic cation transporter, we have analyzed the prognostic value for the different renal, lung, and liver subtypes. Figure 2 shows the hazard ratio for organic anion transporters in the different renal cancer subtypes.

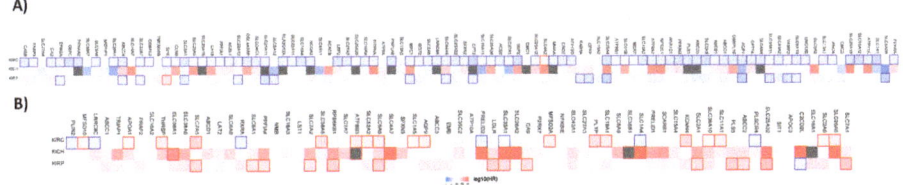

Figure 2. Hazard ratio of the organic anion transporter expression in different renal cancer subtypes. The hazard ratio (HR) was calculated for (**A**) the favorable and (**B**) unfavorable list of genes separately for renal clear cell carcinoma (KIRC), renal papillary cell carcinoma (KIRP), and chromophobe renal cell carcinoma (KICH). The red and blue colors denote higher and lower risk, respectively. The rectangle with frames represents the statistically significant HR ($p < 0.05$).

Out of the 96 favorable prognostic genes in renal cancer, 80 genes have a prognostic value for patients with clear cell renal carcinoma. Interestingly, *SLC4A2* have an unfavorable value for patients with clear cell renal carcinoma when analyzed separately. Out of the 96 genes, none has a prognostic value for patients with chromophobe renal carcinoma. In papillary renal cell carcinoma, 17 of the genes have a favorable and one gene an unfavorable prognostic value. The pattern for the unfavorable set of genes (69 in total) looks different. Only 25 have a prognostic value in clear cell renal carcinoma, while 7 of them have favorable prognostic value. In the chromophobe renal cancer cohort 10 genes and in the papillary renal cell carcinoma cohort 15 genes have a prognostic value.

A similar pattern is also evident for the liver and lung cancer subtypes. Most of the genes have prognostic value only for one cancer type (Figure 3).

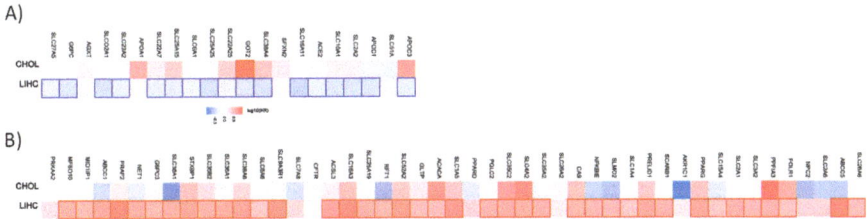

Figure 3. Hazard ratio of the organic anion transporter expression in different liver cancer subtypes. The hazard ratio (HR) was calculated for (**A**) the favorable and (**B**) unfavorable list of genes in liver cancer for cholangiocarcinoma (CHOL) and liver hepatocellular carcinoma (LIHC). The red and blue color denote higher and lower risk, respectively. The rectangles with frames represent the statistically significant HR ($p < 0.05$).

From the 21 favorable genes, 17 have a prognostic value in the liver hepatocellular carcinoma cohort. Interestingly, the expression of *GOT2* has an unfavorable prognostic value in cholangiocarcinoma. Out of the 47 genes with an unfavorable prognostic value, 39 have a prognostic impact in the liver hepatocellular carcinoma (LIHC). None has a prognostic value in the cholangiocarcinoma cohort.

For lung cancer, 5 out of 7 genes have a favorable prognostic value in the lung adenocarcinoma cohort. None are prognostic for lung squamous cell carcinoma. Within the unfavorable set of genes, 6 out of 9 have a prognostic value in the LUAD cohort and none of them in the LUSC cohort (Figure 4).

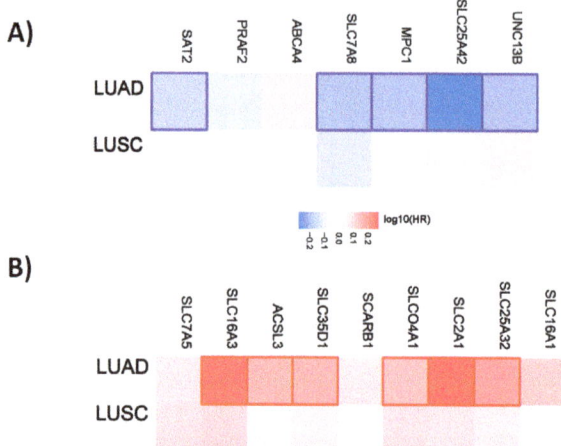

Figure 4. Hazard ratio of organic anion transporter expression in different lung cancer subtypes. The hazard ratio (HR) was calculated for (**A**) the favorable and (**B**) unfavorable list of genes in liver cancer for lung adenocarcinoma (LUAD) and lung squamous cell carcinoma (LUSC). The red and blue colors denote higher and lower risk, respectively. The rectangles with frames represent the statistically significant HR ($p < 0.05$).

In the same way as shown in Table 1, the lists of organic anion transporters were analyzed to identify a common set of genes separately for the unfavorable and favorable list of genes. Figure S3 shows the number of genes that are common between the different tumor entities.

The number of prognostic genes is the highest in renal cancer (96 genes) and at least two (breast and lung cancer) and a maximum of ten (pancreatic cancer) genes are common in renal cancer. We have also identified genes that are common in more than two tumor entities. *UNC13B* is prognostic in five and *SFXN2* in four different tumor entities as shown in Table 3. The whole common gene list is provided as Table S1.

Table 3. Top ten favorable organic anion transporters common between different tumor entities.

Gene ID	Present in
UNC13B	Renal, Lung, Head and Neck, Pancreatic, Colon
SFXN2	Renal, Urothelial, Cervical, Liver
SIT1	Head and Neck, Cervical, Endometrial, Melanoma
MMAA	Renal, Urothelial, Colon
MPC1	Renal, Lung, Cervical
PITPNA	Renal, Endometrial, Pancreatic
PLA2G2D	Cervical, Breast, Endometrial
PRAF2	Lung, Cervical, Pancreatic
SAT2	Lung, Endometrial, Pancreatic
SLC16A11	Renal, Liver, Pancreatic

While *UNC13B* and *SFXN2* are present in five and four tumor entities, respectively, only for renal cancer are both *UNC13B* and *SFXN2* favorable.

In the same way we have analyzed the lists of unfavorable organic anion transporters (Figure S4).

In renal cancer the number of prognostic genes (69) is the highest. Similar to organic cation transporters, the intersection between renal cancer and other tumor entities starts with 1 (breast) and goes up to 19 (liver) genes. One gene, *SLC2A1*, is present in five tumor entities (renal, urothelial, lung, liver and pancreatic cancer) and *PLS3*, *SLC16a1*, and *SLC16A3* are present in four tumor entities (Table 4).

Table 4. Top ten unfavorable organic anion transporters common between different tumor entities.

Gene ID	Present in
SLC2A1	Renal, Urothelial, Lung, Liver, Pancreatic
PLS3	Renal, Urothelial, Head and Neck, Pancreatic
SLC16A1	Renal, Lung, Endometrial, Pancreatic
SLC16A3	Renal, Lung, Cervical, Liver
LDLR	Kidney, Urothelial, Pancreatic
SCARB1	Kidney, Lung, Liver
SLC15A4	Kidney, Head and Neck, Liver
SLC16A2	Kidney, Urothelial, Breast
SLC25A32	Kidney, Lung, Endometrial
SLC52A2	Kidney, Cervical, Liver

With our approach we have identified organic anion transporters and organic cation transporters that are prognostic for a given tumor entity. We were also able to identify genes that are prognostic in several tumor entities. The highest numbers of genes were identified for the organic anion transporter. *UNC13B* is favorable in five and *SFXN2* in four tumor entities, implicating that these genes might have a general prognostic value. We have used the UCSC Xena platform to analyze if these genes have an prognostic value in the TCGA-PANCAN cohort with more than 12,800 samples derived from 17 different tumor entities [14]. We generated Kaplan–Meier plots and calculated overall survival probability for *SFXN2* and *UNC13B* (Figure 5).

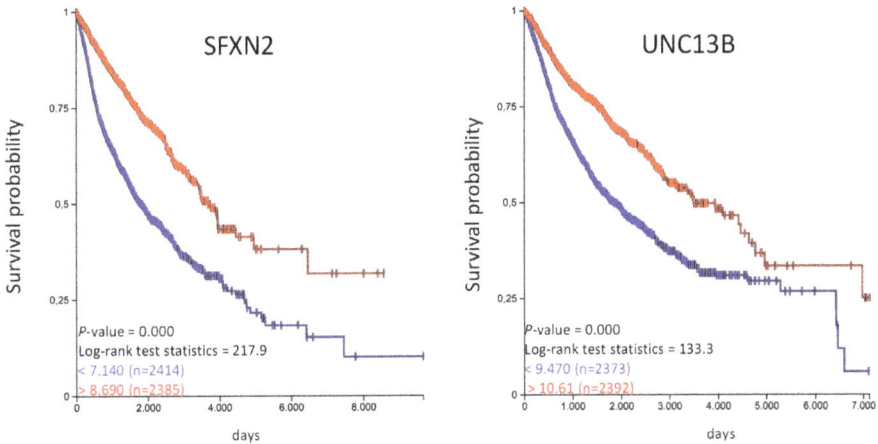

Figure 5. High *SFXN2* and *UNC13B* expression is associated with longer overall survival in the PANCAN cohort. The TCGA-PANCAN cohort was queried for *SFXN2* and *UNC13B* if they have an impact on survival probability. We filtered the data for primary tumor samples and generated Kaplan–Meier plots using the quartiles of gene expression level to separate high (red) and low (blue) expression level.

The Kaplan–Meier analysis shows that high expression of *SFX2* and *UNC13B* are associated with a significantly longer overall survival probability. In the same way we have analyzed the unfavorable genes listed in Table 4 and calculated the overall survival probability in the TCGA-PANCAN cohort (Figure 6).

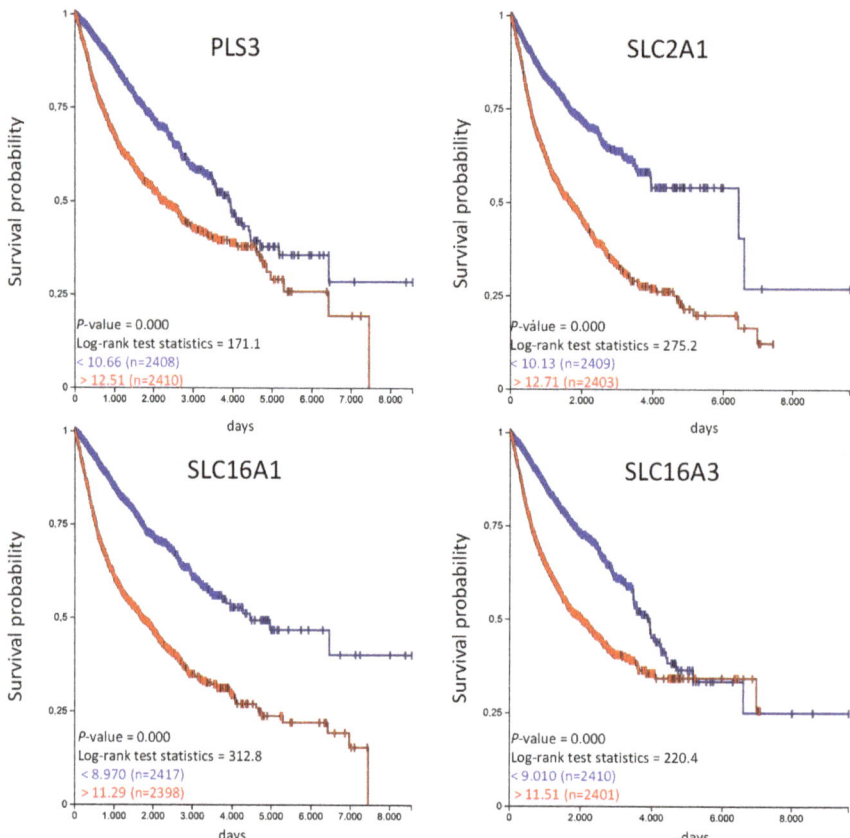

Figure 6. High *PLS3*, *SLC2A1*, *SLC16A1*, and *SLC16A3* expression is associated with shorter overall survival in the TCGA-PANCAN cohort. The TCGA-PANCAN cohort was queried for *PLS3*, *SLC2A1*, *SLC16A1*, and *SLC16A3* if they have an impact on survival probability. We filtered the data for primary tumor samples and calculated survival probability by Kaplan–Meier plots using the quartiles of gene expression level to separate high (red) and low (blue) expression.

Similar to the favorable organic anion transporter, high expression of unfavorable organic anion transporter correlates with a poor overall probability in the TCGA PANCAN cohort. Unfortunately, the TCGA data does not provide information regarding the treatment strategy (medication used, etc.) for the individual patients. We have used the available information from the PANCAN cohort and analyzed if patients in the "treatment_outcome_first_course" indicated with "complete remission/response," have a different expression of the above mentioned genes in comparison to patients qualified as "progressive disease" in the TCGA PANCAN cohort [15]. And indeed, the expression of *SFXN2* and *UNC13B* was significantly higher in patients with "complete remission/response" compared to patients with "progressive disease" (Figure S5). This was vice versa for *PLS3*, *SLC2A1* and *SLC16A1*, lower expression in patients with "complete remission/response" but higher in patients with "progressive disease". There were no significant differences for *SLC16A3* (Figure S6). This data also shows that the expression level has influence on treatment outcome.

3. Discussion

Due to next generation sequencing (NGS) data from different tumor entities deposited in TCGA together with clinical data of patients, it is possible to identify genes that correlate with patients' clinical outcome. The Human Pathology Atlas provides lists of genes where high expression is either favorable or unfavorable [10]. Highest number of prognostic genes is detected in renal cancer. One explanation could be that due to the different cell types involved in the physiological function of the kidney, a complex expression of genes is associated with each cell type [16]. Within this study we analyzed the prognostic value of organic anion and organic cation transport related genes. Regarding Gene Ontology classification, 29 genes are classified as organic cation transporters. While 7 of them have an unfavorable prognostic value, 17 have a favorable prognostic value, indicating that organic cation transporter gene expression is beneficial. Further support is given by the significant enrichment of organic cation transporter within the favorable set of genes in renal and lung cancer. No significant enrichment was observed within the unfavorable set of genes. For example, *OCT1* (*SLC22A2*) and *Mate-1* (*SLC47A1*) play important physiological roles in the proximal tubule of the kidneys [17]. Both genes are prognostic favorable in renal cancer and the high expression level might present less differentiation of the proximal tubule cells toward a tumor cell. This could be also an explanation for the prognostic value of *OCT1* (*SLC22A1*) expression in liver cancer. It is the main *OCT* in the liver and high expression could represent less differentiation toward a tumor cell.

The analysis of the different renal, liver, or lung cancer subtypes showed that the majority of the genes have a prognostic value only for one cancer subtype. In renal cancer most of the genes are prognostic in the clear cell renal carcinoma, in lung cancer in lung adenocarcinoma, and in liver cancer in liver hepatocellular carcinoma cohort.

In contrast to *OCT1* and *OCT2*, *OCT3* (*SLC22A3*) has a broad expression pattern [18] and is able to transport a variety of substances including drugs and chemotherapeutics and high expression has an unfavorable prognostic value in cervical and urothelial cancer. In contrast, for colon cancer patients' receiving 5-fluorouracil, folinic acid, and oxaliplatin as therapy, the survival probability was higher when organic cation transporter-3 expression is high [19]. This was also evident for patients with head and neck tumors receiving cisplatin [20]. In both cases, high organic cation transporter-3 expression increased transport of the chemotherapeutic drugs. In pancreatic cancer, high *OCT3* protein expression correlated with better clinical outcome of the patients [21]. *SLC25A19* is the mitochondrial thiamine pyrophosphate transporter and mice deficient for this protein are embryonic lethal [22]. Studies showing an involvement in tumor diseases are missing.

In lung and renal cancer, we observe an enrichment of organic cation transporter in the favorable set of genes. For both cancer types, high expression of *MATE1* is favorable. *MATE1* is involved in the luminal excretion of organic compounds from cells that have been, for example, imported by basolateral expressed organic cation transporters. It has been shown that *MATE1* can transport a wide variety of endogenous and exogenous substrates (reviewed in [23]). *MATE1* is also able to transport cisplatin and to a higher content, oxaliplatin [24]. This would prevent accumulation of these drugs, for example in the cells of proximal tubulus, and thereby reduce the nephrotoxic effect of these compounds. On the other hand, reduced *MATE1* would have the opposite effect [23]. It has also been shown that *MATE1* expression is associated with better uptake of the tyrosine kinase inhibitor imatinib in chronic myeloid leukemia cells [25]. In this case *MATE1* has a beneficial role by providing sufficient uptake into the cells. There are studies missing that show a specific function of *MATE1* in treatment or progression of renal and lung cancer. We can only speculate if there is only a correlation of *MATE1* expression with patients' survival or if there is a link with *MATE1* function.

Based on Gene Ontology classification more genes are classified as organic anion transporter related genes compared to organic cation transporter. But we have only an enrichment of organic anion transporter in the favorable set of genes in renal and liver cancer. Out of the classical *OATs* only *OAT2* (*SLC22A7*) has a favorable prognostic value in renal and liver cancer. These are also the main organs for *OAT2* expression [26] and similar to *OCT1* and *OCT2*, high expression of *OAT2* might represent less differentiation toward a cancer cell.

In contrast to organic cation transporter in renal cancer, some of the organic anion transport related genes are also prognostic for papillary and chromophobe renal cell cancer but the majority is prognostic for clear cell renal carcinoma. Interestingly, some of the unfavorable genes in renal cancer have a favorable prognostic value for patients with clear cell renal carcinoma. For example, high *SLC35A1* expression is favorable for clear cell renal carcinoma but unfavorable for papillary and chromophobe renal cell carcinoma. *SLC35A1* encodes for the CMP-Sia transporter and so far studies related to renal function are missing [27]. For the different lung and liver cancer subtypes, the majority of the genes are prognostic for one subtype, lung adenocarcinoma and liver hepatocellular carcinoma.

We have identified sets of genes that are prognostic in different cancer entities. For example, high expression of *UNC13B* is favorable in five and *SFXN2* in four different cancer types. Both genes together are cover nine different tumor entities. *UNC13B* also known as mammalian homologs of *Caenorhabditis elegans uncoordinated gene 13* (*MUNC13*) and it has been shown that it is involved in regulated exocytosis of vesicles [28]. *UNC13B* is not a classical organic anion transporter since it does not directly transport any substances. So far, no function has been described for *UNC13B* in cancer. *SFXN2*, or *sideroflexin 2*, is an evolutionary conserved protein that is expressed in outer mitochondrial membrane and is involved in iron homeostasis [29]. Similar to *UNC13B*, studies showing any functional correlation of *SFXN2* with cancer progression, developments, etc. are missing. Since the expression of both genes is associated with a significant better overall survival in the TCGA PANCAN cohort, further studies analyzing the cellular function of both proteins could be promising.

Within the unfavorable organic anion transporters, *SLC2A1* is present in five tumor entities. *SLC2A1*, also known as *GLUT1*, belongs to the members of glucose transporters which are involved in the transport of glucose across the cell membrane [30]. Since tumor cells have an increased metabolic rate, the expression of *SLC2A1* is often deregulated in different cancer types [31] and since they are involved in the support of tumor cells with energy, they present therapeutic targets [31].

PLS3, also known as T-plastin, is an actin binding protein and not a classical organic anion transporter [32]. High *PLS3* expression has been shown to have poor prognosis in pancreatic cancer, acute myeloid leukemia, gastric cancer, and colorectal cancer [33–36]. A direct function of PLS3 as transport protein is not known in the analyzed cancer entities.

SLC16A1, also known as MCT1 (monocarboxylate transporter 1) and SLC16A3, also known as MCT4, are involved in the proton coupled transport of lactate, pyruvate or ketone bodies and their predominant role is the transport of these substances in and out of the cell [37]. They can also act as drug transporters. MCT1 is able to transport valproic acid, nicotinic acid, nateglinide, and gamma-hydroxybutyrate across the plasma membranes [38]. They served also as targets for drugs. For example the inhibition of MCT1 activity in T cells inhibited effective immune response by reducing the rapid T cell division during activation process [39].

The unique pH characteristics in tumor cells provides development of treatments that target pH-related mechanisms to selectively kill cancer cells [40]. Cancer cells have a more alkaline pH compared to normal cells and this is even more evident in aggressive tumor cells [41,42]. This is mediated by transporters, like MCTs, that mediate proton transport out of the cells and might explain why high expression of *MCT1* and *MCT4* is associated with an unfavorable clinical outcome [42]. Targeting CD147, a MCT chaperone, by siRNA induced a decrease in *MCT1* and *MCT4* expression which was associated with reduced glycolysis, pH, and ATP production in melanoma [43]. MCT4 plays also an important role in cell migration [44] and targeting *MCT1* and *MCT4* expression has been shown to reduce the malignant potential of pancreatic cancer [45].

Similar to *UNC13B* and *SFXN2*, high expression of *SLC2A1*, *PLS3*, *SLC16A1*, and *SLC16A3* is associated with a significant reduced overall survival of the patients in the PANCAN cohort. While for *SLC2A1* this could be explained by the functional support of the tumor cells with glucose, there is no explanation if PLS3 is functionally associated with tumor progression.

Within this in silico analysis, we have tried to identify organic anion transporters and organic cation transporters that have a prognostic value for patients with different tumor types. This study however also has limitations. The Human Pathology Atlas provides data that show if the expression of a given gene is prognostic for a patient's overall survival. The expression data is obtained at the time of diagnosis/biopsy/surgery and information about the individual treatment strategy is missing. It is important to analyze why, for example, *SLC22A3* expression is unfavorable. It has been shown that *SLC22A3* is involved in the uptake of cisplatin, and in head and neck or colorectal cancer upregulated *SLC22A3* expression improved cisplatin uptake and survival of the patients [20,46]. This one example shows that beside gene expression, also the treatment regime, including the used drugs, has to be included for a better understanding why a given organic anion transporter or organic cation transporter expression is prognostic and if there might be a functional interaction of the used drugs with the transporters.

It is also important to know if the observed expression of a gene derived from TCGA is derived from the tumor cell, the surrounding stroma cells or from infiltrating tumor cells. The cytotoxic T cells are the main tumor targeting cells and checkpoint inhibitors are widely used to keep activity of T cells at a high level [47]. The expression of *MCT1* is unfavorable in different tumor entities. Specific inhibitors could be used to down regulate the function of MCT1. As described above, MCT1 function is also important for the immune response of T cells. In this case, the functional inhibition of MCT1 could also counteract the T cell against tumor cell response. Therefore, it is important to know if a given deregulated expression pattern of a gene is mediated by the tumor cell itself or is derived from infiltrating immune cells.

4. Materials and Methods

For this study we have used free publicly available databases and online analysis tools. The lists of favorable and unfavorable genes for a given tumor entity were downloaded from the Human Pathology Atlas [10]. To identify organic anion transporters and organic cation transporters within the list of genes, the Gene Ontology classification was used [11]. For organic anion transporters, all genes classified in the GO:0015711 were used and for organic cation transporters, genes classified in the GO:0015695 were used. For classification, the list of genes were analyzed with the PANTHER classification system [12]. This helped to identify genes classified as organic anion transporters and organic cation transporters. In the next step, an enrichment analysis was performed to identify if organic anion transporters or organic cation transporters are either enriched or reduced in a given tumor entity [12]. The multiple list comparator was used to identify genes that are present in multiple tumor entities (http://www.molbiotools.com/listcompare.html). Survival heat maps and hazard ratio calculation were performed using the GEPIA2 web tool [13]. Single gene survival query using the TCGA PANCAN cohort and Kaplan–Meier analysis were performed with the Xena-Browser [14].

Supplementary Materials: Supplementary materials can be found at http://www.mdpi.com/1422-0067/21/12/4491/s1. Figure S1. Number of prognostic genes identified in the different tumor entities. Figure S2. Number of prognostic organic anion transporter organic anion transporter identified in the different tumor entities. Figure S3. Intersection of prognostic organic anion transporter organic anion transporter identified in the different tumor entities. Figure S4. Intersection of prognostic unfavorable organic anion transporter organic anion transporter identified in the different tumor entities. Figure S5. Expression level of *SFXN2* and *UNC13b* in relation to treatment outcome in the TCGA PANCAN cohort. Figure S6. Expression level of PLS3, SLC2A1, SLC16A1 and SLC16A3 in relation to treatment outcome in the TCGA PANCAN cohort. Table S1. OAT Gene Names.

Author Contributions: The work was completely performed by B.E. The author has read and agreed to the published version of the manuscript

Funding: Funding was received from the DFG ED 181/9-1. We acknowledge the financial support within the funding programme Open Access Publishing by the German Research Foundation (DFG).

Conflicts of Interest: The author declares no conflict of interest.

References

1. Roth, M.; Obaidat, A.; Hagenbuch, B. OATPs, OATs and OCTs: The organic anion and cation transporters of the SLCO and SLC22A gene superfamilies. *Br. J. Pharmacol.* **2012**, *165*, 1260–1287. [CrossRef] [PubMed]
2. Burckhardt, G. Drug transport by Organic Anion Transporters (OATs). *Pharmacol. Ther.* **2012**, *136*, 106–130. [CrossRef] [PubMed]
3. Ciarimboli, G. Organic cation transporters. *Xenobiotica* **2008**, *38*, 936–971. [CrossRef] [PubMed]
4. Li, T.-T.; An, J.-X.; Xu, J.-Y.; Tuo, B.-G. Overview of organic anion transporters and organic anion transporter polypeptides and their roles in the liver. *World J. Clin. Cases* **2019**, *7*, 3915–3933. [CrossRef]
5. Koepsell, H. The SLC22 family with transporters of organic cations, anions and zwitterions. *Mol. Asp. Med.* **2013**, *34*, 413–435. [CrossRef]
6. Pelis, R.M.; Wright, S.H. Chapter Six—SLC22, SLC44, and SLC47 Transporters—Organic Anion and Cation Transporters: Molecular and Cellular Properties. In *Current Topics in Membranes*; Bevensee, M.O., Ed.; Elsevier Inc. Academic Press: Cambridge, MA, USA, 2014; Volume 73, pp. 233–261.
7. Dobson, P.D.; Kell, D.B. Carrier-mediated cellular uptake of pharmaceutical drugs: An exception or the rule? *Nat. Rev. Drug Discov.* **2008**, *7*, 205–220. [CrossRef]
8. Sprowl, J.A.; Sparreboom, A. Uptake carriers and oncology drug safety. *Drug Metab. Dispos.* **2014**, *42*, 611–622. [CrossRef]
9. Chin, L.; Hahn, W.C.; Getz, G.; Meyerson, M. Making sense of cancer genomic data. *Genes Dev.* **2011**, *25*, 534–555. [CrossRef]
10. Uhlen, M.; Zhang, C.; Lee, S.; Sjostedt, E.; Fagerberg, L.; Bidkhori, G.; Benfeitas, R.; Arif, M.; Liu, Z.; Edfors, F.; et al. A pathology atlas of the human cancer transcriptome. *Science* **2017**, *357*. [CrossRef]
11. Ashburner, M.; Ball, C.A.; Blake, J.A.; Botstein, D.; Butler, H.; Cherry, J.M.; Davis, A.P.; Dolinski, K.; Dwight, S.S.; Eppig, J.T.; et al. Gene Ontology: Tool for the unification of biology. *Nat. Genet.* **2000**, *25*, 25–29. [CrossRef]
12. Mi, H.; Muruganujan, A.; Ebert, D.; Huang, X.; Thomas, P.D. PANTHER version 14: More genomes, a new PANTHER GO-slim and improvements in enrichment analysis tools. *Nucleic Acids Res.* **2018**, *47*, D419–D426. [CrossRef] [PubMed]
13. Tang, Z.; Kang, B.; Li, C.; Chen, T.; Zhang, Z. GEPIA2: An enhanced web server for large-scale expression profiling and interactive analysis. *Nucleic Acids Res.* **2019**, *47*, W556–W560. [CrossRef]
14. Goldman, M.; Craft, B.; Hastie, M.; Repečka, K.; McDade, F.; Kamath, A.; Banerjee, A.; Luo, Y.; Rogers, D.; Brooks, A.N.; et al. The UCSC Xena platform for public and private cancer genomics data visualization and interpretation. *bioRxiv* **2019**, 326470.
15. Liu, J.; Lichtenberg, T.; Hoadley, K.A.; Poisson, L.M.; Lazar, A.J.; Cherniack, A.D.; Kovatich, A.J.; Benz, C.C.; Levine, D.A.; Lee, A.V.; et al. An Integrated TCGA Pan-Cancer Clinical Data Resource to Drive High-Quality Survival Outcome Analytics. *Cell* **2018**, *173*, 400–416.e11. [CrossRef] [PubMed]
16. Park, J.; Shrestha, R.; Qiu, C.; Kondo, A.; Huang, S.; Werth, M.; Li, M.; Barasch, J.; Susztak, K. Single-cell transcriptomics of the mouse kidney reveals potential cellular targets of kidney disease. *Science* **2018**, *360*, 758–763. [CrossRef] [PubMed]
17. Koepsell, H. Organic Cation Transporters in Health and Disease. *Pharm. Rev.* **2020**, *72*, 253–319. [CrossRef] [PubMed]
18. Chen, L.; Hong, C.; Chen, E.C.; Yee, S.W.; Xu, L.; Almof, E.U.; Wen, C.; Fujii, K.; Johns, S.J.; Stryke, D.; et al. Genetic and epigenetic regulation of the organic cation transporter 3, SLC22A3. *Pharm. J.* **2013**, *13*, 110–120. [CrossRef]
19. Lee, W.K.; Thevenod, F. Oncogenic PITX2 facilitates tumor cell drug resistance by inverse regulation of hOCT3/SLC22A3 and ABC drug transporters in colon and kidney cancers. *Cancer Lett.* **2019**, *449*, 237–251. [CrossRef]
20. Hsu, C.M.; Lin, P.M.; Chang, J.G.; Lin, H.C.; Li, S.H.; Lin, S.F.; Yang, M.Y. Upregulated SLC22A3 has a potential for improving survival of patients with head and neck squamous cell carcinoma receiving cisplatin treatment. *Oncotarget* **2017**, *8*, 74348–74358. [CrossRef]
21. Cervenkova, L.; Vycital, O.; Bruha, J.; Rosendorf, J.; Palek, R.; Liska, V.; Daum, O.; Mohelnikova-Duchonova, B.; Soucek, P. Protein expression of ABCC2 and SLC22A3 associates with prognosis of pancreatic adenocarcinoma. *Sci. Rep.* **2019**, *9*, 19782. [CrossRef]

22. Lindhurst, M.J.; Fiermonte, G.; Song, S.; Struys, E.; De Leonardis, F.; Schwartzberg, P.L.; Chen, A.; Castegna, A.; Verhoeven, N.; Mathews, C.K.; et al. Knockout of Slc25a19 causes mitochondrial thiamine pyrophosphate depletion, embryonic lethality, CNS malformations, and anemia. *Proc. Natl. Acad. Sci. USA* **2006**, *103*, 15927–15932. [CrossRef] [PubMed]
23. Nies, A.T.; Damme, K.; Kruck, S.; Schaeffeler, E.; Schwab, M. Structure and function of multidrug and toxin extrusion proteins (MATEs) and their relevance to drug therapy and personalized medicine. *Arch. Toxicol.* **2016**, *90*, 1555–1584. [CrossRef] [PubMed]
24. Yonezawa, A.; Masuda, S.; Yokoo, S.; Katsura, T.; Inui, K. Cisplatin and oxaliplatin, but not carboplatin and nedaplatin, are substrates for human organic cation transporters (SLC22A1-3 and multidrug and toxin extrusion family). *J. Pharmacol. Exp. Ther.* **2006**, *319*, 879–886. [CrossRef] [PubMed]
25. Harrach, S.; Schmidt-Lauber, C.; Pap, T.; Pavenstadt, H.; Schlatter, E.; Schmidt, E.; Berdel, W.E.; Schulze, U.; Edemir, B.; Jeromin, S.; et al. MATE1 regulates cellular uptake and sensitivity to imatinib in CML patients. *Blood Cancer J.* **2016**, *6*, e470. [CrossRef]
26. Shen, H.; Lai, Y.; Rodrigues, A.D. Organic Anion Transporter 2: An Enigmatic Human Solute Carrier. *Drug Metab. Dispos.* **2017**, *45*, 228–236. [CrossRef]
27. Hadley, B.; Litfin, T.; Day, C.J.; Haselhorst, T.; Zhou, Y.; Tiralongo, J. Nucleotide Sugar Transporter SLC35 Family Structure and Function. *Comput. Struct. Biotechnol. J.* **2019**, *17*, 1123–1134. [CrossRef]
28. Li, Y.; Wang, S.; Li, T.; Zhu, L.; Ma, C. Tomosyn guides SNARE complex formation in coordination with Munc18 and Munc13. *FEBS Lett.* **2018**, *592*, 1161–1172. [CrossRef]
29. Mon, E.E.; Wei, F.Y.; Ahmad, R.N.R.; Yamamoto, T.; Moroishi, T.; Tomizawa, K. Regulation of mitochondrial iron homeostasis by sideroflexin 2. *J. Physiol. Sci.* **2019**, *69*, 359–373. [CrossRef] [PubMed]
30. Lizak, B.; Szarka, A.; Kim, Y.; Choi, K.S.; Nemeth, C.E.; Marcolongo, P.; Benedetti, A.; Banhegyi, G.; Margittai, E. Glucose Transport and Transporters in the Endomembranes. *Int. J. Mol. Sci.* **2019**, *20*, 5898. [CrossRef]
31. Ancey, P.B.; Contat, C.; Meylan, E. Glucose transporters in cancer - from tumor cells to the tumor microenvironment. *FEBS J.* **2018**, *285*, 2926–2943. [CrossRef]
32. Delanote, V.; Vandekerckhove, J.; Gettemans, J. Plastins: Versatile modulators of actin organization in (patho)physiological cellular processes. *Acta Pharmacol. Sin.* **2005**, *26*, 769–779. [CrossRef]
33. Xin, Z.; Li, D.; Mao, F.; Du, Y.; Wang, X.; Xu, P.; Li, Z.; Qian, J.; Yao, J. PLS3 predicts poor prognosis in pancreatic cancer and promotes cancer cell proliferation via PI3K/AKT signaling. *J. Cell. Physiol.* **2020**. [CrossRef] [PubMed]
34. Velthaus, A.; Cornils, K.; Hennigs, J.K.; Grub, S.; Stamm, H.; Wicklein, D.; Bokemeyer, C.; Heuser, M.; Windhorst, S.; Fiedler, W.; et al. The Actin Binding Protein Plastin-3 Is Involved in the Pathogenesis of Acute Myeloid Leukemia. *Cancers* **2019**, *11*, 1663. [CrossRef] [PubMed]
35. Kurashige, J.; Yokobori, T.; Mima, K.; Sawada, G.; Takahashi, Y.; Ueo, H.; Takano, Y.; Matsumura, T.; Uchi, R.; Eguchi, H.; et al. Plastin3 is associated with epithelial-mesenchymal transition and poor prognosis in gastric cancer. *Oncol. Lett.* **2019**, *17*, 2393–2399. [CrossRef]
36. Yokobori, T.; Iinuma, H.; Shimamura, T.; Imoto, S.; Sugimachi, K.; Ishii, H.; Iwatsuki, M.; Ota, D.; Ohkuma, M.; Iwaya, T.; et al. Plastin3 is a novel marker for circulating tumor cells undergoing the epithelial-mesenchymal transition and is associated with colorectal cancer prognosis. *Cancer Res.* **2013**, *73*, 2059–2069. [CrossRef] [PubMed]
37. Halestrap, A.P. The SLC16 gene family—Structure, role and regulation in health and disease. *Mol. Asp. Med.* **2013**, *34*, 337–349. [CrossRef] [PubMed]
38. Halestrap, A.P.; Wilson, M.C. The monocarboxylate transporter family—Role and regulation. *IUBMB Life* **2012**, *64*, 109–119. [CrossRef]
39. Murray, C.M.; Hutchinson, R.; Bantick, J.R.; Belfield, G.P.; Benjamin, A.D.; Brazma, D.; Bundick, R.V.; Cook, I.D.; Craggs, R.I.; Edwards, S.; et al. Monocarboxylate transporter MCT1 is a target for immunosuppression. *Nat. Chem. Biol.* **2005**, *1*, 371–376. [CrossRef]
40. Parks, S.K.; Chiche, J.; Pouyssegur, J. pH control mechanisms of tumor survival and growth. *J. Cell. Physiol.* **2011**, *226*, 299–308. [CrossRef]
41. Gillies, R.J.; Raghunand, N.; Karczmar, G.S.; Bhujwalla, Z.M. MRI of the tumor microenvironment. *J. Magn. Reson. Imaging* **2002**, *16*, 430–450. [CrossRef]

42. Cardone, R.A.; Casavola, V.; Reshkin, S.J. The role of disturbed pH dynamics and the Na+/H+ exchanger in metastasis. *Nat. Rev. Cancer* **2005**, *5*, 786–795. [CrossRef] [PubMed]
43. Su, J.; Chen, X.; Kanekura, T. A CD147-targeting siRNA inhibits the proliferation, invasiveness, and VEGF production of human malignant melanoma cells by down-regulating glycolysis. *Cancer Lett.* **2009**, *273*, 140–147. [CrossRef]
44. Gallagher, S.M.; Castorino, J.J.; Philp, N.J. Interaction of monocarboxylate transporter 4 with beta1-integrin and its role in cell migration. *Am. J. Physiol. Cell Physiol.* **2009**, *296*, C414–C421. [CrossRef] [PubMed]
45. Schneiderhan, W.; Scheler, M.; Holzmann, K.H.; Marx, M.; Gschwend, J.E.; Bucholz, M.; Gress, T.M.; Seufferlein, T.; Adler, G.; Oswald, F. CD147 silencing inhibits lactate transport and reduces malignant potential of pancreatic cancer cells in in vivo and in vitro models. *Gut* **2009**, *58*, 1391–1398. [CrossRef] [PubMed]
46. Gu, J.; Dong, D.; Long, E.; Tang, S.; Feng, S.; Li, T.; Wang, L.; Jiang, X. Upregulated OCT3 has the potential to improve the survival of colorectal cancer patients treated with (m)FOLFOX6 adjuvant chemotherapy. *Int. J. Colorectal. Dis.* **2019**, *34*, 2151–2159. [CrossRef]
47. Farhood, B.; Najafi, M.; Mortezaee, K. CD8(+) cytotoxic T lymphocytes in cancer immunotherapy: A review. *J. Cell. Physiol.* **2019**, *234*, 8509–8521. [CrossRef]

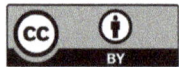

© 2020 by the author. Licensee MDPI, Basel, Switzerland. This article is an open access article distributed under the terms and conditions of the Creative Commons Attribution (CC BY) license (http://creativecommons.org/licenses/by/4.0/).

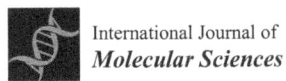

Article

Drosophila SLC22 Orthologs Related to OATs, OCTs, and OCTNs Regulate Development and Responsiveness to Oxidative Stress

Darcy C. Engelhart [1], Priti Azad [2], Suwayda Ali [2], Jeffry C. Granados [3], Gabriel G. Haddad [2] and Sanjay K. Nigam [2,4,*]

1 Department of Biology, University of California San Diego, San Diego, CA 92093, USA; dengelha@ucsd.edu
2 Department of Pediatrics, University of California San Diego, San Diego, CA 92093, USA; pazad@ucsd.edu (P.A.); saa023@ucsd.edu (S.A.); ghaddad@ucsd.edu (G.G.H.)
3 Department of Bioengineering, University of California San Diego, San Diego, CA 92093, USA; j6granad@ucsd.edu
4 Department of Medicine, University of California San Diego, San Diego, CA 92093, USA
* Correspondence: snigam@ucsd.edu

Received: 11 February 2020; Accepted: 13 March 2020; Published: 15 March 2020

Abstract: The SLC22 family of transporters is widely expressed, evolutionarily conserved, and plays a major role in regulating homeostasis by transporting small organic molecules such as metabolites, signaling molecules, and antioxidants. Analysis of transporters in fruit flies provides a simple yet orthologous platform to study the endogenous function of drug transporters in vivo. Evolutionary analysis of *Drosophila melanogaster* putative SLC22 orthologs reveals that, while many of the 25 SLC22 fruit fly orthologs do not fall within previously established SLC22 subclades, at least four members appear orthologous to mammalian SLC22 members (SLC22A16:CG6356, SLC22A15:CG7458, CG7442 and SLC22A18:CG3168). We functionally evaluated the role of SLC22 transporters in *Drosophila melanogaster* by knocking down 14 of these genes. Three putative SLC22 ortholog knockdowns—*CG3168*, *CG6356*, and *CG7442/SLC22A*—did not undergo eclosion and were lethal at the pupa stage, indicating the developmental importance of these genes. Additionally, knocking down four SLC22 members increased resistance to oxidative stress via paraquat testing (*CG4630*: $p < 0.05$, *CG6006*: $p < 0.05$, *CG6126*: $p < 0.01$ and *CG16727*: $p < 0.05$). Consistent with recent evidence that SLC22 is central to a Remote Sensing and Signaling Network (RSSN) involved in signaling and metabolism, these phenotypes support a key role for SLC22 in handling reactive oxygen species.

Keywords: solute carrier 22 (SLC22); Remote Sensing and Signaling Theory; interorgan communication; organic anion transporter; organic cation transporter; SLC22A15; SLC22A16; SLC22A18; kidney; Malpighian tubule

1. Introduction

SLC (solute carrier) proteins are the second largest family of membrane proteins in the human genome after G protein-coupled receptors (GPCRs) and are relatively understudied given how much of the genome they represent. SLC22 has been identified as a central hub of coexpression with almost every other SLC family and appears to be one of the major hubs of coexpression amongst SLCs, ATP-binding cassette proteins (ABCs), and drug-metabolizing enzymes (DMEs) as well as the predominant hub for coexpression with phase I and phase II DMEs [1,2]. This central position within coexpression analyses of healthy, non-drug-treated tissues highlights the crucial role that these transporters likely play in endogenous physiology, as proposed in the Remote Sensing and Signaling Theory [3]. The Remote Sensing and Signaling Theory proposes that transporters and enzymes expressed in several organs function together to maintain homeostasis via inter-organ and intra-organ communication through movement of small molecules. To better understand the systemic functionality of the SLC22 family using a highly conserved but simpler model organism than mice, we chose to disrupt this central metabolic hub in *Drosophila*. Our observation of both developmental and oxidative stress phenotypes further underscores the importance of these transporters as developmental regulators and mediators of exogenous stressors.

We utilized *Drosophila melanogaster* as a model system to gain insight into the potential physiological reasons for evolutionary conservation of SLC22 and to investigate their role in mediation of oxidative stress. Evolutionary studies suggest that, in addition to animals, the SLC22 family is conserved in members of the fungi kingdom, such as the unicellular eukaryote *S. cerevisiae*, as well as *A. thaliana* of the plant kingdom. However, these species lack physiologically "parallel" systems that could provide insight into the function of human SLC22 transporters [4]. Due to the similarities between *Drosophila melanogaster* physiology and human systems, such as shared functions of the *Drosophila* hindgut and Malpighian tubules and the human intestines and kidneys, the fruit fly serves as a valuable model for human renal and intestinal disease states. Approximately 65% of human disease-associated genes have putative orthologs in *Drosophila* and within functional regions, these fly genes can share up to 90% amino acid or DNA sequence identity with their human orthologs [5]. With identification of 25 SLC22 proteins in the *Drosophila* genome and the availability of reliable RNAi lines for many of these genes from the Bloomington Drosophila Stock Center (BDSC), the fruit fly provides a feasible platform for our overall developmental and physiological inquiry [5–7].

Although there are no established SLC22 orthologs between fly and human, there is evidence that some SLC22 fly genes share substrates and possibly functionality with human SLC22 members. Two of these genes, *CarT*/carcinine transporter (*CG9317*) and *BalaT*/β-alanine transporter (*CG3790*), play major roles in histamine recycling. In *Drosophila* photoreceptor neurons, *CarT* mediates the uptake of carcinine, an inactive metabolite that results from the conjugation of β-alanine and histamine [8]. Carcinine has been detected in mammalian tissues such as the human intestine and is transported by human OCT2 (SLC22A2) in both in vitro and in vivo studies [8,9]. *BalaT* mediates the recycling of β-alanine, which is necessary for histamine homeostasis in *Drosophila* photoreceptor synapses [10]. In addition to the imperative role of histamine in *Drosophila* neurotransmission, histamine and histamine receptors (HRs) have broad physiological and regulatory functionality in both the cardiovascular and central nervous systems. OCT2 and OCT3 (SLC22A3) which share high homology with CarT and BalaT, are expressed in higher order species, such as mice and humans [8,10–13]. This relationship is supported by shared substrate specificity for monoamines, such as carcinine and other neurotransmitters, as well as similar neuronal expression patterns of fly and human genes [9,14,15]. Despite *CarT* knockdowns in flies resulting in blindness and complete loss of photoreceptor transmission and *BalaT* knockdowns in flies severely disrupting vision and inhibiting photoreceptor synaptic transmission, both *Oct2* and *Oct3* knockout mice show no phenotypic abnormalities [8,10,16,17]. To better utilize *Drosophila* as a model of human SLC22 proteins and direct future studies, a homology-based analysis was performed with all fruit fly putative SLC22 orthologs in the frame of well-established SLC22 members from human, mouse, and other common model organisms. This analysis found at least 10 of the putative fruit fly orthologs within the previously defined SLC22 subclades [18]. Four of these fly genes share common ancestry with single SLC22 members which is characteristic of a direct, functional ortholog.

SLC22 members in mice, such as OAT1 (SLC22A6), OCT1 (SLC22A1), and OAT2 (SLC22A7), are transiently expressed throughout development in tissues that show minimal or no expression in adulthood [19]. *Oct1-3* (*Slc22a1-3*), *Octn1* (*Slc22a4*), *Oat1*, *Oat3* and *Rst* (*Slc22a12*) knockout (KO) mice are fertile, viable and show no general phenotypic abnormalities except for the *Oat3* KO's decreased blood pressure, serum metabolite changes, and the *Octn1* KO's increased susceptibility to intestinal inflammation [6,16,17,20–25]. The only SLC22 knockout mouse line with a reported clear developmental phenotype is the *Octn2* (*Slc22a5*) KO [24]. OCTN2 (SLC22A5) is the main transporter of carnitine in the bodies of both humans and mice and mutations in this gene are associated with systemic carnitine deficiency [26,27]. The *Octn2* KO line is also referred to as the JVS (juvenile visceral steatosis) line because of the defects in fatty acid oxidation due to carnitine deficiency that results in the abnormal accumulation of lipids. Without carnitine supplementation, *Octn2* KO mice develop dilated cardiomyopathy, fatty livers and steatosis of other organs, and expire in 3–4 weeks [24]. Although *Oat* KO's (including *Slc22a12*) and *Oct* KO's have abnormal levels of metabolites and signaling molecules, with only one clear developmental phenotype observed thus far in mice, determining the functional importance of these genes in *Drosophila* could provide insight for orthologous developmental roles in mice and humans given their interesting developmental expression patterns [19,28–31]. As an initial developmental screen, we created ubiquitous RNAi knockdowns driven by a ubiquitous *da-GAL4* driver of 14 of the putative SLC22 orthologs and observed their development. A ubiquitous driver was chosen due to the diverse expression patterns of human SLC22 members [32]. Fruit flies have distinct, easily observable developmental stages of which the egg and pupa stage are the most sensitive to environmental stressors and RNAi knockdowns [33,34]. We show that, of the 14 RNAi knockdowns, three are lethal at the pupa stage, for the first time implicating *Slc22a15*, *Slc22a16*, and *Slc22a18* genes in development. 14 out of the 24 putative SLC22 orthologs were readily available from BDSC.

Paraquat (PQ) resistance tests were performed on ubiquitously expressing knock-down SLC22 lines that progressed to the adult stage. Paraquat is an herbicide and neurotoxicant that is known to cause Parkinson's disease [35]. Low levels of this herbicide can induce redox cycling that yields high levels of reactive oxygen species (ROS), causing systemic oxidative stress [36]. Because of this, it is used as a tool for investigation of acquired resistance to oxidative stress in *Drosophila melanogaster* [37]. As a major contributor to the pathogenesis of a multitude of human diseases, such as cardiovascular disease, metabolic syndrome, neurological disorders, and general cell and tissue degradation associated with aging, oxidative stress, and the mechanisms with which we manage free radicals, are of extreme interest [38]. Ubiquitous RNAi knockdowns of at least some SLC22 members might be predicted to affect resistance to oxidative stress because many SLC22 members transport or affect serum levels of antioxidants. Some examples observed in both mice and humans are OCTN1 (SLC22A4) and ergothioneine (EGT), URAT1 (SLC22A12) and uric acid, and OAT1/OAT3 and uric acid, dietary flavonoids, as well as TCA (tricarboxylic acid) intermediates such as the oxoacid, α-ketoglutarate [6,22,39,40]. Additionally, carcinine, the characteristic substrate of the fly SLC22 member, CarT, is transported by hOCT2 and has antioxidant properties [41]. Strikingly, our studies revealed that ubiquitous RNAi knockdown of four SLC22 genes resulted in significantly increased oxidative stress resistance at one or more time points.

2. Results

2.1. Drosophila Melanogaster SLC22 Phylogenetic and Genomic Analysis

As in mammalian genomes, fly SLC22 genes exist in clusters. The majority of SLC22 genes in *Drosophila* are found on chromosome 3R with many members found in tandem with other putative SLC22 orthologs. One notably large cluster consists of 6 SLC22 genes (*CG7333*, *CG7342*, *CG17751*, *CG17752*, *CG16727*, and *CG6231*) (Table 1). Inclusion of *D. melanogaster* orthologous genes in a homology-based analysis of all SLC22 members across a multitude of species (Table 2; Figure 1) resulted in the observation of at least four members that appear orthologous to mammalian SLC22 members (CG6356: Slc22a16, CG7458, SLC22A/CG7442:Slc22a15 and CG3168:Slc22a18) and an additional six members that can be preliminarily assigned to the individual subclades. The subclades of SLC22 are based on phylogenetic relatedness and functional characterization. They exist within two major clades—OAT and OCT. Although recently revised [42] the original definitions still stand here: Oat, Oat-like, Oat-related, Oct, Octn, and Oct/Octn-related [17]. When a GUIDANCE 2.0 alignment was performed and all sequences with a GUIDANCE score of <0.6 were removed, the only topology change observed was the omission of all SLC22A18 sequences and the reassignment of CG3168 to the large fly SLC22 transporter group, indicating that it may have sequence homology with SLC22A18, but not the other members of the

Oat-related subclade. Interestingly, *CG3168* is the only putative SLC22 ortholog that is localized to the X chromosome in flies. CG6006 and CG8654 fall within the Oat-related subclade and CG6126, CG8654, Orct/CG6331, and Orct2/CG13610 appear to be part of the Oct subclade. The remaining 15 orthologs form their own group outside of the SLC22 subclades and are considered to be mostly organic cation transporters [5,18]. In summary, in flies, SLC22 appears to have at least some orthologous genes that, based off of sequence analysis, may prove to be useful models for their relatively understudied human counterparts.

Table 1. Overview of SLC22 in *Drosophila melanogaster*. The following table describes all known and putative orthologs of SLC22 in *D. melanogaster*. Genes are ordered by chromosomal location and those which appear in tandem are bolded. Tissue expression was collected from FlyAtlas [15].

Gene ID	Genomic Loci	Expression Patterns Tissue/Sexual Dimorphism	Phenotypic Data Physiological Role	Substrates
CG3168	X: 6,720,004–6,739,986	CNS, glial specific, ubiquitously expressed in other tissues		
CarT/CG9317	2L: 20,727,151–20,730,282	head, brain, eye, salivary gland	histamine recycling in photoreceptor neurons	carcinine, neurotransmitters
BalaT/CG3790	2R: 12,872,787–2,875,012	head, brain, eye, midgut	histamine recycling in photoreceptor neurons	Beta-alanine
CG4630	2R: 13,215,659–13,219,247	ubiquitously expressed, except for ovary and testis		
CG8654	2R: 19,979,242–19,984,895	ubiquitously expressed, except for larval and adult midgut and ovaries		
CG5592	3L: 5,897,638–5,899,395	Testis, males only		
CG10486	3L: 5,904,211–5,906,699	testis		
CG42269	3L: 6,066,296–6,071,545	head, hindgut		
CG7458	3L: 21,955,110–21,958,041	ubiquitously expressed, lower expression in larval CNS and adult brain		
SLC22A/CG7442	3L: 21,934,704–21,938,636	ubiquitously expressed, except for ovary and testis	memory suppressor gene	MPP, Choline, Acetylcholine, Dopamine, Histamine, Serotonin, TEA, Betaine, L-carnitine
CG14855	3R: 14,796,305–14,798,474	CNS, brain		
CG14856	3R: 14,798,986–14,801,163	hindgut, midgut, heart, higher expression in larva		
CG6006	3R: 16,154,982–16,171,766	head, brain, eye, hindgut		
CG8925	3R: 16,171,991–16,180,475	head, eye, salivary gland, midgut, hindgut		
CG6126	3R: 16,198,000–16,203,083	ubiquitously expressed, except for testis		
CG7333	3R: 19,600,635–19,602,629	testis		
CG7342	3R: 19,603,375–19,606,475	CNS, midgut, Malpighian tubule, hindgut, testis		
CG17751	3R: 19,607,254–19,609,322	Malpighian tubule, heart		
CG17752	3R: 19,607,254–19,609,322	Malpighian tubule		
CG16727	3R: 19,613,381–19,615,784	Malpighian tubule, testis		
CG6231	3R: 19,616,024–19,632,718	Ubiquitously expressed, lower expression in adult midgut		
CG7084	3R: 22,298,805–22,304,420	CNS, midgut, Malpighian tubule, hindgut		
Orct2/CG13610	3R: 24,273,029–24,275,728	ubiquitously expressed, except for Malpighian tubules		
Orct/CG6331	3R: 24,276,260–24,278,792	ubiquitously expressed, lower expression in ovaries		
CG6356	3R: 24,283,955–24,288,617	CNS, testis	putative A16 ortholog/carnitine transporter	

Table 2. Sequence alignment and functional analysis of SLC22 in *Drosophila Melanogaster*. ✓ addresses column title.

Gene ID	Phylogenetic Relationship		RNAi BDSC Stock ID	Tested	Phenotypes	
	Subgroup/Subclade	Transporter			Pupa Stage Arrest	PQR
CG3168	Oat-related	A18	29301	✓	✓	
CarT/CG9317	neither Oct or Oat Major Clade					
BalaT/CG3790	neither Oct or Oat Major Clade		67274	✓		
CG4630	neither Oct or Oat Major Clade		61249	✓		✓
CG8654	Oct subclade		57428	✓		
CG5592	neither Oct or Oat Major Clade					
CG10486	neither Oct or Oat Major Clade					
CG42269	neither Oct or Oat Major Clade					
CG7458	Octn-related	A15				
SLC22A/CG7442	Octn-related	A15	35817	✓	✓[43] confirmed in this study	
CG14855	neither Oct or Oat Major Clade					
CG14856	neither Oct or Oat Major Clade					
CG6006	Oat related, A16 *		55282	✓		✓
CG8925	Oat related, A16 *					
CG6126	Oct subclade		56038	✓		✓
CG7333	neither Oct or Oat Major Clade		57433	✓		
CG7342	neither Oct or Oat Major Clade					
CG17751	neither Oct or Oat Major Clade					
CG17752	neither Oct or Oat Major Clade					
CG16727	neither Oct or Oat Major Clade		57434	✓		✓
CG6231	neither Oct or Oat Major Clade		63013	✓		
CG7084	neither Oct or Oat Major Clade		42767	✓		
Orct2/CG13610	Oct subclade		57583	✓		
Orct/CG6331	Oct subclade		60125	✓		
CG6356	Octn	A16	28745	✓	✓	

Our analysis consists of a phylogenetic analysis (performed with both ClustalOmega and MAFFT alignments), observational developmental phenotypes as well as Paraquat sensitivity testing, both denoted by a check mark. Each cross that arrested at the pupa stage was repeated on three separate occasions. Paraquat tests were performed on the F1 generation of a cross between SLC22 RNAi knock-down lines (obtained from BDSC) and *da-GAL4* driver parent lines. Percent survival of F1 flies was compared to both parent lines as controls. Each test consisted of 3 replicates of 10 male flies per line. * indicates a topology seen with ClustalOmega alignment only. Genes are ordered by chromosomal location and those which appear in tandem are bolded. PQR: positive paraquat resistance phenotype.

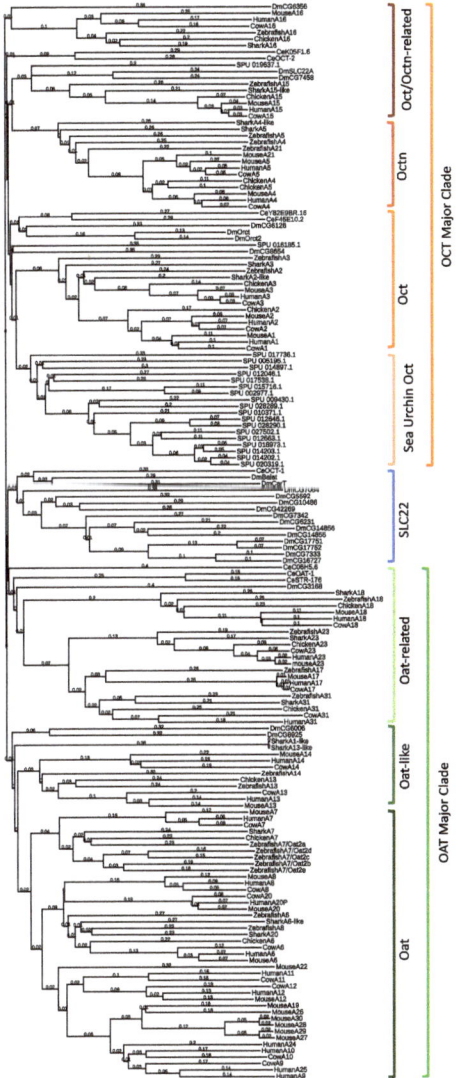

Figure 1. Guide tree of the SLC22 Transporter Family Using 167 Sequences. Sequences from human, mouse, cow, chicken, shark, zebrafish, sea urchin (SPU), *C. elegans* (Ce), and fruit fly (Dm) were aligned and tree was generated using Clustal Omega (using default parameters). The tree was viewed using Interactive Tree of Life (iTOL). Branch length values are calculated via the Kimura method [44]. Large sea urchin expansion within the Oct Major clade is labeled "Sea Urchin Oct". Sequences that fall between the Oat Major Clade (green) and Oct Major Clade (orange) are denoted as SLC22 (blue).

2.2. Developmental Phenotypes of D. melanogaster SLC22 Knockdowns

One of the many advantages of using *Drosophila melanogaster* as a model organism is its distinct, easily visualized developmental stages. Additionally, RNAi knockdowns of any gene in *Drosophila* show pupal lethality at a rate of about 15% [34]. These developmental observations provide valuable information regarding the developmental function of orthologous genes that may have compensatory mechanisms in higher-order species. Three SLC22 ubiquitous knockdowns (*CG7442/SLC22A*, *CG3168*, and *CG6356*) proved to be lethal at the pupa stage when crossed with the ubiquitous *da-GAL4* driver line. Crosses were repeated three times to confirm phenotypes. CG6356 appears to be a direct ortholog of SLC22A16, a carnitine transporter related to OCTNs. In addition, *CG3168*, which also arrests at the pupa stage is a putative ortholog of the poorly understood SLC22 member, SLC22A18. To our knowledge, the murine knockouts of these genes have not been reported.

2.3. PQ Resistance Test of D. melanogaster SLC22 Knockdowns

Paraquat testing is commonly used in *Drosophila* to determine oxidative stress resistance in which increased survival is correlated to increased resistance to oxidative stress [36,37]. Previous studies have established reliable dose-response curves for paraquat testing in *D. melanogaster* [45]. SLC22 transport proteins in the proximal tubule cells of the kidney take small molecules, such as the antioxidants and SLC22 characteristic substrates uric acid and ergothioneine, into cells to be later excreted [39,40,46,47]. By blocking this route of excretion, levels of these small molecules, such as antioxidants (including dietary flavonoids), are expected to increase in the *Drosophila* hemolymph and increased hemolymph levels of antioxidants would confer resistance to oxidative stress. Through paraquat testing, we show that knocking down SLC22 members in *Drosophila* significantly increases resistance to oxidative stress at different time points in at least four knock-down lines (CG4630: $p < 0.05$, CG6006: $p < 0.05$, CG6126: $p < 0.01$ and *CG16727*: $p < 0.05$) when compared to parent and *da-GAL4* control lines (Figure 2, Figure S1–S4). The most apparent oxidative stress resistant phenotype is observed for the knock-down of *CG6126*, showing statistically significant increased survival at 36-, 48- and 60-h time points with 100% survival of the RNAi knockdown flies for all three time points – and an average of about 40% at 36 h, 20% at 48 h, and 10% at 60 h for the parent lines which were used as a control ($p < 0.01$). In mice, it is known that SLC22 transporters like OAT1, OAT3, RST, and OCTN1 directly regulate key antioxidants such as uric acid, EGT, flavonoids, and TCA intermediates [6,25,48]. Whether or not these fly transporters directly or indirectly regulate redox states will be explored in future studies.

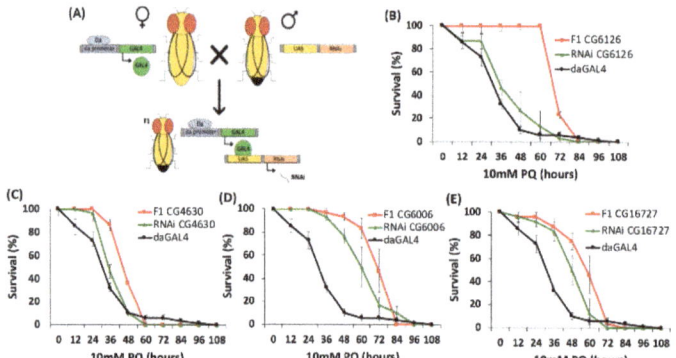

Figure 2. Four RNAi knockdown lines show resistance to oxidative stress. All tested lines were observed for 108 h. For each line, there is at least one time point in which the RNAi knockdown flies survived at statistically significant higher rates than both parent lines. Further information regarding statistical significance can be found in Supplementary Figures S1–S4. (**A**) Schematic of GAL4/UAS system used to generate RNAi knockdown lines. (**B**) Survival of *CG6126* knockdowns compared to parent lines (**C**) Survival of *CG4630* knockdowns compared to parent lines. (**D**) Survival of *CG6006* knockdowns compared to parent lines. (**E**) Survival of *CG16727* knockdowns compared to parent lines.

3. Discussion

Out of the seven transporters chosen by the International Transporter Consortium and the FDA for evaluation during drug development, three (OAT1, OAT3, and OCT2) are members of the SLC22 family [49]. 17 SLC22 members are also identified as drug transporters by the VARIDT database [50]. In addition to their pharmacological importance, many of these transporters transport metabolites that play a role in the response to endogenous stressors such as oxidative stress induced by reactive oxygen species. Using *Drosophila melanogaster* as a model organism, we sought to better understand the role of SLC22 in response to oxidative stress and development. Due to the lack of information regarding SLC22 fruit fly orthologs, we attempted to characterize and classify them utilizing multiple sequence alignments and RNAi knockdowns. Because there are minimal developmental phenotypes (apart from *Octn2*) for single *SLC22* knockouts in mice despite developmentally interesting and highly dynamic expression patterns, developmental phenotypes observed in *Drosophila* could help further our understanding of how SLC22 contributes to development in other organisms as well [19,28–31]. Prior to our analysis, only three (BalaT, CarT and SLC22A) out of the 25 fruit fly SLC22 orthologs were functionally investigated beyond global tissue expression screens and homology studies [5,10,15,43,51,52].

Alignment of fly orthologs with the SLC22 family shows at least ten members that fall within the established Oct, Octn, Oct/Octn-related, or Oat-related subclades. There appear to be four putative orthologs to individual SLC22 members, three of which proved to be lethal in ubiquitous RNAi knockdowns. The *Drosophila* protein CG6356 shares distinct homology with SLC22A16 and RNAi knockdown of this gene resulted in arrest at the pupa stage. Based on what is known about SLC22A16 transport function and its membership in the Oct/Octn-related subclade, it is possible that this arrest is due to a systemic imbalance of both carnitine and choline. Previous *Drosophila* developmental studies have found that proper levels of either carnitine or choline are necessary for flies to reach eclosion [53]. Although SLC22A16 (FLIPT2/OCT6/CT2) has not yet been evaluated for the ability to transport choline, it is an established carnitine transporter [54]. SLC22A16 is homologous to two carnitine transporters of the SLC22 family, OCTN1 and OCTN2, which have been shown to transport acetylcholine and choline, respectively, in addition to acetylcarnitine and carnitine [55–58].

We observed that ubiquitous knockdown of *SLC22A/CG7442* caused arrest at the pupa stage, confirming observations made in previous studies [43]. The fly protein SLC22A/CG7442, which shares homology with human SLC22A15, has been confirmed as a transporter of characteristic OCT and OCTN metabolites MPP+, dopamine, serotonin, carnitine, TEA, choline, and acetylcholine [43]. The fly protein CG7458 also groups with SLC22A15 but lacks any phenotypic data to infer function. With further analysis, these associations could provide a basis for investigation of the endogenous function of the orphan transporter SLC22A15. Developmental tissue expression studies show transiently high expression of SLC22A15 in vital organs such as the heart, liver, and kidneys [59]. This transporter is also known to be highly expressed in white blood cells in humans, which are present at the highest concentration at birth and decrease to normal, adult levels by two years of age [55]. In combination with the observed *SLC22A/CG7442* developmental phenotype, it appears likely that putative CG7442 orthologs (such as SLC22A15) in other species may play a developmental role.

CG3168 groups with the Oat-related subclade, appearing to share direct ancestry with the orphan transporter, SLC22A18. Previous studies have observed high levels of CG3168 expression in glial cells during embryogenesis [60]. SLC22A18 has been shown to be expressed in low levels in the adult brain in the Human Protein Atlas, GTEx, and FANTOM5 RNA-seq studies [59]. It also has low expression levels in the human fetal brain [61]. Between the adult and fetal brain, there is a pattern of consistent expression of SLC22A18 in the cerebral cortex. The cerebral cortex consists of ~75% glial cells which could represent partly orthologous expression patterns between CG3168 and Slc22a18 in different species. Further investigation of CG3168 and its relationship to the orphan SLC22 member, SLC22A18, could build an understanding of how both of these genes are implicated in development.

In addition to phylogenetic and developmental functional screens, RNAi knockdown fly lines that progressed to adulthood were examined for resistance to oxidative stress via paraquat resistance testing. Four knock-down lines (*CG4630*: $p < 0.05$, *CG6006*: $p < 0.05$, *CG6126*: $p < 0.01$ and *CG16727*: $p < 0.05$) showed significantly greater resistance to oxidative stress. CG16727 has no phenotypic or phylogenetic associations other than increased paraquat survival for crosses with two separate *da-GAL4* driver lines. However, it is specifically expressed in the Malpighian tubules, which are often considered somewhat analogous to the mammalian kidneys, where excretion of the antioxidant-acting oxoacids of the TCA cycle, uric acid, and flavonoids normally occurs via OATs [15,62–64]. TCA intermediates pyruvate, oxaloacetate, and α-ketoglutarate are known to mediate oxidative stress responses, due to direct interaction of their α-ketoacid structure with reactive oxygen species such as H_2O_2 [48,65,66]. Due to the conservation of metabolites between *Drosophila* and humans, we raise the possibility that RNAi knockdowns of potential OAT orthologs would be more resistant to PQ due to increased systemic levels of metabolites with antioxidant properties. The removal of the excretory route for these metabolites would result in increased serum levels, which would protect against oxidative stress. Further, investigation of a Malpighian tubule-specific knockdown of this gene would be necessary to assess this phenotype and hypothetical functionality. *CG4630*, *CG6006* and *CG6126* knockdowns showed similar oxidative stress resistant phenotypes when crossed with one *da-GAL4* driver line. All three of these transporters are expressed within the *Drosophila* excretory system but have a wider range of tissue expression than CG16727. Resistance to oxidative stress exhibited by these RNAi knockdown lines must be further examined by hemolymph analysis for classical SLC22 antioxidants such as urate, EGT, and the oxoacids of the TCA. Oxidative stress resistance is of particular interest in the search for SLC22 organic anion transporters in fruit flies. Our homology-based analyses show no unambiguous OAT orthologs in fruit flies. However, it is possible that some SLC22 fly genes transport organic anions but do not share enough sequence similarity for multiple sequence alignment programs to determine their functions.

Although some SLC22 RNAi knockdown lines may not show a significant phenotype, it has been shown that knocking down specific organic anion transporters in *D. melanogaster* can affect the expression patterns of other transporters with similar functionality, indicating a mechanism of sensing and signaling tied to organic anion, cation, and zwitterion transporters (OATs, OCTs, and OCTNs) [67,68]. Changes of expression levels of functionally similar transporters could provide further support for the Remote Sensing and Signaling Theory, in which drug-related proteins (e.g., drug transporters and drug metabolizing enzymes) and signaling molecules mediate inter-organ communication to maintain physiological balance [69,70]. For mammalian organs, a transporter and DME gene remote sensing and signaling network (RSSN) has recently been proposed [47].

Our findings show that the fruit fly is a useful model system to investigate understudied transporters, specifically SLC22A15, SLC22A16, and SLC22A18, as well as to gain functional insight into the SLC22 gene family as a whole. Additionally, confirmation of apparently strong phylogenetic relationships could result in viable models to better understand the functionality and developmental role of SLC22A16 and SLC22A18 through CG6356 and CG3168, respectively. While further study is necessary to understand the mechanism of oxidative stress resistance in certain RNAi knockdown lines, it will also be interesting to determine if there are increased levels of antioxidants in these lines and what those antioxidants might be. Given the substantial genetic and physiological conservation between mammals and *Drosophila*, these findings may support, in certain contexts, the use of fruit flies as a pre-clinical model organism for select SLC22 transporters, for instance, in elucidating their role in handling oxidative stress.

4. Materials and Methods

4.1. Data Collection

SLC22 human and mouse sequences were collected manually from the NCBI protein database. Sea Urchin and *C. elegans* sequences were collected manually from EchinoBase (http://www.echinobase.org/Echinobase/) and WormBase (https://www.wormbase.org/#012-34-5), respectively [71,72]. Sequences were confirmed using the UCSC genome browser by searching within each available species on the online platform (https://genome.ucsc.edu/cgi-bin/hgGateway) [73]. The NCBI BLASTp web-based program was used to find sequences similar to those that were searched for manually [74]. BLASTp was run with default parameters using query SLC22 sequences from human or mouse. The database chosen was non-redundant protein sequence (nr), and no organisms were excluded. SLC22 fruit fly orthologs were determined from FlyBase (http://flybase.org/reports/FBgg0000667.html), and sequences were collected manually from the NCBI protein database [75]. Genomic locations of all transporters in question for fruit fly were determined from FlyBase. Drosophila tissue expression data was collected from FlyAtlas (http://flyatlas.org/atlas.cgi) [15].

4.2. Phylogenetic Analysis

Sequences for SLC22 were aligned using Clustal-Omega (Clustal-W) and MAFFT (Multiple alignment using fast Fourier transform) with default parameters via the online platform provided by the European Bioinformatics Institute (EMBL-EBI) (https://www.ebi.ac.uk/Tools/msa/clustalo/) [76–78]. Clustal-W and MAFFT produced similar topologies. These alignments were then visualized using The Interactive Tree of Life (http://itol.embl.de/) [79]. Topology confidence was additionally confirmed by branch length values, which are a result of the neighbor-joining method which calculates the number of amino acid changes between the organism at the end of the branch and the common ancestor from which it branched to visually display relatedness [80].

4.3. Drosophila Strains and Genetics

Drosophila stocks were fed on standard cornmeal-molasses-yeast diet and kept at room temperature [45]. *Gal4* and RNAi lines were obtained from the Bloomington Drosophila Stock Center (Indiana University, Bloomington, IN, USA) [81]. Ubiquitous RNAi via the *GAL4/UAS* was used to downregulate the following putative SLC22 transporters: *BalaT* (*CG3790*), *CG6231*, *CG4630*, *Orct* (*CG6331*), *Orct2* (*EP1027, CG13610*), *SLC22A* (*CG7442*), *CG16727*, *CG7333*, *CG8654*, *CG6126*, *CG6006*, *CG7084*, *CG3168*, *CG6356* [5,51]. Male SLC22 RNAi stocks were crossed to *da-GAL4* female virgins to produce an F1 generation with ubiquitous downregulation of the specific SLC22 transporters [82].

4.4. RNAi Developmental Screens and Paraquat Exposure

F1 offspring were observed from the egg stage through eclosion. Developmental phenotypes were defined as normal development of the F1 generation up until the failure to reach eclosion and surpass the pupa stage. Male F1 flies aged two to seven days after eclosion were tested for paraquat sensitivity as defined by survival. Both parent lines were tested in parallel as controls. Three replicates of 10 flies each were tested per strain. Flies were fed on a 3 mm Whatmann paper soaked with 10 mM paraquat (N,N'-dimethyl-4,4'-bipyridinium dichloride, Sigma) in 10% sucrose. Fresh paraquat was added daily. For the initial 60 h, the number of dead flies were recorded every 12 h. All tests were performed at room temperature. In order to avoid unnecessary stress, flies were not starved before adding paraquat. The significance of survival trends was assessed using one-way ANOVA followed by a post hoc Tukey's *t*-test.

Supplementary Materials: Supplementary Materials can be found at http://www.mdpi.com/1422-0067/21/6/2002/s1.

Author Contributions: (Contributor Roles Taxonomy-CRediT); Conceptualization, D.C.E., J.C.G., S.K.N.; methodology, D.C.E., P.A.; validation, G.G.H., S.K.N.; formal analysis, D.C.E., S.A., D.S.; resources, G.G.H., P.A. S.K.N.; data curation, D.C.E., S.A.; supervision, P.A., S.K.N.; writing—original draft preparation, D.C.E., J.C.G.; writing—review and editing, D.C.E., J.C.G., and S.K.N.; visualization, D.C.E.; funding acquisition, S.K.N. All authors have read and agreed to the published version of the manuscript.

Funding: This work was supported by the National Institutes of Health (NIH), granted to S.K.N. from the National Institute of Diabetes and Digestive and Kidney Diseases (NIDDK) [R01DK109392], National Institute of General Medical Sciences (NIGMS) [R01GM132938], and the Eunice Kennedy Shriver National Institute of Child Health and Human Development (NICHD) [U54HD090259]. Support for J.C.G. is from the training grant T32EB009380. Support for G.G.H.'s group comes from the National Heart, Lung, and Blood Institute (NHLBI) [R01HL146530-01].

Conflicts of Interest: The authors declare no conflict of interest.

Abbreviations

SLC22	Solute Carrier Family 22
OAT	Organic Anion Transporter
OCT	Organic Cation Transporter
OCTN	Organic Zwitterion Transporter
EGT	Ergothioneine
MSA	Multiple Sequence Alignment
MPP+	1-methyl-4-phenylpyridinium
PQ	Paraquat, N,N'-dimethyl-4,4'-bipyridinium dichloride
TEA	Tetraethylammonium
RSST	Remote Sensing and Signaling Theory
RSSN	Remote Sensing and Signaling Network
DME	Drug Metabolizing Enzyme
GPCR	G Protein Coupled Receptor
ABC	ATP-Binding Cassette
BDSC	Bloomington Drosophila Stock Center
HR	Histamine Receptor
KO	Knockout
URAT1	Uric Acid Transporter
JVS	Juvenile Visceral Steatosis
UAS	Upstream Activation Sequence
RNAi	Interfering RNA
ROS	Reactive Oxygen Species
CarT	Carcinine Transporter
BalaT	Beta Alanine Transporter
SPU	Strongylocentrotus Purpuratus
TCA	Tricarboxylic Acid Cycle

References

1. César-Razquin, A.; Snijder, B.; Frappier-Brinton, T.; Isserlin, R.; Gyimesi, G.; Bai, X.; Reithmeier, R.A.F.; Hepworth, D.; Hediger, M.A.; Edwards, A.M.; et al. A Call for Systematic Research on Solute Carriers. *Cell* **2015**, *162*, 478–487. [CrossRef]
2. Rosenthal, S.; Bush, K.T.; Nigam, S. A Network of SLC and ABC Transporter and DME Genes Involved in Remote Sensing and Signaling in the Gut-Liver-Kidney Axis. *Sci. Rep.* **2019**, *9*, 11879. [CrossRef] [PubMed]
3. Nigam, S. What do drug transporters really do? *Nat. Rev. Drug Discov.* **2014**, *14*, 29–44. [CrossRef] [PubMed]
4. Höglund, P.J.; Nordström, K.; Schiöth, H.B.; Frediksson, R. The solute carrier families have a remarkably long evolutionary history with the majority of the human families present before divergence of Bilaterian species. *Mol. Biol. Evol.* **2010**, *28*, 1531–1541. [CrossRef] [PubMed]
5. Limmer, S.; Weiler, A.; Volkenhoff, A.; Babatz, F.; Klämbt, C. The Drosophila blood-brain barrier: Development and function of a glial endothelium. *Front. Mol. Neurosci.* **2014**, *8*, 365. [CrossRef] [PubMed]
6. Eraly, S.A.; Vallon, V.; Rieg, T.; Gangoiti, J.A.; Wikoff, W.R.; Siuzdak, G.; Barshop, B.A.; Nigam, S. Multiple organic anion transporters contribute to net renal excretion of uric acid. *Physiol. Genom.* **2008**, *33*, 180–192. [CrossRef] [PubMed]
7. Pandey, U.B.; Nichols, C.D. Human disease models in Drosophila melanogaster and the role of the fly in therapeutic drug discovery. *Pharmacol. Rev.* **2011**, *63*, 411–436. [CrossRef]
8. Xu, Y.; An, F.; Borycz, J.A.; Borycz, J.; Meinertzhagen, I.A.; Wang, T. Histamine Recycling Is Mediated by CarT, a Carcinine Transporter in Drosophila Photoreceptors. *PLoS Genet.* **2015**, *11*, e1005764. [CrossRef]
9. Ogasawara, M.; Yamauchi, K.; Satoh, Y.-I.; Yamaji, R.; Inui, K.; Jonker, J.W.; Schinkel, A.H.; Maeyama, K. Recent advances in molecular pharmacology of the histamine systems: Organic cation transporters as a histamine transporter and histamine metabolism. *J. Pharmacol. Sci.* **2006**, *101*, 24–30. [CrossRef]
10. Han, Y.; Xiong, L.; Xu, Y.; Tian, T.; Wang, T. The β-alanine transporter BalaT is required for visual neurotransmission in Drosophila. *eLife* **2017**, *6*, e29146. [CrossRef]

11. Hattori, Y.; Hattori, K.; Matsuda, N. Regulation of the Cardiovascular System by Histamine. In *Handbook of Experimental Pharmacology*; Springer Science and Business Media LLC: Berlin, Germany, 2016; Volume 241, pp. 239–258.
12. Hu, W.; Chen, Z. The roles of histamine and its receptor ligands in central nervous system disorders: An update. *Pharmacol. Ther.* **2017**, *175*, 116–132. [CrossRef] [PubMed]
13. Wang, Y.; Moussian, B.; Schaeffeler, E.; Schwab, M.; Nies, A.T. The fruit fly Drosophila melanogaster as an innovative preclinical ADME model for solute carrier membrane transporters, with consequences for pharmacology and drug therapy. *Drug Discov. Today* **2018**, *23*, 1746–1760. [CrossRef] [PubMed]
14. Mayer, F.; Schmid, D.; Owens, W.A.; Gould, G.; Apuschkin, M.; Kudlacek, O.; Salzer, I.; Boehm, S.; Chiba, P.; Williams, P.H.; et al. An unsuspected role for organic cation transporter 3 in the actions of amphetamine. *Neuropsychopharmacology* **2018**, *43*, 2408–2417. [CrossRef] [PubMed]
15. Chintapalli, V.R.; Wang, J.; Dow, J.A.T. Using FlyAtlas to identify better Drosophila melanogaster models of human disease. *Nat. Genet.* **2007**, *39*, 715–720. [CrossRef] [PubMed]
16. Zwart, R.; Verhaagh, S.; Buitelaar, M.; Popp-Snijders, C.; Barlow, D.P. Impaired Activity of the Extraneuronal Monoamine Transporter System Known as Uptake-2 in Orct3/Slc22a3-Deficient Mice. *Mol. Cell. Biol.* **2001**, *21*, 4188–4196. [CrossRef]
17. Jonker, J.W.; Wagenaar, E.; van Eijl, S.; Schinkel, A.H. Deficiency in the Organic Cation Transporters 1 and 2 (Oct1/Oct2 [Slc22a1/Slc22a2]) in Mice Abolishes Renal Secretion of Organic Cations. *Mol. Cell. Biol.* **2003**, *23*, 7902–7908. [CrossRef]
18. Zhu, C.; Nigam, K.B.; Date, R.C.; Bush, K.T.; Springer, S.A.; Saier, M.H.; Wu, W.; Nigam, S.K. Evolutionary Analysis and Classification of OATs, OCTs, OCTNs, and Other SLC22 Transporters: Structure-Function Implications and Analysis of Sequence Motifs. *PLoS ONE* **2015**, *10*, e0140569. [CrossRef]
19. Pavlova, A.; Sakurai, H.; Leclercq, B.; Beier, D.R.; Yu, A.S.; Nigam, S. Developmentally regulated expression of organic ion transporters NKT (OAT1), OCT1, NLT (OAT2), and Roct. *Am. J. Physiol.-Ren. Physiol.* **2000**, *278*, F635–F643. [CrossRef]
20. Vallon, V.; Eraly, S.A.; Wikoff, W.R.; Rieg, T.; Kaler, G.; Truong, D.M.; Ahn, S.-Y.; Mahapatra, N.R.; Mahata, S.K.; Gangoiti, J.A.; et al. Organic Anion Transporter 3 Contributes to the Regulation of Blood Pressure. *J. Am. Soc. Nephrol.* **2008**, *19*, 1732–1740. [CrossRef]
21. Bush, K.T.; Wu, W.; Lun, C.; Nigam, S. The drug transporter OAT3 (SLC22A8) and endogenous metabolite communication via the gut–liver–kidney axis. *J. Biol. Chem.* **2017**, *292*, 15789–15803. [CrossRef]
22. Eraly, S.A.; Vallon, V.; Vaughn, D.A.; Gangoiti, J.A.; Richter, K.; Nagle, M.; Monte, J.C.; Rieg, T.; Truong, D.M.; Long, J.M.; et al. Decreased Renal Organic Anion Secretion and Plasma Accumulation of Endogenous Organic Anions in OAT1 Knock-out Mice. *J. Biol. Chem.* **2005**, *281*, 5072–5083. [CrossRef] [PubMed]
23. Sweet, D.; Miller, D.S.; Pritchard, J.B.; Fujiwara, Y.; Beier, D.R.; Nigam, S. Impaired Organic Anion Transport in Kidney and Choroid Plexus of Organic Anion Transporter 3 (Oat3(Slc22a8)) Knockout Mice. *J. Biol. Chem.* **2002**, *277*, 26934–26943. [CrossRef] [PubMed]
24. Ahn, S.-Y.; Jamshidi, N.; Mo, M.L.; Wu, W.; Eraly, S.A.; Dnyanmote, A.; Bush, K.T.; Gallegos, T.F.; Sweet, D.; Palsson, B.Ø.; et al. Linkage of Organic Anion Transporter-1 to Metabolic Pathways through Integrated "Omics"-driven Network and Functional Analysis. *J. Biol. Chem.* **2011**, *286*, 31522–31531. [CrossRef] [PubMed]
25. Kato, Y.; Kubo, Y.; Iwata, D.; Kato, S.; Sudo, T.; Sugiura, T.; Kagaya, T.; Wakayama, T.; Hirayama, A.; Sugimoto, M.; et al. Gene Knockout and Metabolome Analysis of Carnitine/Organic Cation Transporter OCTN1. *Pharm. Res.* **2010**, *27*, 832–840. [CrossRef]
26. Nezu, J.-I.; Tamai, I.; Oku, A.; Ohashi, R.; Yabuuchi, H.; Hashimoto, N.; Nikaido, H.; Sai, Y.; Koizumi, A.; Shoji, Y.; et al. Primary systemic carnitine deficiency is caused by mutations in a gene encoding sodium ion-dependent carnitine transporter. *Nat. Genet.* **1999**, *21*, 91–94. [CrossRef]
27. Urban, T.J.; Gallagher, R.C.; Brown, C.; Castro, R.A.; Lagpacan, L.L.; Brett, C.M.; Taylor, T.R.; Carlson, E.J.; Ferrin, T.; Burchard, E.G.; et al. Functional Genetic Diversity in the High-Affinity Carnitine Transporter OCTN2 (SLC22A5). *Mol. Pharmacol.* **2006**, *70*, 1602–1611. [CrossRef]
28. Momper, J.D.; Nigam, S. Developmental regulation of kidney and liver solute carrier and ATP-binding cassette drug transporters and drug metabolizing enzymes: The role of remote organ communication. *Expert Opin. Drug Metab. Toxicol.* **2018**, *14*, 561–570. [CrossRef]

29. Momper, J.D.; Yang, J.; Gockenbach, M.; Vaida, F.; Nigam, S.K. Dynamics of Organic Anion Transporter-Mediated Tubular Secretion during Postnatal Human Kidney Development and Maturation. *Clin. J. Am. Soc. Nephrol.* **2019**, *14*, 540–548. [CrossRef]
30. Sweeney, D.E.; Vallon, V.; Rieg, T.; Wu, W.; Gallegos, T.F.; Nigam, S. Functional Maturation of Drug Transporters in the Developing, Neonatal, and Postnatal Kidney. *Mol. Pharmacol.* **2011**, *80*, 147–154. [CrossRef]
31. Martovetsky, G.; Tee, J.B.; Nigam, S. Hepatocyte nuclear factors 4α and 1α regulate kidney developmental expression of drug-metabolizing enzymes and drug transporters. *Mol. Pharmacol.* **2013**, *84*, 808–823. [CrossRef]
32. Uhlén, M.; Fagerberg, L.; Hallström, B.M.; Lindskog, C.; Oksvold, P.; Mardinoglu, A.; Sivertsson, Å.; Kampf, C.; Sjöstedt, E.; Asplund, A.; et al. Tissue-based map of the human proteome. *Science* **2015**, *347*, 1260419. [CrossRef] [PubMed]
33. Bainbridge, S.P.; Bownes, M. Staging the metamorphosis of Drosophila melanogaster. *J. Embryol. Exp. Morphol.* **1981**, *66*, 57–80. [PubMed]
34. Chen, Y.-W.; Song, S.; Weng, R.; Verma, P.; Kugler, J.-M.; Buescher, M.; Rouam, S.; Cohen, S. Systematic Study of Drosophila MicroRNA Functions Using a Collection of Targeted Knockout Mutations. *Dev. Cell* **2014**, *31*, 784–800. [CrossRef] [PubMed]
35. McCormack, A.L.; Mona, T.; Amy, B.M.-B.; Christine, T.J.; William, L.; Deborah, A.C.-S.; Donato, A.D.M. Environmental risk factors and Parkinson's disease: Selective degeneration of nigral dopaminergic neurons caused by the herbicide paraquat. *Neurobiol. Dis.* **2002**, *10*, 119–127. [CrossRef]
36. Cohen, G.M.; Doherty, M.D. Free radical mediated cell toxicity by redox cycling chemicals. *Br. J. Cancer* **1987**, *8*, 46–52.
37. Bus, J.S.; Gibson, J.E. Paraquat: Model for oxidant-initiated toxicity. *Environ. Health Perspect.* **1984**, *55*, 37–46. [CrossRef]
38. Roberts, C.K.; Sindhu, K.K. Oxidative stress and metabolic syndrome. *Life Sci.* **2009**, *84*, 705–712. [CrossRef]
39. Ames, B.N.; Cathcart, R.; Schwiers, E.; Hochstein, P. Uric acid provides an antioxidant defense in humans against oxidant- and radical-caused aging and cancer: A hypothesis. *Proc. Natl. Acad. Sci. USA* **1981**, *78*, 6858–6862. [CrossRef]
40. Cheah, I.K.; Halliwell, B. Ergothioneine; antioxidant potential, physiological function and role in disease. *Biochim. Biophys. Acta (BBA)-Mol. Basis Dis.* **2012**, *1822*, 784–793. [CrossRef]
41. Marchette, L.D.; Wang, H.; Li, F.; Babizhayev, M.A.; Kasus-Jacobi, A. Carcinine Has 4-Hydroxynonenal Scavenging Property and Neuroprotective Effect in Mouse Retina. *Investig. Opthalmol. Vis. Sci.* **2012**, *53*, 3572–3583. [CrossRef]
42. Engelhart, D.C.; Granados, J.; Shi, D.; Milton, H.S., Jr.; Baker, M.E.; Abagyan, R.; Nigam, S. Systems Biology Analysis Reveals Eight SLC22 Transporter Subgroups, Including OATs, OCTs, and OCTNs. *Int. J. Mol. Sci.* **2020**, *21*, 1791. [CrossRef] [PubMed]
43. Gai, Y.; Liu, Z.; Cervantes-Sandoval, I.; Davis, R.L. Drosophila SLC22A Transporter Is a Memory Suppressor Gene that Influences Cholinergic Neurotransmission to the Mushroom Bodies. *Neuron* **2016**, *90*, 581–595. [CrossRef] [PubMed]
44. Kimura, M. A simple method for estimating evolutionary rates of base substitutions through comparative studies of nucleotide sequences. *J. Mol. Evol.* **1980**, *16*, 111–120. [CrossRef] [PubMed]
45. Huang, H.; Haddad, G.G. Drosophila dMRP4 regulates responsiveness to O2 deprivation and development under hypoxia. *Physiol. Genom.* **2007**, *29*, 260–266. [CrossRef]
46. Nigam, S. The SLC22 Transporter Family: A Paradigm for the Impact of Drug Transporters on Metabolic Pathways, Signaling, and Disease. *Annu. Rev. Pharmacol. Toxicol.* **2018**, *58*, 663–687. [CrossRef]
47. Nigam, A.K.; Li, J.G.; Lall, K.; Shi, D.; Bush, K.T.; Bhatnagar, V.; Abagyan, R.; Nigam, S.K. Unique metabolite preferences of the drug transporters OAT1 and OAT3 analyzed by machine learning. *J. Biol. Chem.* **2020**, *295*, 1829–1842. [CrossRef]
48. Andrae, U.; Singh, J.; Ziegler-Skylakakis, K. Pyruvate and related α-ketoacids protect mammalian cells in culture against hydrogen peroxide-induced cytotoxicity. *Toxicol. Lett.* **1985**, *28*, 93–98. [CrossRef]
49. Huang, S.-M.; Zhang, L.; Giacomini, K.M. The International Transporter Consortium: A Collaborative Group of Scientists from Academia, Industry, and the FDA. *Clin. Pharmacol. Ther.* **2010**, *87*, 32–36. [CrossRef]

50. Yin, J.; Yin, J.; Sun, W.; Li, F.; Hong, J.; Li, X.; Zhou, Y.; Lu, Y.; Liu, M.; Zhang, X.; et al. VARIDT 1.0: Variability of drug transporter database. *Nucleic Acids Res.* **2020**, *48*, D1042–D1050. [CrossRef]
51. Eraly, S.A.; Monte, J.C.; Nigam, S. Novel slc22 transporter homologs in fly, worm, and human clarify the phylogeny of organic anion and cation transporters. *Physiol. Genom.* **2004**, *18*, 12–24. [CrossRef]
52. Stenesen, E.; Moehlman, A.; Krämer, H. The carcinine transporter CarT is required in Drosophila photoreceptor neurons to sustain histamine recycling. *eLife* **2015**, *4*, e10972. [CrossRef] [PubMed]
53. Geer, B.W.; Vovis, G.F. The effects of choline and related compounds on the growth and development of Drosophila melanogaster. *J. Exp. Zool.* **1965**, *158*, 223–236. [CrossRef] [PubMed]
54. Enomoto, A.; Wempe, M.; Tsuchida, H.; Goto, A.; Sakamoto, A.; Cha, S.H.; Anzai, N.; Niwa, T.; Kanai, Y.; Endou, H.; et al. Molecular Identification of a Novel Carnitine Transporter Specific to Human Testis. *J. Biol. Chem.* **2002**, *277*, 36262–36271. [CrossRef] [PubMed]
55. Eraly, S.A.; Nigam, S. Novel human cDNAs homologous to Drosophila Orct and mammalian carnitine transporters. *Biochem. Biophys. Res. Commun.* **2002**, *297*, 1159–1166. [CrossRef]
56. Pochini, L.; Scalise, M.; Di Silvestre, S.; Belviso, S.; Pandolfi, A.; Arduini, A.; Bonomini, M.; Indiveri, C. Acetylcholine and acetylcarnitine transport in peritoneum: Role of the SLC22A4 (OCTN1) transporter. *Biochim. Biophys. Acta (BBA)-Biomembr.* **2016**, *1858*, 653–660. [CrossRef] [PubMed]
57. Wu, X.; Huang, W.; Prasad, P.D.; Seth, P.; Rajan, D.P.; Leibach, F.H.; Chen, J.; Conway, S.J.; Ganapathy, V. Functional characteristics and tissue distribution pattern of organic cation transporter 2 (OCTN2), an organic cation/carnitine transporter. *J. Pharmacol. Exp. Ther.* **1999**, *290*, 1482–1492.
58. Tamai, I.; Ohashi, R.; Nezu, J.; Sai, Y.; Kobayashi, D.; Oku, A.; Shimane, M.; Tsuji, A. Molecular and Functional Characterization of Organic Cation/Carnitine Transporter Family in Mice. *J. Biol. Chem.* **2000**, *275*, 40064–40072. [CrossRef]
59. Papatheodorou, I.; Fonseca, N.A.; Keays, M.; Tang, A.; Barrera, E.; Bazant, W.; Burke, M.; Füllgrabe, A.; Fuentes, A.M.-P.; George, N.; et al. Expression Atlas: Gene and protein expression across multiple studies and organisms. *Nucleic Acids Res.* **2018**, *46*, D246–D251. [CrossRef]
60. Altenhein, B.; Becker, A.; Busold, C.; Beckmann, B.; Hoheisel, J.D.; Technau, G.M. Expression profiling of glial genes during Drosophila embryogenesis. *Dev. Biol.* **2006**, *296*, 545–560. [CrossRef]
61. Lindsay, S.; Xu, Y.; Lisgo, S.N.; Harkin, L.F.; Copp, A.J.; Gerrelli, D.; Clowry, G.J.; Talbot, A.; Keogh, M.J.; Coxhead, J.; et al. HDBR Expression: A Unique Resource for Global and Individual Gene Expression Studies during Early Human Brain Development. *Front. Neuroanat.* **2016**, *10*, 86. [CrossRef]
62. Berridge, M.J.; Oschman, J.L. A structural basis for fluid secretion by malpighian tubules. *Tissue Cell* **1969**, *1*, 247–272. [CrossRef]
63. Yee, S.W.; Stecula, A.; Chien, H.-C.; Zou, L.; Feofanova, E.V.; Van Borselen, M.; Cheung, K.W.K.; Yousri, N.A.; Suhre, K.; Kinchen, J.M.; et al. Unraveling the functional role of the orphan solute carrier, SLC22A24 in the transport of steroid conjugates through metabolomic and genome-wide association studies. *PLoS Genet.* **2019**, *15*, e1008208. [CrossRef] [PubMed]
64. Nigam, S.K.; Bush, K.T.; Martovetsky, G.; Ahn, S.-Y.; Liu, H.C.; Richard, E.; Bhatnagar, V.; Wu, W. The organic anion transporter (OAT) family: A systems biology perspective. *Physiol. Rev.* **2015**, *95*, 83–123. [CrossRef] [PubMed]
65. Fork, C.; Bauer, T.; Golz, S.; Geerts, A.; Weiland, J.; Del Turco, D.; Schomig, E.; Gründemann, D. OAT2 catalyses efflux of glutamate and uptake of orotic acid. *Biochem. J.* **2011**, *436*, 305–312. [CrossRef] [PubMed]
66. Sawa, K.; Uematsu, T.; Korenaga, Y.; Hirasawa, R.; Kikuchi, M.; Murata, K.; Zhang, J.; Gai, X.; Sakamoto, K.; Koyama, T.; et al. Krebs Cycle Intermediates Protective against Oxidative Stress by Modulating the Level of Reactive Oxygen Species in Neuronal HT22 Cells. *Antioxidants* **2017**, *6*, 21. [CrossRef] [PubMed]
67. Chahine, S.; Campos, A.; O'Donnell, M.J. Genetic knockdown of a single organic anion transporter alters the expression of functionally related genes in Malpighian tubules of Drosophila melanogaster. *J. Exp. Biol.* **2012**, *215*, 2601–2610. [CrossRef]
68. Chahine, S.; Seabrooke, S.; O'Donnell, M.E. Effects of genetic knock-down of organic anion transporter genes on secretion of fluorescent organic ions by malpighian tubules of drosophila melanogaster. *Arch. Insect Biochem. Physiol.* **2012**, *81*, 228–240. [CrossRef]
69. Ahn, S.-Y.; Nigam, S. Toward a systems level understanding of organic anion and other multispecific drug transporters: A remote sensing and signaling hypothesis. *Mol. Pharmacol.* **2009**, *76*, 481–490. [CrossRef]

70. Wu, W.; Dnyanmote, A.V.; Nigam, S. Remote communication through solute carriers and ATP binding cassette drug transporter pathways: An update on the remote sensing and signaling hypothesis. *Mol. Pharmacol.* **2011**, *79*, 795–805. [CrossRef]
71. Cary, G.; Cameron, R.A.; Hinman, V.F. *EchinoBase: Tools for Echinoderm Genome Analyses*; Humana Press Inc.: New York, NY, USA, 2018; Volume 1757, pp. 349–369.
72. Lee, R.; Howe, K.L.; Harris, T.; Arnaboldi, V.; Cain, S.; Chan, J.; Chen, W.J.; Davis, P.; Gao, S.; Grove, C.; et al. WormBase 2017: Molting into a new stage. *Nucleic Acids Res.* **2018**, *46*, D869–D874. [CrossRef]
73. Casper, J.; Zweig, A.S.; Villarreal, C.; Tyner, C.; Speir, M.L.; Rosenbloom, K.R.; Raney, B.J.; Lee, C.M.; Lee, B.T.; Karolchik, D.; et al. The UCSC Genome Browser database: 2018 update. *Nucleic Acids Res.* **2018**, *46*, D762–D769. [PubMed]
74. Altschul, S.F.; Gish, W.; Miller, W.; Myers, E.W.; Lipman, D.J. Basic local alignment search tool. *J. Mol. Biol.* **1990**, *215*, 403–410. [CrossRef]
75. Marygold, S.J.; Crosby, M.A.; Goodman, J.L. *Using FlyBase, a Database of Drosophila Genes and Genomes*; Humana Press Inc.: New York, NY, USA, 2016; Volume 1478, pp. 1–31.
76. Sievers, F.; Wilm, A.; Dineen, D.; Gibson, T.J.; Karplus, K.; Li, W.; López, R.; McWilliam, H.; Remmert, M.; Soeding, J.; et al. Fast, scalable generation of high-quality protein multiple sequence alignments using Clustal Omega. *Mol. Syst. Biol.* **2011**, *7*, 539. [CrossRef] [PubMed]
77. Katoh, K.; Standley, D.M. MAFFT multiple sequence alignment software version 7: Improvements in performance and usability. *Mol. Biol. Evol.* **2013**, *30*, 772–780. [CrossRef]
78. Madeira, F.; Park, Y.M.; Lee, J.; Buso, N.; Gur, T.; Madhusoodanan, N.; Basutkar, P.; Tivey, A.R.N.; Potter, S.; Finn, R.D.; et al. The EMBL-EBI search and sequence analysis tools APIs in 2019. *Nucleic Acids Res.* **2019**, *47*, W636–W641. [CrossRef]
79. Letunic, I.; Bork, P. Interactive Tree Of Life (iTOL) v4: Recent updates and new developments. *Nucleic Acids Res.* **2019**, *47*, W256–W259. [CrossRef]
80. Saitou, N.; Nei, M. The neighbor-joining method: A new method for reconstructing phylogenetic trees. *Mol. Biol. Evol.* **1987**, *4*, 406–425.
81. Perkins, L.A.; Holderbaum, L.; Tao, R.; Hu, Y.; Sopko, R.; McCall, K.; Yang-Zhou, N.; Flockhart, I.; Binari, R.; Shim, H.-S.; et al. The Transgenic RNAi Project at Harvard Medical School: Resources and Validation. *Genetics* **2015**, *201*, 843–852. [CrossRef]
82. Piccin, A. Efficient and heritable functional knock-out of an adult phenotype in Drosophila using a GAL4-driven hairpin RNA incorporating a heterologous spacer. *Nucleic Acids Res.* **2001**, *29*, e55. [CrossRef]

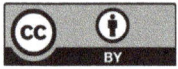

© 2020 by the authors. Licensee MDPI, Basel, Switzerland. This article is an open access article distributed under the terms and conditions of the Creative Commons Attribution (CC BY) license (http://creativecommons.org/licenses/by/4.0/).

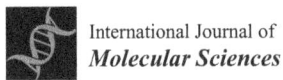

Article

Systems Biology Analysis Reveals Eight SLC22 Transporter Subgroups, Including OATs, OCTs, and OCTNs

Darcy C. Engelhart [1], Jeffry C. Granados [2], Da Shi [3], Milton H. Saier Jr. [4], Michael E. Baker [5], Ruben Abagyan [3] and Sanjay K. Nigam [5,6,*]

[1] Department of Biology, University of California San Diego, San Diego, CA 92093, USA; dengelha@ucsd.edu
[2] Department of Bioengineering, University of California San Diego, San Diego, CA 92093, USA; j6granad@ucsd.edu
[3] School of Pharmacy and Pharmaceutical Sciences, University of California San Diego, San Diego, CA 92093, USA; das046@ucsd.edu (D.S.); rabagyan@ucsd.edu (R.A.)
[4] Department of Molecular Biology, Division of Biological Sciences, University of California San Diego, San Diego, CA 92093, USA; msaier@ucsd.edu
[5] Department of Medicine, University of California San Diego, San Diego, CA 92093, USA; mbaker@ucsd.edu
[6] Department of Pediatrics, University of California San Diego, San Diego, CA 92093, USA
* Correspondence: snigam@ucsd.edu

Received: 11 February 2020; Accepted: 3 March 2020; Published: 5 March 2020

Abstract: The SLC22 family of OATs, OCTs, and OCTNs is emerging as a central hub of endogenous physiology. Despite often being referred to as "drug" transporters, they facilitate the movement of metabolites and key signaling molecules. An in-depth reanalysis supports a reassignment of these proteins into eight functional subgroups, with four new subgroups arising from the previously defined OAT subclade: OATS1 (SLC22A6, SLC22A8, and SLC22A20), OATS2 (SLC22A7), OATS3 (SLC22A11, SLC22A12, and Slc22a22), and OATS4 (SLC22A9, SLC22A10, SLC22A24, and SLC22A25). We propose merging the OCTN (SLC22A4, SLC22A5, and Slc22a21) and OCT-related (SLC22A15 and SLC22A16) subclades into the OCTN/OCTN-related subgroup. Using data from GWAS, in vivo models, and in vitro assays, we developed an SLC22 transporter-metabolite network and similar subgroup networks, which suggest how multiple SLC22 transporters with mono-, oligo-, and multi-specific substrate specificity interact to regulate metabolites. Subgroup associations include: OATS1 with signaling molecules, uremic toxins, and odorants, OATS2 with cyclic nucleotides, OATS3 with uric acid, OATS4 with conjugated sex hormones, particularly etiocholanolone glucuronide, OCT with neurotransmitters, and OCTN/OCTN-related with ergothioneine and carnitine derivatives. Our data suggest that the SLC22 family can work among itself, as well as with other ADME genes, to optimize levels of numerous metabolites and signaling molecules, involved in organ crosstalk and inter-organismal communication, as proposed by the remote sensing and signaling theory.

Keywords: transporters; endogenous metabolism; functional subgroups; SLC22; remote sensing and signaling; drug transporters; gut microbiome; chronic kidney disease

1. Introduction

The SLC (solute carrier) gene family includes 65 families with over 400 transporter genes. In humans, 52 of these families are expressed, encompassing more than 395 genes and it has been estimated that 2000 (10% of the genome) human genes are transporter-related [1]. Various solute carrier 22 (SLC22) members are expressed on both the apical and basolateral surfaces of epithelial cells where they direct small molecule transport between body fluids and vital organs, such as the kidney, liver, heart, and brain [2]. SLC22 transporters are also found in circulating cell types such as erythrocytes (e.g., SLC22A7), monocytes, and macrophages (e.g., SLC22A3, SLC22A4, SLC22A15, and SLC22A16) [3,4]. With recent calls for research on solute carriers, there has been a large influx of data over the past five years, including novel roles in remote sensing and signaling, leading to the need for a more comprehensive understanding of the functional importance of transporters [5].

The SLC22 family is comprised of at least 31 transporters and is found in species ranging from *Arabidopsis thaliana* of the plant kingdom to modern day humans [6,7]. Knowledge surrounding this family of proteins has expanded greatly since its proposed formation in 1997, when SLC22A6 (OAT1, originally known as novel kidney transporter or NKT) was first cloned [8]. Its homology to SLC22A1 (OCT1) and SLC22A7 (OAT2/NLT) led to the establishment of a new family (SLC22, TC# 2.A.1.19) of transport proteins within the major facilitator superfamily (TC# 2.A.1, MFS) as classified by the IUBMB-approved transporter classification (TC) system [8,9]. These proteins all share 12 α-helical transmembrane domains (TMD), a large extracellular domain (ECD) between TMD1 and TMD2, and a large intracellular domain (ICD) between TMD6 and TMD7 [10]. Research has shown these transporters to be integral participants in the movement of drugs, toxins, and endogenous metabolites and signaling molecules, such as prostaglandins, urate, α-ketoglutarate, carnitine, and cyclic nucleotides across the cell membrane [11].

As key players in small organic molecule transport, SLC22 members are hypothesized to play a role in the remote sensing and signaling theory [12–15]. The remote sensing and signaling theory posits that ADME genes—conventionally viewed as central to the absorption (A), distribution (D), metabolism (M), and elimination (E) of drugs, namely drug transporters and enzymes—aid in maintaining homeostasis through remote communication between organs via metabolites and signaling molecules in the blood that may in turn regulate gene expression [16]. This remote communication is supported by the example of serum uric acid levels. In the setting of the compromised kidney function, the increase in serum uric acid seems to be partly mitigated through a compensatory increase in the expression and/or function of ABCG2 in the intestine, which allows the excretion of uric acid in the feces rather than the urine [17,18]. Current research is focusing on determining the ways in which these transporters collaborate to regulate metabolite levels throughout the body [19].

Rather than maintaining a simple division of SLC22 into organic anion transporters (OATs), organic cation transporters (OCTs), and organic zwitterion/cation transporters (OCTNs), previous evolutionary studies have identified six phylogenetic "subclades"—OAT, OAT-like, OAT-related, OCT, OCTN-related, and OCTN—within the OAT and OCT "major clades" [10]. These subclades consist, on average, of three to four members with the exception of the OAT subclade that claims more than half of the 31 known members of SLC22 [10]. Although these subclades are phylogenetically sound, the endogenous functions of many SLC22 members within the six subclades remain ill-defined or unknown. With the emergence of new functional data, we performed a re-analysis of the SLC22 family to better characterize the functional, endogenous grouping of these transporters. Our re-analysis shows eight apparent subgroups, with four of these subgroups arising out of the previously defined (but very large) OAT subclade. Since these groupings are more closely related to well-known OATs rather than OCTs, OCTNs, or other subclades, we refer to these as OAT subgroups (OATS1, OATS2, OATS3, and OATS4).

We considered many factors in our re-analysis of SLC22 and subsequent designation of functionally based subgroups. To better describe the subgroups while still highlighting the nuances of each individual transporter, we utilized data from genomic loci, tissue expression, sequence similarity searches, proteomic motif searches, and functional transporter-metabolite data from GWAS, in vitro assays, and in vivo models. In place of phylogenetic studies, we performed multiple sequence alignments (MSA) and generated guide-trees that are based on sequence similarity or homology and thus provide more insight into function than solely phylogenetic studies. While the SLC22 family is composed of putative transporters, some members, like Slc22a20 and Slc22a17, have proposed mechanisms that differ from those of classic transporters [20,21]. To that effect, we explored the sequence similarities between SLC22 transporters and non-transport related proteins. We also used systems biology tools to develop an SLC22 transporter-metabolite networks as well as networks for each subgroup. This analysis elucidates the diversity of the endogenous functions of SLC22 transporters in various tissues and provides an updated functional framework for assigning each transporter to a subgroup. Considering the importance of SLC22 transporters, forming functional groups that incorporate endogenous substrates and tissue expression patterns can help better define their roles in intra-organ, inter-organ, and inter-organismal communication.

2. Results

Emerging data continue to indicate the centrality of the SLC22 family (particularly OATs, OCTs, and OCTNs) in endogenous physiology [5,16]. Our thorough reanalysis of the previously described phylogenetic subclades [10] revealed eight functional subgroups: OATS1, OATS2, OATS3, OATS4, OAT-like, OAT-related, OCT, and OCTN/OCTN-related (Table 1). By thus grouping this large family of proteins, we highlighted differences in substrate selectivity, showing that each member has a unique profile of associated metabolites. Based on the number of different metabolites it interacts with, each SLC22 transporter can be classified as relatively mono-, oligo-, or multi-specific. In what follows, publicly available data from GWAS, in vitro, and in vivo datasets were used to build functional networks that support the subgroups (Figure 1). In addition to these functional data and systems biology analyses, subgroups were also supported by structural, genomic, and other analyses explained below. Since some SLC22 members remain understudied, we also investigated low level sequence identity with non-transport proteins to better characterize these "orphaned" transporters.

Table 1. Updated SLC22 family subgroups. The SLC22 family was previously separated into 6 phylogenetic subclades. We propose a reclassification into 8 subgroups based on functional data and supported by the methods described in the text.

Former Groupings		Updated Groupings	
Subclade	Members	Subgroup	Members
OAT	A6, A7, A8, A9, A10, A11, A12, A19, A20, A22, A24, A25, A26, A27, A28, A29, A30	OATS1	A6, A8, A20
		OATS2	A7
		OATS3	A11, A12, a22
		OATS4 [1]	A9, A10, A24, A25
OAT-like	A13, A14	OAT-like	A13, A14
OAT-related	A17, A18. A23, A31	OAT-related	A17, A18. A23, A31
OCTN-related	A15, A16	OCTN/OCTN related	A4, A5, A15, A16, a21
OCTN	A4, A5		
OCT	A1, A2, A3	OCT	A1, A2, A3

[1] Six rodent-specific transporters are not included due to their species specificity and lack of functional data.

In Figure 1 (in which metabolites linked to only a single transporter are not shown), 24 SLC22 proteins are linked to 79 unique metabolites, highlighting the physiological relevance of this family. This representation also brings attention to the number of shared substrates among SLC22, with 222 total edges present in this highly connected trimmed network. The multi-specific, oligo-specific, and mono-specific nature of different family members suggests how one transporter (e.g., a multi-specific member) may be able to compensate for the reduced function of another transporter (e.g., a mono-specific transporter). Furthermore, several of the metabolites interacting with the transporters (prostaglandins, carnitine derivatives, and bile acids) belong to different metabolic pathways, indicating that many processes, at both the systemic and cellular level, are dependent upon SLC22. In the following sections, the role of each subgroup in regulating metabolites in this larger SLC22 network was discussed in more detail.

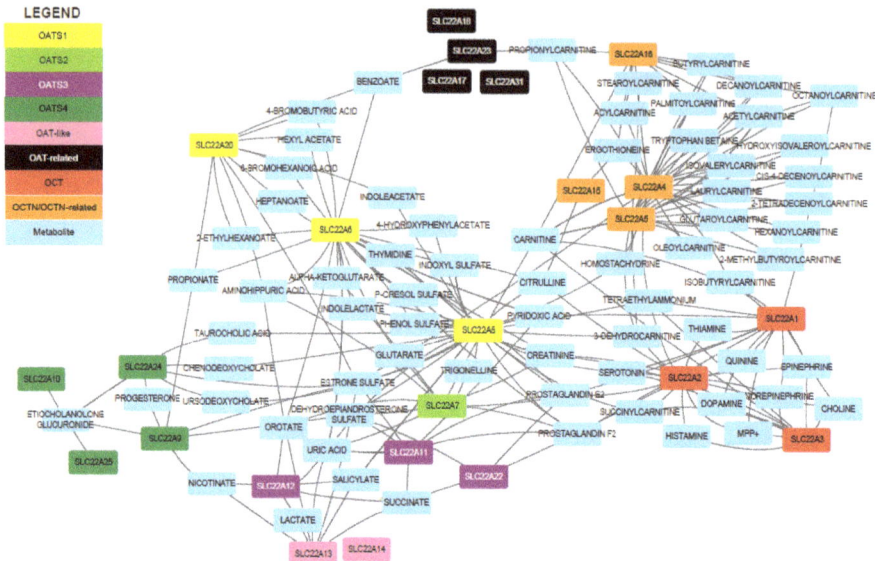

Figure 1. Pruned SLC22 network. All SLC22 transporters with functional data were initially included. Metabolites associated with only one transporter were removed for improved visualization. SLC22 transporters and metabolites are colored nodes. Each edge represents a significant transporter-metabolite association. Multiple edges connecting one metabolite to a specific transporter were bundled (e.g., in vitro and GWAS support).

2.1. Analysis of Substrate Specificity and Selectivity Helps Categorize Mono-, Oligo-, and Multi-Specificity of SLC22 Members

The concept of multi-, oligo-, and mono-specific SLC22 transporters was supported in part based on the number of unique drugs that are known to interact with each SLC22 member (Table 2) [22]. Several SLC22 members (e.g., OAT1 and OCT2) are best known as "drug" transporters and due to this association, many have been extensively tested as potential drug targets. While drugs were not the primary focus of this research, the number of drugs a transporter is linked to is indicative of how many structurally different substrates it can interact with. This may translate to endogenous compounds from different metabolic pathways. As interest in solute carriers has increased over the past decade, there has been a large influx of functional data (Table S1). We used these data to validate our initial specificity assignments, and found that, for the most part, the metabolite data were in agreement with the drug data. A transporter linked to many unique drugs was often linked to many unique metabolites. For example, OATS1 members SLC22A6 and SLC22A8 are linked to 100 or more drugs, respectively. This is reflected in the metabolite data, as each transporter was associated with at least 50 unique metabolites, confirming their multi-specific nature. OATS4 members SLC22A9, SLC22A10, SLC22A24, and SLC22A25 are understudied with respect to drugs. As a group, they are only associated with three drugs, making it difficult to predict their substrate selectivity. Endogenously, the group appears to have relatively mono-specific members that are dedicated to conjugated sex steroids, and oligo-specific members, which are linked to conjugated sex hormones, short chain fatty acids, and bile acids.

2.2. Construction of Functional Networks from Metabolite-Transporter Interaction Data Support the Eight Subgroups

To visualize these transporter-metabolite interactions, which were acquired from a combination of GWAS, in vivo, and in vitro studies, we created networks using Cytoscape [23]. These networks allowed us to see the extent of unique and overlapping substrate specificity between transporters in the SLC22 family and within the proposed subgroups (Figures S1 and S2). The networks also provide, for the first time, a systems biology lens into the subgroup (as opposed to a single transporter) function. In these networks, all edges are undirected and represent a statistically significant result linking an SLC22 member to a metabolite. To give an example, the OATS1 network uses the members (SLC22A6, SLC22A8, and SLC22A20) as central nodes. Each associated metabolite is connected to the member, and the networks are then combined to represent the entire subgroup and demonstrate how a metabolite may be linked to multiple transporters (Figure S1A). Functional data were available for 21 of 31 known SLC22 transporters. The trimmed SLC22 network is displayed in Figure 1, the individual subgroup networks are in Figures S1 and S2, and the total SLC22 network is in Figure S3. The compiled data with transporter, metabolite, study, quantitative metric, and citation are present in Table S1.

Table 2. Number of SLC22 transporter associations with unique drugs from DrugBank and metabolites. SLC22 transporter substrate specificity (mono-, oligo-, or multi) was predicted from the number of drugs each was associated with. Metabolite data were then used to support the predicted assignment. In the absence of drug data, metabolites were used to determine specificity. #: number, n/a: not applicable.

SLC22 Transporter	Common Name	# of Unique Drugs	# of Metabolites	Sum	Specificity	Metabolic Pathways
A1	OCT1	70	15	85	multi	Monoamines, carnitines, PG [1]
A2	OCT2	84	24	108	multi	Monoamines, carnitines, PG, creatinine
A3	OCT3	40	12	52	oligo	Monoamines, carnitines, creatinine
A4	OCTN1	33	25	58	oligo	Carnitines, ergothioneine
A5	OCTN2	55	20	75	oligo	Carnitines
A6	OAT1	99	52	151	multi	Uric acid, PG, gut microbiome derived products, TCA [2]
A7	OAT2	35	16	51	oligo	Cyclic nucleotides, PG, carnitine, creatinine, TCA
A8	OAT3	126	88	214	multi	Uric acid, PG, creatinine, gut microbiome derived products, TCA, bile acids
A9	OAT7	0	9	9	oligo	Conjugated sex steroids, SCFA [3]
A10	OAT5	3	2	5	mono	Conjugated sex steroids
A11	OAT4	42	9	51	oligo	Uric acid, PG, conjugated sex steroids
A12	URAT1	4	7	11	mono	Uric acid, TCA
A13	OAT10, ORCTL3	n/a	13	13	mono	Uric acid, TCA
A14	ORCTL4	n/a	n/a	n/a	n/a	Understudied
A15	FLIPT1	n/a	7	7	mono	EGT, complex lipids
A16	FLIPT2, CT2	2	16	18	oligo	Carnitines, EGT
A17	BOCT1, NGAL, Lcn2-R	n/a	2	2	mono	Lipocalin
A18	SLC22A1L, TSSC5,	n/a	2	2	n/a	Understudied
A20	OAT6	n/a	13	13	oligo	Odorants, SCFA
a21	Octn3, Slc22a9	n/a	1	1	mono	Carnitine
a22	OAT-PG	n/a	12	12	mono	PG, conjugated sex steroids
A23	BOCT2	n/a	12	12	oligo	Fatty acids
A24	n/a	n/a	10	10	oligo	Conjugated sex steroids, bile acids
A25	UST6	n/a	1	1	mono	Conjugated sex steroids
A31	n/a	n/a	n/a	n/a	n/a	Understudied

[1] prostaglandins; [2] citric acid cycle intermediates; [3] short chain fatty acids.

While there is no single metabolite that is associated with all SLC22 transporters, some are linked to multiple family members, and thus may be a hallmark of the subgroup or family as a whole. These metabolites are prostaglandin E2, prostaglandin F2, estrone sulfate, uric acid, carnitine, and creatinine, which are each linked to at least five different SLC22 members, respectively (Figure S3). This result demonstrated that SLC22, as a group, is involved in regulating several metabolic processes, ranging from blood vessel dilation through prostaglandins to cellular energy production through carnitine [24,25]. This also implies that the particular structural features of the SLC22 family in general (12 TMD, large ECD between TMD1 and TMD2, and large ICD between TMD6 and TMD7) lend itself well to interacting with these compounds. This is further supported by the subgroup-specific network analyses and motif analysis we performed (Figure 1).

2.3. OATS1 (SLC22A6, SLC22A8, and SLC22A20) Handles a Wide Variety of Metabolites, Signaling Molecules, Uremic Toxins, and Odorants

Several metabolites have been identified as substrates of SLC22A6 (OAT1) and SLC22A8 (OAT3). While many are unique, there is notable overlap. Both OAT1 and OAT3 interact with uremic toxins (indoxyl sulfate, p-cresol sulfate, and uric acid) and gut microbiome derived products (indolelactate and 4-hydroxyphenylacetate), as well as many of the more general SLC22 metabolites, like prostaglandin E2, prostaglandin F2, uric acid, and creatinine [26–30]. SLC22A20 (OAT6), while not as well-studied, has affinity for several odorants and short chain fatty acids that are also associated with OAT1 [31]. OAT1 and OAT3 are clearly multi-specific, and OAT6 appears to be oligo-specific, as it handles both odorants and some short chain fatty acids. With respect to remote signaling, the shared metabolites among these transporters (Figure S1A) were noteworthy because of their tissue localization (Table 3). OAT1 and OAT3 were primarily expressed in the kidney proximal tubule, with some expression in other tissues, like the choroid plexus and retina (Table 3). OAT6, however, is expressed in the olfactory mucosa of mice, presumably reflecting its affinity for odorants [21,31,32]. In the kidney, OAT1 and OAT3, along with many other SLC22 transport proteins, help regulate the urine levels of many metabolites and signaling molecules, which may potentially facilitate inter-organismal communication. For example, a volatile compound in one organism may be excreted into the urine through OAT1 and then somehow sensed by another individual of the same or different species through a mechanism involving OAT6 in the olfactory mucosa [12].

Table 3. Genomic localization and tissue expression of the SLC22 family. The following table describes the genomic localization and tissue expression patterns of all SLC22 members excluding the mouse-specific Slc22a19, Slc22a26, Slc22a27, Slc22a28, Slc22a29, and Slc22a30. Slc22a22 and Slc22a21 expression patterns described are from mouse [33,34]. (m) denotes expression patterns observed exclusively in mice. Tissue expression data in humans were collected from various sources and databases [4,24,34]. Expression is assumed from mRNA expression analysis, unless confirmed experimentally. A checkmark represents the presence of the specific transporter in a specific tissue. n/a: not applicable.

Subgroup	SLC22 Transporter	Common Name	Genomic Loci Human Chr.	Genomic Loci Mouse Chr.	Liver	Kidney	Brain	Gut	Heart	Lung	Testis	Immune Cell	Bone Marrow	Placenta
OATS1	SLC22A6	OAT1	11	19		✓	✓							
	SLC22A8	OAT3	11	19		✓	✓							
	SLC22A20	OAT6	11	19			✓				✓(m)		✓	
OATS2	SLC22A7	OAT2	6	17	✓	✓					✓			✓
OATS3	SLC22A11	OAT4	11	n/a		✓								
	SLC22A12	URAT1	11	19		✓								
	Slc22a22	OAT-PG	-	15		✓(m)								
OATS4	SLC22A9	OAT7	11	-	✓		✓						✓	
	SLC22A10	OAT5	11	-	✓		✓							
	SLC22A24	n/a	11	-		✓	✓	✓			✓			
	SLC22A25	UST6	11	-	✓									
OAT-like	SLC22A13	OAT10, ORCTL3	3	9		✓	✓	✓	✓		✓			
	SLC22A14	ORCTL4	3	9		✓	✓				✓			
OAT-related	SLC22A17	BOCT1, NGAL, Lcn2-R	14	14	✓	✓	✓	✓	✓		✓			
	SLC22A18	SLC22A1L, TSSC5	11	7	✓	✓	✓	✓						
	SLC22A23	BOCT2	6	13	✓	✓	✓	✓		✓				
	SLC22A31	n/a	16	-						✓	✓			
OCTN/OCTN-related	SLC22A4	OCTN1	5	11	✓	✓	✓	✓		✓		✓	✓	
	SLC22A5	OCTN2	5	11	✓	✓	✓	✓		✓	✓	✓	✓	✓
	SLC22A15	FLIPT1	6	10		✓	✓	✓	✓	✓	✓	✓		
	SLC22A16	FLIPT2, CT2	1	3	✓	✓	✓	✓			✓			✓
	Slc22a21	Octn3, Slc22a9	-	11		✓	✓	✓			✓			✓
OCT	SLC22A1	OCT1	6	17	✓	✓	✓	✓	✓	✓		✓		✓
	SLC22A2	OCT2	6	17	✓	✓	✓	✓		✓				
	SLC22A3	OCT3	6	17	✓	✓	✓	✓	✓	✓		✓		✓

2.4. OATS2 (SLC22A7) is a Systemically-Expressed Transporter of Organic Anions and Cyclic Nucleotides

SLC22A7 (OAT2) is the only member of the OATS2 subgroup and is associated with prototypical SLC22 substrates, such as prostaglandins, carnitine, creatinine, and uric acid [29,35–37]. Evolutionarily, OAT2 appeared to be single member subgroup with a distinct branching pattern and single common ancestor within our generated guide trees (Figure 2, Figures S5 and S6). OAT2 was also linked to cyclic nucleotides and dicarboxylic acids, which when taken with the previous metabolites, created a unique profile worthy of its own subgroup (Figure S1B) [38]. Another distinguishing feature of OAT2 was its tissue expression patterns (Table 3). While its expression in the liver and kidney are common to many SLC22 members, it has been localized to circulating red blood cells, where it may function in cyclic nucleotide transport [3]. Its expression in a mobile cell type and transport of cyclic nucleotides raises the possibility that it may act as an avenue for signaling.

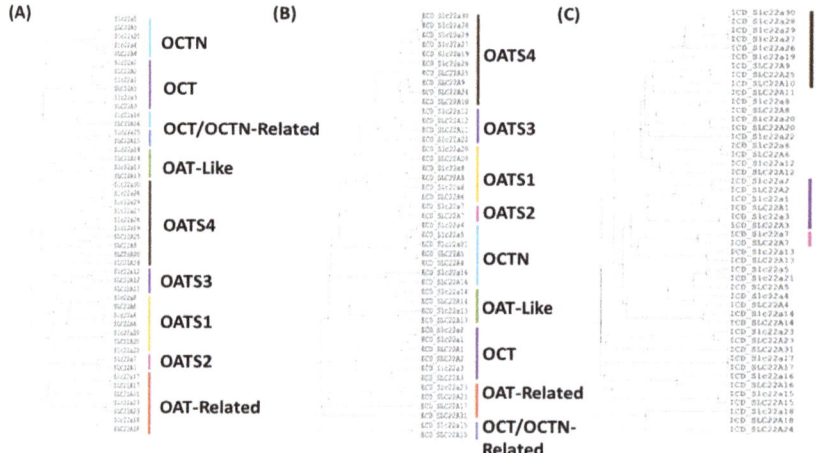

Figure 2. Multiple sequence alignment using ICM-Pro v3.8-7c tree of SLC22 members implies function. All known mouse and human SLC22 sequences, excluding Slc22a18, were aligned using ICM-Pro v3.8-7c sequence similarity-based alignment. (**A**) Full sequence. (**B**) Extracellular loop (not including Slc22a18, due to its lack of a characteristic large extracellular loop between TMD1 and TMD2). (**C**) Intracellular loop.

2.5. OATS3 (SLC22A11, SLC22A12, and Slc22a22) Functions to Balance Uric Acid and Prostaglandins

In humans, SLC22A11 (OAT4) and SLC22A12 (URAT1) share only two substrates, uric acid and succinate (Figure S1C) [39,40]. Uric acid is a beneficial metabolite in the serum as it is thought to be responsible for more than half of human antioxidant activity in the blood [41]. However, high levels of uric acid can be harmful and are associated with gout [42]. URAT1 is associated with very few metabolites and is best understood for its role in uric acid reabsorption in the kidney proximal tubule, making it relatively mono-specific [39]. OAT4, on the other hand, has been shown to transport prostaglandins and conjugated sex hormones in addition to uric acid, making it oligo-specific [43–45]. URAT1 is almost exclusively expressed in the kidney, and OAT4 is expressed in the kidney, placenta, and epididymis (Table 3). The more diverse tissue expression of SLC22A11 seems consistent with its wider range of substrates. The subgroup differs in rodents because mice do not express Oat4. Instead, the rodent subgroup is composed of Slc22a12, known as the renal-specific transporter (Rst) in mice, and Slc22a22, known as the prostaglandin-specific organic anion transporter (Oat-pg). While Rst and Oat-pg do not share substrate specificity, together, they combine to play the role of URAT1 and OAT4 by handling uric acid and prostaglandins [46].

2.6. OATS4 (SLC22A9, SLC22A10, SLC2A24, and SLC22A25) Members are Specifically Associated with Conjugated Sex Hormones

GWAS analyses support the association of all human members of this subgroup with one common metabolite, etiocholanolone glucuronide, a conjugated sex hormone, with a p-value of 4.12×10^{-27} or lower for all members (Table 3, Table S1) [47]. While this group shares at least one conjugated sex hormone, SLC22A24 and SLC22A9 appear to be more oligo-specific transporters, with SLC22A9 linked to short chain fatty acids and SLC22A24 linked to bile acids [48,49]. SLC22A10 and SLC22A25 are only linked to conjugated sex hormones, making them relatively mono-specific transporters (Figure S1D) [47]. In terms of tissue expression, there is a distinct correlation between patterns and shared function amongst human OATS4 members (Table 4). We predicted that all four members are conjugated sex steroid transporters with SLC22A9, A10, and A25 showing high expression in the liver where conjugation of glucuronides and sulfates to androgens and other gonadal steroids occurs [48]. SLC22A24 has low expression levels in the liver but is highly expressed in the proximal tubule, where it is predicted to reabsorb these conjugated steroids [48]. This subgroup also includes a large rodent-specific expansion, consisting of Slc22a19 and Slc22a26-30. Although the rodent-specific expansion is greatly understudied, transport data for rat Slc22a9/a24 show shared substrate specificity for estrone sulfate with SLC22A24, but not for bile acids or glucuronidated steroids, which is consistent with the lack of glucuronides in rat urine and serum [48]. While sulfatases are extremely highly conserved amongst humans, rats, and mice, the separation of rodent- and nonrodent-specific OATS4 groups may be due to the species differences in expression and function of glucuronidases [50]. Despite their distinct differences from human OATS4 members in sequence similarity studies and minimal functional data, the rodent-specific transporters are also highly expressed in both liver and kidney [51].

2.7. OAT-Like (SLC22A13 and SLC22A14) has Potentially Physiologically Important Roles

Very little functional data are available for the OAT-like subgroup. SLC22A13 (OAT10/ORCTL3) has been well characterized as a transporter of both urate and nicotinate, but SLC22A14 has no available transport data [52]. However, N'-methyl nicotinate is increased in the plasma levels of self-reported smokers, and GWAS studies have implicated SNPs in the SLC22A14 gene to be associated with success in smoking cessation [53,54]. Although these data do not directly relate SLC22A14 to nicotinate, it suggests a possible route of investigation into the functional role of this transporter, one that may, in some ways, overlap with that of OAT10. SLC22A13 is primarily expressed in the kidney, and although we found no human protein expression data for SLC22A14, transcripts for this gene are found at low levels in the kidney and notably high levels the testis (Table 4), which is in concordance with its critical role in sperm motility and fertility in male mice [55]. Future studies are required to determine the functional classification of this subgroup; however, our genomic localization and sequence-based analyses provided enough data to support the notion that these two belonged in their own individual subgroup.

2.8. OAT-Related (SLC22A17, SLC22A18, SLC22A23, and SLC22A31) is Anomalous Amongst SLC22 Members but has Interesting Functional Mechanisms and Disease Associations

The OAT-related subgroup was an outlier within the SLC22 family, consisting of the orphan transporters SLC22A17, SLC22A18, SLC22A23, and SLC22A31. SLC22A17 and SLC22A23 were strongly related, with greater than a 30% shared amino acid identity. When these two transporters were initially identified together as BOCT1 (SLC22A17) and BOCT2 (SLC22A23), it was noted that they both show high expression levels in the brain, as well as a nonconserved amino terminus that may negate prototypical SLC22 function [56]. SLC22A17 is known as LCN2-R (Lipocalin receptor 2) and is reported to mediate iron homeostasis through binding and endocytosis of iron-bound lipocalin, as well as exhaustive protein clearance from the urine as shown by high affinities for proteins such as calbindin [20,57]. SLC22A23 has no confirmed substrates, but SNPs and mutations within this gene have medically relevant phenotypic associations such as QT elongation, inflammatory bowel disease, endometriosis-related infertility, and the clearance of antipsychotic drugs [58–60]. SLC22A31 is the most understudied transporter of the SLC22 family but has been associated with right-side colon cancer [33]. SLC22A18 remains an outlier and lacks the characteristic SLC22 large ECD. Its membership within the SLC22 family is arguable due to high sequence similarity with the DHA H^+-antiporter family (Figure S4) [10]. Further study is required to confirm if the OAT-related members share substrates as a group or if their sequence diversity and deviations from classical physical SLC22 member characteristics are the reason for their phylogenetic association.

Table 4. Combined functional data for OATS4. These data were manually curated and collected from genome-wide association, in vitro, and in vivo studies. Only statistically significant results from each study are included. Column A is the SLC22 transporter, column B is the metabolite, column C is the source of these data (rsid for GWAS, cell line for in vitro, and the physiological measurement for in vivo), column D is the quantitative metric (p value for GWAS, Km, Ki, IC50, or inhibition percentage compared to control for in vitro, and p value for in vivo), and column E is the citation.

Gene	Metabolite	Source	Metrics	Citation
SLC22A9	butyrate	in vitro, *Xenopus* oocytes	trans-stimulates transport $p < 0.001$	[37]
SLC22A9	dehydroepiandrosterone sulfate	in vitro, *Xenopus* oocytes	Km: 2.2 uM	[37]
SLC22A9	estrone sulfate	in vitro, *Xenopus* oocytes	Km: 8.7 uM	[37]
SLC22A9	etiocholanolone glucuronide	GWAS, rs113747568	$p = 5.27 \times 10^{-28}$	[47]
SLC22A9	nicotinate	in vitro, *Xenopus* oocytes	trans-stimulates transport $p < 0.01$	[37]
SLC22A9	progesterone	GWAS, rs112295236	$p = 8.00 \times 10^{-12}$	[47]
SLC22A9	propionate	in vitro, *Xenopus* oocytes	trans-stimulates transport $p < 0.01$	[37]
SLC22A9	tyramine o-sulfate	GWAS, rs397740636	$p = 2.06 \times 10^{-6}$	[47]
SLC22A9	valerate	in vitro, *Xenopus* oocytes	trans-stimulates transport $p < 0.001$	[37]
SLC22A10	epiandrosterone sulfate	GWAS, rs1939769	$p = 2.06 \times 10^{-7}$	[37]
SLC22A10	etiocholanolone glucuronide	GWAS, rs112753913	$p = 1.88 \times 10^{-27}$	[47]
SLC22A24	androstanediol glucuronide	in vitro, HEK293 Flp-In	IC50: 21 ± 11 uM	[48]
SLC22A24	chenodeoxycholate	in vitro, HEK293 Flp-In	IC50: 2.6 ± 1.0 uM	[48]
SLC22A24	estradiol glucuronide	in vitro, HEK293 Flp-In	3-5 fold over vector control	[48]
SLC22A24	estrone sulfate	in vitro, HEK293 Flp-In	5-10 fold over vector control	[48]
SLC22A24	etiocholanolone glucuronide	in vitro, HEK293 Flp-In	IC50: 29 ± 4.7 uM	[48]
SLC22A24	etiocholanolone glucuronide	GWAS, rs113532193	$p = 5.90 \times 10^{-37}$	[47]
SLC22A24	pregnanediol-3-glucuronide	in vitro, HEK293 Flp-In	IC50: >200 uM	[48]
SLC22A24	pregnanediol-3-glucuronide	GWAS, rs202187460	$p = 5.91 \times 10^{-7}$	[47]
SLC22A24	pregnenolone sulfate	in vitro, HEK293 Flp-In	IC50: 1.4 ± 0.1 uM	[48]
SLC22A24	progesterone	in vitro, HEK293 Flp-In	IC50: 7.4 ± 3.0 uM	[48]
SLC22A24	taurocholic acid	in vitro, HEK293 Flp-In	10–20 fold over vector control	[48]
SLC22A24	ursodeoxycholate	in vitro, HEK293 Flp-In	IC50: 7.6 ± 1.2 uM	[48]
SLC22A25	etiocholanolone glucuronide	GWAS, rs113950742	$p = 4.12 \times 10^{-27}$	[47]

2.9. OCT (SLC22A1, SLC22A2, and SLC22A3) Members Are Characteristic Organic Cation Transporters with High Affinities for Monoamine Neurotransmitters and Other Biologically Important Metabolites and Signaling Molecules

The OCT subclade of SLC22A1 (OCT1), SLC22A2 (OCT2), and SLC22A3 (OCT3) has ample data to support its formation and has been widely accepted and utilized as the prototypical subgroup of organic cation transporters. All three members of this subgroup transport monoamine neurotransmitters, carnitine derivatives, creatinine and the characteristic OCT substrates, MPP+, and TEA (Figure S2A) [34,37,61–64]. All three members of this subgroup were expressed in the liver, kidney, and brain (Table 4). When considered together with the transport of neurotransmitters, this subgroup serves as an example of inter-organ communication between the brain and the kidney–liver axis via transporters. The systemic levels of these neurotransmitters and thus, their availability to the brain can be regulated by the expression of OCT subgroup members in the

2.10. OCTN/OCTN-Related (SLC22A4, SLC22A5, SLC22A15, and SLC22A16) Subgroup Consists of Prototypical Carnitine and Ergothioneine Transporters

The OCTN/OCTN-Related subgroup is a combination of two previously established subclades, OCTN and OCTN-related [10]. Previous studies have mistakenly named SLC22A15 as CT1 (carnitine transporter 1), but this name actually belongs to SLC22A5 (OCTN2) [13]. GWAS data show that SLC22A4 (OCTN1), SLC22A5 (OCTN2/CT1), and SLC22A16 (FLIPT2/CT2) are heavily linked to carnitine and its derivatives [37]. This is consistent with in vitro data showing that OCTN2 and FLIPT2 are carnitine transporters [65,66]. Although OCTN1 has lower affinity for carnitine than OCTN2 and FLIPT2, it has high affinity for the endogenous antioxidant ergothioneine, which GWAS data suggest may be a shared metabolite with both SLC22A15 (FLIPT1) and FLIPT2 (SLC22A16; Figure 2B) [37,67]. SLC22A15 is associated with many complex lipids that are not characteristic of any other SLC22 transporter [47]. Although data are very limited, this anomalous SLC22 member so far appears to only share one potential substrate with this subgroup, but its inclusion is supported by multiple sequence alignments focusing on the intracellular loop and tissue expression patterns. Most other subgroups in this family are limited to a few tissues, mainly the liver and kidney, but the members of the OCTN/OCTN-Related subgroup are all expressed in at least five tissues as well as circulating immune cells (Table 4) [4,7]. This broad tissue expression pattern, in conjunction with our network analysis, supports the notion that these transporters' main task is transporting carnitine derivatives, as carnitine metabolism is an energy producing mechanism in nearly every cell. It may also play a role in regulating levels of the antioxidant ergothioneine, which appears to be a unique substrate of this subgroup [24,68].

2.11. Multiple Sequence Alignment Further Supports the Classification of Subgroups

Our new subgroupings are primarily based on the endogenous function of the transporters, but they are also supported by additional analyses. These analyses are necessary, as structural and evolutionary similarities can predict functional traits that have yet to be discovered. Though the previously established phylogenetic subclades remain sound, our re-analysis includes new and updated amino acid sequences that support the proposed subgroups with more confidence, especially when investigating similarities within functional regions [10]. MSA programs were favored over phylogenetics because MSA searches are based upon structural similarities rather than evolutionary relatedness [69]. These structural similarities, especially in the large ECD (extracellular domain) and large ICD (intracellular domain) of SLC22 proteins, may indicate shared function.

Full length sequence analysis via Clustal-Omega, MAFFT, and ICM-Pro v3.8-7 supported the division of SLC22 into eight subgroups (Figure 2A, Figures S5 and S6). While the OATS1, OATS2, OATS4, OAT-like, OAT-related, and OCT subgroups were supported by full-length sequence analyses, OATS3 and OCTN/OCTN-Related required a more rigorous investigation. To further clarify "borderline" subgroup assignments from the full-length sequence analysis, sequence similarity between the ECDs and ICDs of all human and mouse SLC22 members was determined using ICM-Pro v3.8-7, and the results were visualized via guide trees (Figure 2B,C). ECD alignment preserved all eight subgroups, with the exception of SLC22A15 in the OCTN/OCTN-Related subgroup. In contrast, ICD alignment preserved only the OATS4, OATS2, and OCT subgroups.

The branching pattern of OATS3 member Oat-pg (Slc22a22) differs between tree variations. These analyses consistently indicate a similar relationship between Oat-pg and OATS3, as well as OATS4. However, in an analysis of the SLC22 ECDs, it is most closely associated with OATS3 over any other subgroup. This, in conjunction with shared substrate specificity with both SLC22A12 and SLC22A11, and not OATS4 members, supports its membership within the OATS3 subgroup [29,39,40,46].

In full-length sequence alignments, the grouping of SLC22A4, SLC22A5, and Slc22a21 is consistently conserved, while the topology of both SLC22A15 and SLC22A16 is irregular. Despite this, analysis of the large ECD shows similarity between all OCTN/OCTN-related members other than SLC22A15. Previous analyses have noted the large difference between the ECD of SLC22A15 and all other SLC22 members, which is supported by our analysis in Figure 2B [10]. Interestingly, there appears to be some similarity between the large intracellular domains of SLC22A16 and SLC22A15. Although much of the support for the establishment of the OCTN/OCTN-related subgroup comes from functional data (Figure S2B), the described MSA analyses highlight shared structural, and possibly functional, regions.

2.12. Analysis of Genomic Localization Highlights Evolutionary Relatedness of Subgroup Members and Suggests Basis of Coregulation

Genomic clustering within the SLC22 family has been previously described [10]. Specifically, genes found in tandem on the chromosome, such as OAT-like members SLC22A13 and SLC22A14, are predicted to have arisen from duplication events, indicating a strong evolutionary relationship. Despite the majority of the OAT subclade being found on chromosome 11 in humans and chromosome 19 in mice, clustering within the chromosome supports the division of the OAT subclade into smaller subgroups. For example, OATS4 members SLC22A9, SLC22A10, SLC22A24, and SLC22A25 appear in tandem on human chromosome 11 within the UST (Unknown Substrate Transporter) region of the genome. This region is analogous to the UST region within the mouse genome on chromosome 19, where the mouse-specific OATS4 members Slc22a19, Slc22a26, Slc22a27, Slc22a28, Slc22a29, and Slc22a30 reside as well as the rat UST region on chromosome 1 that contains Slc22a9/a24, Slc22a9/a25, Ust4r, and Ust5r (Table 3) [70,71]. It has been proposed that genes within clusters, to some degree, are coordinately regulated and thus are predicted to have similar overall tissue expression patterns [70,72,73]. Support for shared regulatory mechanisms of subgroup members within genomic clusters can be inferred from similar patterns of tissue expression or by expression of subgroup members along a common axis of metabolite transport such as the gut–kidney–liver axis. Genomic localization from the UCSC Genome browser and resultant tissue expression patterns for all SLC22 members are shown in Table 3.

2.13. Analysis of OAT Subgroup Specific Motifs Highlight Patterns Potentially Involved in Specificity

Motif analyses revealed subgroup specific motifs within functionally important regions, such as the large ICD, large ECD, and the region spanning TMD9 and TMD10, for all novel OAT subgroups [10,74]. However, the number of unique residues appears to be correlated to the range of substrate specificity.

Of the newly proposed OAT subgroups, OATS2 claims the smallest number of subgroup-specific amino acid motifs and is the only subgroup without a specific motif in TMD9 (Figure 3B). The lack of multiple subgroup-specific regions is interesting not only because this subgroup consists of a single transporter but also because this may be indicative of a more promiscuous transporter with a wide range of substrates, which is substantiated by the functional data, as described earlier in "*OATS2 (SLC22A7) is a Systemically-Expressed Transporter of Organic Anions and Cyclic Nucleotides*". This pattern is also seen in OATS1, which consists of multi- and oligo-specific transporters OAT1, OAT3, and OAT6. In addition to having few subgroup-specific motifs, the multi/oligo-specific nature of this subgroup is reflected by the shared evolutionary conservation of the large extracellular domain with other OAT subclade members (Figure 3A).

To further clarify the membership of Oat-pg in OATS3, evolutionarily conserved motifs were determined between all three members, as well as just Slc22a11 and Slc22a12. This analysis revealed a total of ten evolutionarily conserved amino acid motifs between all three members, eight of which were present in the analysis of only OAT4 and URAT1 (Figure 3, Tables S4 and S5). Specifically, both analyses exhibited a notably large motif in the large intracellular loop found at D313-Q332 on URAT1 and

Q312-G331 on OAT-PG (Figure 3C,D). This larger number of conserved regions seems consistent with a more limited range of substrates (e.g., uric acid and prostaglandins) [43].

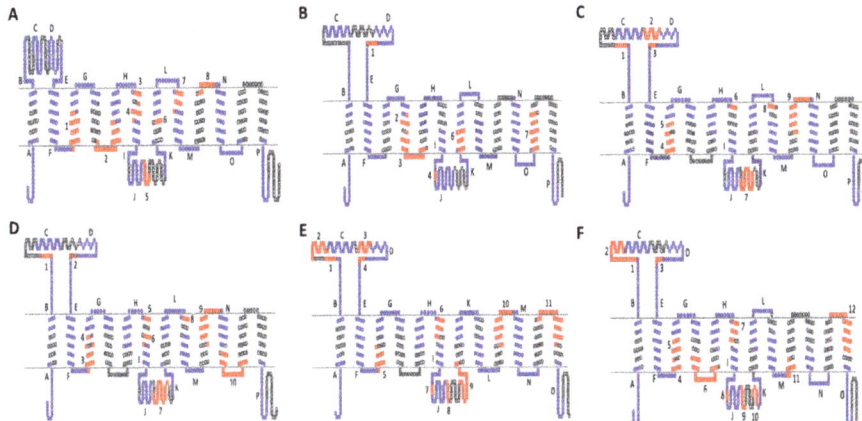

Figure 3. Evolutionarily conserved motifs for each subgroup within the OAT major subgroup mapped onto 2D topology of prototypical members. (**A**) OATS1 mapped onto SLC22A6 (OAT1). (**B**) OATS2 mapped onto hSLC22A7 (OAT2). (**C**) OATS3 mapped onto hSLC22A12 (URAT1). (**D**) OATS3 mapped onto mSlc22a22 (OAT-PG). (**E**) OATS4 mapped onto hSLC22A9 (OAT7). (**F**) OATS4 mapped onto mSlc22a7. In each panel, red sequences are subgroup specific motifs, blue sequences are OAT-major subgroup motifs. Conserved OAT-major subgroup motifs are assigned letters and specific, conserved OAT subgroup motifs are numbered. Data, including motif sequence identities, exact locations, and p-values can be found in Tables S2–S7.

Motif analysis was performed separately on the OATS4 rodent and non-rodent specific subgroups and the entirety of the OATS4 subgroup members. In all analyses, OATS4 claims the largest number of evolutionarily conserved and subgroup-specific amino acid residues amongst the OAT subgroups, supporting selective substrate specificity, possibly for conjugated sex steroids (Figure 3E,F). In the case of non-rodent transporters, a unique motif spanned the sixth extracellular domain and TMD12. This region is predicted to govern substrate specificity of transporters of the MFS, to which the SLC22 family belongs [74]. Recent publications defining the substrate specificity of SLC22A24 point to a more narrow range of substrates and conservation of this specific region amongst OATS4 members may explain the association of conjugated steroid hormones with SLC22A9, SLC22A10, SLC22A24, and SLC22A25 in GWAS studies [47,48]. Although further analysis was required to fully understand the relationship between the structure and substrate specificity in SLC22 transporters, we provided a basis for investigation into specific regions that might determine functional patterns. The sequences and p-values for each motif are in Tables S2–S7.

2.14. Sequence Similarity Study Suggests Novel Potential Functions to Explore and Possible Tertiary Structure of SLC22

Each SLC22 member is a putative transporter, but there is evidence that suggests some members may have alternative mechanisms of action [31,57]. To further explore this possibility and to potentially find sequence similarity to other proteins, the specific amino acid sequences for the extracellular and intracellular loops of each SLC22 member were compared to all proteins in the ICM-Pro v3.8-7c database. The large extracellular loop of the OCT subclade (hSLC22A1-A3) showed notable homologies to human, cow, mouse, and rat SCO-spondin, a glycoprotein secreted by the subcommissural organ in the brain. In all of these species, SCO-spondin contains two potent binding sites for glycosaminoglycan (BBXB) and cytokines (TXWSXWS) as well as LDL receptor type A repeats. Human SCO-spondin shares 28.97% (pP = 5.47) and 27.43% (pP = 5.33) sequence identity with human SLC22A1 ECD and SLC22A3 ECD, respectively. The extracellular loop of mouse Slc22a16 shares 26% sequence identity (pP = 5.4) with chicken beta-crystallin B3 (CRBB3). Beta-crystallin is a structural protein mainly comprised of beta sheets [75]. The similarity between the ECD of mouse Slc22a16 and CRBB3 could point to potential for a beta sheet like configuration. Since none of the SLC22 family members have been crystallized, any insight into tertiary structure is of interest.

SLC22A31, a member of the divergent OAT-Related subclade, is the most ambiguous member of the SLC22 family with no functional data available. An investigation of the human SLC22A31 large ECD shows at least 30% shared sequence identity with RNA-binding protein 42 (RBM42) in mouse, rat, cow, and human. This analysis also showed a 37% sequence identity (pP = 5.5) shared between the ECD of hSLC22A31 and human heterochromatinization factor BAHD1. These and other interesting sequence similarities to proteins, including those involved in signaling, are noted in Table 5.

Table 5. ICM finds significant similarities with SLC22 members. The following table shows significant amino acid similarities found between full-length and the ECD sequences of SLC22 members and other known proteins from human (*Homo sapiens*, h), cow (*Bos taurus*, b), chicken (*Gallus gallus*, g), mouse (*Mus musculus*, m), and rat (*rattus norvegicus*, r). No significant similarities were found for SLC22 ICDs. pP value is the log of the *p*-value and is described in the methods.

Subclade	SLC22 Family Member	Common Name	Non-SLC22 Protein	Identity Shared (%)	pP Value
OCT	hSLC22A1 ECD	OCT1	hSCO-spondin	28.97	5.47
			bSCO-spondin	30.84	5.35
			mSCO-spondin	24.3	6.24
			rSCO-spondin	24.3	6.16
	hSLC22A2 ECD	OCT2	bSCO-spondin	30.84	5.29
			mSCO-spondin	25.23	5.92
			rSCO-spondin	24.3	5.61
	hSLC22A3 ECD	OCT3	hSCO-spondin	27.43	5.33
			bSCO-spondin	22.12	5.49
			mSCO-spondin	27.43	5.89
			rSCO-spondin	25.66	5.81
OAT-related	hSLC22A31 ECD	n/a	hRBM42	30.95	5.95
			bRBM42	32.14	6.05
			mRBM42	30.95	5.95
			rRBM42	30.95	5.95
			hBAHD1	36.9	5.39
OCTN	mSlc22a16 ECD	FLIPT2, CT2	gCRBB3	26	5.4
	hSLC22A16		hTAS2R41	20	5.3
	hSLC22A5	OCTN2	GPR160	21	6.1

3. Discussion

In the years following the establishment of the previous SLC22 subclades, there has been a notable increase in functional data, particularly with respect to endogenous substrates, concerning these transporters and their substrates [10]. With these data, we are now in a position to better characterize the biology of these transporters, which play important physiological roles and are implicated in certain diseases. However, our newly proposed subgroups are not entirely dependent on functional data, as we have considered multiple approaches including phylogenetics, multiple sequence alignments, evolutionarily conserved motifs, sequence homology, and both tissue and genomic localization. Each of these approaches has individual value in that they reveal unique characteristics of each transporter; yet it is the combination of multiple approaches that ensures the full variety of available data (though still incomplete) for these transporters is considered when forming functional subgroups. We support the subgroups with a thorough literature search of metabolites associated with SLC22 proteins.

Although the functional data were inherently biased due to the high level of interest in some SLC22 members, particularly the "drug" transporters OAT1, OAT3, OCT1, and OCT2, for the majority of the transporters, there are enough data to create functional subgroups that play distinct and overlapping roles in metabolism (Figure 1, Table S1). Genomic localization reveals evolutionary information and provides insight on how genes may arise from duplication events. Phylogenetic analysis determines the evolutionary relatedness of these proteins, while MSA, motif analysis, and sequence homology focus on structural similarities, which can be indicative of function. We often see that members of a subgroup are expressed in the same tissues or along functional axes. For example, substrates transported from the liver via SLC22 transporters (e.g., SLC22A1/OCT1) can be either excreted into or retrieved from the urine by other SLC22 members (SLC22A2/OCT2) of the same subgroup. Establishment of these functional subgroups may also inform future virtual screenings for metabolites of understudied transporters.

Protein families are established based on shared ancestry and structural similarity, which is commonly considered grounds for shared functionality. This is exemplified amongst SLC22 members with the generally shared structural characteristics of 12 TMDs, a large extracellular loop between TMD1 and TMD2, and a smaller intracellular loop between TMD6 and TMD7. Despite these shared features, we show here that there are many functional differences between these transporters. Although our analyses mostly align with previous evolutionary studies when considering ancestry, here, we show that phylogenetic grouping is not always reflective of a similar structure and function. For example, although the previously established OCTN subclade of SLC22A4, SLC22A5, and Slc22a21 does not share common ancestry with Slc22a16, the newly proposed group shares functional similarity and ECD homology. Thus, by expanding our investigation beyond phylogenetic relationships, we can now more appropriately group proteins from the same family and better understand their roles in endogenous physiology.

An important concept in the remote sensing and signaling network is that of multi-specific, oligo-specific, and relatively mono-specific transporters working in a coordinated function [16]. Multi-specific transporters are able to interact with a wide variety of structurally different compounds, oligo-specific with a smaller variety, and relatively mono-specific transporters are thought to interact with only one or a few substrates. Existing functional data suggest that it is unlikely that any truly mono-specific transporters exist within the SLC22 family, yet the different subgroups we have formed imply that multi-specific, oligo-specific, and relatively mono-specific transporters are more likely to form subgroups with transporters that share substrate specificity. Multi-specific transporters, like those in the OATS1 and OCT subgroups, handle a diverse set of drugs, toxins, endogenous metabolites, and signaling molecules [14,61]. Conversely, the OATS4 subgroup appears to be a collection of relatively mono-specific transporters with an affinity for conjugated sex steroid hormones, specifically etiocholanolone glucuronide, which is also supported by a recent study focused on SLC22A24, a member of the OATS4 subgroup [47,48]. Previous evolutionary studies have suggested that multi-specific transporters arose before the mono-specific transporters [10]. As evolution has progressed, more specific transporters have developed to handle the burden of changing metabolism. The multi-specific transporters have been more extensively characterized because of their importance in pharmaceuticals, but in the case of endogenous metabolic diseases, the oligo and mono-specific transporters may be more appropriate targets for drugs or therapies.

One of the best examples of multi-specific transporters working in concert with oligo, and mono-specific transporters is the regulation of uric acid [17,18]. Handling of uric acid mainly occurs in the kidney, but when renal function is compromised, multi-specific transporters regulate their expression to compensate. Two proteins, SLC22A12 (URAT1) and SLC2A9, are expressed in the proximal tubule and are nearly exclusively associated with uric acid. The multi-specific transporters SLC22A6 (OAT1) and SLC22A8 (OAT3) are also present in the proximal tubule and are able to transport uric acid. When the kidney is damaged, one would expect serum uric acid levels to increase because most of the proteins involved in its elimination are in the kidney. However, this is partly mitigated due to the increased expression of ABCG2 and/or functional activity in the intestine [17,18]. SLC2A9 is a relatively mono-specific transporter and ABCG2 (BCRP) is a multi-specific ABC transporter, and other uric acid transporters can be considered oligo-specific (e.g., SLC22A11). The example of uric acid serves to illustrate how, when certain mono-, oligo-, and multi-specific transporters are unable to perform their primary function, multi-specific transporters of the same or different function (even of the ABC superfamily) can use their shared substrate specificity to mitigate the consequences. It is generally assumed that all SLC22 family members are transporters. However, Slc22a17, a member of the outlier OAT-related subclade, functions as an endocytosed iron-bound lipocalin receptor and some SLC22 members have been suggested to function as "transceptors" due to homology with GPCR odorant receptors and shared odorant substrates [20,21]. Thus, to better understand the SLC22 family members' individually unique functions and their placement into subgroups/subclades, we compared the full-length amino acid sequences, large ECDs, and large ICDs of all SLC22 family members to a database of known proteins.

When considering such a large number of proteins, the function on both local and systemic levels of metabolites is likely to be impacted. The SLC22 family is a central hub of coexpression for ADME (absorption, distribution, metabolism, excretion)-related genes in non-drug treated conditions, which underscores their importance in regulating endogenous metabolism through the transport of small molecules [16]. In the context of the remote sensing and signaling theory (RSST), it is essential to understand substrate specificity of different SLC22 members and the eight subgroups.

The RSST proposes that a network of ADME genes (drug transporters, drug metabolizing enzymes, and various regulation proteins) regulates the levels of hundreds if not thousands of small organic molecules with "high informational content" including key metabolites and signaling molecules involved in intra-organ, inter-organ, and inter-organismal remote communication. The RSST would seem to imply that organisms are constantly solving a multi-objective optimization problem, where balancing each particular compound's serum concentration represents a single objective. Each compound present in the blood has a range of healthy concentrations, and when the concentration is outside of that range, the body must address it, in part through the regulation of transporters and enzymes. Due to their wide range of tissue expression and diverse functional roles at body fluid interfaces, the particular combination of transporters and enzymes are critical variables necessary for solving this multi-objective optimization problem. Transporters regulate the entry and exit of substrates to and from cells, but enzymes are responsible for the altering of these compounds. To use a simple hypothetical example, if a metabolite's serum concentration is too high, a transporter with high affinity for that metabolite can move it into the cell, where an enzyme with high affinity for the substrate can change it so that it may re-enter the circulation or be more readily cleared from the body. The existence of abundant multi-specific and oligo-specific transporters and enzymes, in addition to relatively mono-specific ones, expressed differentially in tissues and at body fluid interfaces, allows for a highly flexible and responsive complex adaptive system that not only maintains homeostasis in blood, tissue, and body fluid compartments (e.g., cerebrospinal fluid), but also helps restore it after acute or chronic perturbations.

Thus, together, transporters and enzymes have tremendous potential to manage levels of metabolites, signaling molecules, and antioxidants in the circulation and in specific tissues. By developing functional groupings for the SLC22 family, we could better understand the metabolic networks in which they function and how their expression is utilized to regulate concentrations of metabolites, signaling molecules (e.g., cyclic nucleotides, prostaglandins, short chain fatty acids, and sex steroids), antioxidants (ergothioneine, uric acid), and other molecules affecting diverse aspects of homeostasis (e.g., lipocalin). Although this analysis focuses on the SLC22 family, a similar approach can be applied to develop a deeper understanding of other families of transporters and enzymes.

In the past, the majority of functional data have come from transport assays using cells overexpressing a specific SLC22 transporter and a single metabolite of interest. These assays lack uniformity and, as the OAT knockouts have shown, are not necessarily reflective of endogenous physiology [26,28,30]. Recently, GWAS studies have linked many metabolites to polymorphisms in SLC22 genes, and in vivo metabolomic studies using knockout models have also identified several metabolites that may be substrates of transporters [26,28,30,47]. In upcoming years, the integration of multiple types of omics data related to SLC22 family members with functional studies of transporters and evolutionary analyses will likely produce a more fine-grained picture of the roles of these and other transporters in inter-organ and inter-organismal remote sensing and signaling.

4. Materials and Methods

4.1. Data Collection

SLC22 human and mouse sequences were collected from the National Center for Biotechnology Information (NCBI) protein database. Sequences were confirmed and genomic loci were recorded using the University of California Santa Cruz (UCSC) genome browser by searching within each available species on the online platform (https://genome.ucsc.edu/cgi-bin/hgGateway) [76]. The NCBI BLASTp web-based program was used to find similar sequences to those from the NCBI protein database. BLASTp was run with default parameters using query SLC22 sequences from human or mouse. The database chosen was "non-redundant protein sequence" (nr) and no organisms were excluded [77]. Tissue expression of all human SLC22 members was collected from the Human Protein Atlas, GTEx dataset, Illumina Body Map, ENCODE dataset, and RNA-seq datasets available on the EMBL-EBI Expression Atlas (https://www.ebi.ac.uk/gxa/home) [78]. Tissue expression data were also collected via extensive literature search.

4.2. Sequence Alignment and Guide-Trees

Sequences for SLC22 were aligned using Clustal-Omega with default parameters via the online platform provided by the European Bioinformatics Institute (EMBL-EBI) (https://www.ebi.ac.uk/Tools/msa/clustalo/), as well as MAFFT (multiple alignment using fast Fourier transform) and ICM-Pro v3.8-7c [79–82]. Clustal-Omega, MAFFT, and ICM-Pro v3.8-7c produced similar topologies. These alignments were then visualized using The Interactive Tree of Life (http://itol.embl.de/) [83]. Topology was analyzed by branch length values, which are a result of the neighbor-joining method. This method calculates the number of amino acid changes between each organism and the common ancestor from which it branched. It then adopts the minimum-evolution criteria (ME) by building a tree, which minimizes the sum of all branch lengths to visually display relatedness [84]. SSearch36 was utilized to compare representative sequences of all members of the Drug:H+ Antiporter-1 (12 Spanner) (DHA1) Family (2.A.1.2) and the SLC22A family (2.A.1.19) from the Transporter Classification Database (http://www.tcdb.org/) with the Cyanate Porter (CP) Family (2.A.1.17) as an outgroup to further investigate the belongingness of SLC22A18 in either the SLC22 or DHA1 family [9,85]. SSearch36 is an exhaustive comparison method that uses the Smith–Waterman (SW) algorithm to compare FASTA files find sequence similarities [85,86].

ICM-Pro v3.8-7c was used to align sequences in FASTA format as well as perform homology searches of all human and mouse SLC22 sequences against ICM-Pro's curated database of all known proteins [82]. Threshold for homology significance was determined by the probability of structural insignificance (pP), defined as the negative log of the probability value of a homology comparison. Alignments were discarded if the pP value was less than 5.0, indicating that the homology shared between two sequences is likely not due to random sequence similarities.

4.3. Motif Analysis

Motif comparisons were performed on the subgroups of the OAT subclade using the multiple expectation-maximum for motif elicitation (MEME; http://meme-suite.org/tools/meme) suite [87]. A threshold of 20 motifs containing a range of 6–20 amino acid length was set with the normal discovery mode. This detection method yielded a set of evolutionarily conserved motifs within all OAT subclade sequences ($n = 57$) as well as a set of evolutionarily conserved motifs for each of the four proposed OAT subgroups. These motifs were then mapped onto 2D topologies of one member from each of the newly proposed OAT subgroups (SLC22A6 for OATS1, SLC22A7 for OATS2, SLC22A12 for OATS3, and SLC22A9 for OATS4). A separate motif analysis was also performed for the rodent expansion consisting of Slc22a19, and Slc22a26-30 and was mapped onto mouse Slc22a27. Transmembrane domains (TMDs) of these transporters were predicted by the constrained consensus topology prediction server (CCTOP; http://cctop.enzim.ttk.mta.hu/) [88]. TMD locations and the motif locations were entered into TOPO2 (http://www.sacs.ucsf.edu/TOPO2/) to visualize the 2D representation of the transporters with the OAT subclade's evolutionarily conserved motifs shown in blue and each subgroup's evolutionarily conserved motifs shown in red [89].

4.4. SNP, Mutation, In-Vitro, Knockout, and Drug Transport Data

To determine the diversity of substrate specificity, the number of drugs that list SLC22 members as a target on DrugBank were recorded [22]. The Metabolomics GWAS server was utilized to determine SNPs within all SLC22 members. The dataset produced by Shin et al. (2014) with the cohort KORA+TwinsUK (blood) and the association of single metabolites was chosen. This dataset was searched by gene symbol (e.g., SLC22A6) [37,90]. The EMBL GWAS Catalog and Metabolomix's table of all published GWAS with metabolomics (http://www.metabolomix.com/list-of-all-published-gwas-with-metabolomics/) were also utilized in searching for SNPs and their effect on metabolite transport by SLC22 members [91]. Current literature available on the NCBI gene database under gene references into functions (Gene RIFs; https://www.ncbi.nlm.nih.gov/gene/about-generif) was used to search for non-synonymous mutations that did not affect protein expression yet affected transport of metabolites and/or drugs. These methods were accompanied by an extensive literature search for in-vitro transport and knockout data. Most in-vitro data come from tissue culture assays from a variety of cell lines while most in-vivo data comes from genetic or chemical knockout mice. Metabolite data were abstracted from the aforementioned databases and confirmed via literature review. The import from table feature on Cytoscape 3.7.2 was used to generate functional networks for the entire SLC22 family and the subgroups [23]. A spring embedded layout was applied to the networks and the subgroups were color coded manually.

Supplementary Materials: Supplementary materials can be found at http://www.mdpi.com/1422-0067/21/5/1791/s1.

Author Contributions: (Contributor Roles Taxonomy-CRediT); Conceptualization, D.C.E., J.C.G., S.K.N.; methodology, D.C.E., J.C.G.; validation, M.H.S.J., M.E.B.; formal analysis, D.C.E., J.C.G., D.S.; resources, R.A., M.H.S.J., S.K.N.; data curation, D.C.E.; supervision, M.H.S.J., M.E.B. and S.K.N.; writing—original draft preparation, D.C.E., J.C.G.; writing—review and editing, D.C.E., J.C.G. and S.K.N.; visualization, D.C.E., J.C.G.; funding acquisition, S.K.N. All authors have read and agreed to the published version of the manuscript.

Funding: This work was supported by the National Institutes of Health by grants R01DK109392 and R01GM132938 awarded to S.K.N. and the training grant T32EB009380 awarded to J.C.G. Support for R.A.'s group came from the National Institutes of Health grant R35GM131881.

Conflicts of Interest: The authors declare no conflict of interest.

Abbreviations

SLC22	Solute Carrier Family 22
OAT	Organic Anion Transporter
OCT	Organic Cation Transporter
OCTN	Organic Zwitterion Transporter
GWAS	Genome Wide Association Study
SNP	Single Nucleotide Polymorphism
EGT	Ergothioneine
TMD	Transmembrane Domain
ECD	Extracellular Domain

ICD	Intracellular Domain
MFS	Major Facilitator Superfamily
ABCG2	ATP-Binding Cassette Subfamily G, Member 2
MSA	Multiple Sequence Alignment
MPP+	1-methyl-4-phenylpyridinium
TEA	tetraethylammonium
RSST	Remote Sensing and Signaling Theory

References

1. Hediger, M.A.; Clémençon, B.; Burrier, R.E.; Bruford, E.A. The ABCs of membrane transporters in health and disease (SLC series): Introduction. *Mol. Asp. Med.* **2013**, *34*, 95–107. [CrossRef]
2. Lamhonwah, A.M.; Hawkins, C.E.; Tam, C.; Wong, J.; Mai, L.; Tein, I. Expression patterns of the organic cation/carnitine transporter family in adult murine brain. *Brain Dev.* **2008**, *30*, 31–42. [CrossRef]
3. Sager, G.; Smaglyukova, N.; Fuskevaag, O.M. The role of OAT2 (SLC22A7) in the cyclic nucleotide biokinetics of human erythrocytes. *J. Cell. Physiol.* **2018**, *233*, 5972–5980. [CrossRef]
4. Minuesa, G.; Purcet, S.; Erkizia, I.; Molina-Arcas, M.; Bofill, M.; Izquierdo-Useros, N.; Casado, J.F.; Clotet, B.; Pastor-Anglada, M.; Martinez-Picado, J. Expression and functionality of anti-human immunodeficiency virus and anticancer drug uptake transporters in immune cells. *J. Pharmacol. Exp. Ther.* **2008**, *324*, 558–567. [CrossRef]
5. César-Razquin, A.; Snijder, B.; Frappier-Brinton, T.; Hediger, M.A.; Edwards, A.M.; Superti-Furga, G. A Call for Systematic Research on Solute Carriers. *Cell* **2015**, *162*, 478–487.
6. Lelandais-Brière, C.; Jovanovic, M.; Torres, G.A.M.; Perrin, Y.; Lemoine, R.; Corre-Menguy, F.; Hartmann, C. Disruption of AtOCT1, an organic cation transporter gene, affects root development and carnitine-related responses in Arabidopsis. *Plant J.* **2007**, *51*, 154–164. [CrossRef]
7. Uhlén, M.; Fagerberg, L.; Hallström, B.M.; Lindskog, C.; Oksvold, P.; Mardinoglu, A.; Sivertsson, Å.; Kampf, C.; Sjöstedt, E.; Asplund, A.; et al. Tissue-based map of the human proteome. *Science* **2015**, *347*, 1260419.
8. Lopez-Nieto, C.E.; You, G.; Bush, K.T.; Barros, E.J.G.; Beier, D.R.; Nigam, S.K. Molecular cloning and characterization of NKT, a gene product related to the organic cation transporter family that is almost exclusively expressed in the kidney. *J. Biol. Chem.* **1997**, *272*, 6471–6478. [CrossRef]
9. Saier, M.H.; Reddy, V.S.; Tamang, D.S.; Västermark, Å. The transporter classification database. *Nucleic Acids Res.* **2014**, *42*, D251–D258. [CrossRef]
10. Zhu, C.; Nigam, K.B.; Date, R.C.; Bush, K.T.; Springer, S.A.; Saier, M.H.; Wu, W.; Nigam, S.K. Evolutionary analysis and classification of OATs, OCTs, OCTNs, and other SLC22 transporters: Structure-function implications and analysis of sequence motifs. *PLoS ONE* **2015**, *10*, e0140569. [CrossRef]
11. Nigam, S.K. The SLC22 Transporter Family: A Paradigm for the Impact of Drug Transporters on Metabolic Pathways, Signaling, and Disease. *Annu. Rev. Pharmacol. Toxicol.* **2018**, *58*, 663–687. [CrossRef]
12. Ahn, S.Y.; Nigam, S.K. Toward a systems level understanding of organic anion and other multispecific drug transporters: A remote sensing and signaling hypothesis. *Mol. Pharmacol.* **2009**, *76*, 481–490. [CrossRef]
13. Wu, W.; Dnyanmote, A.V.; Nigam, S.K. Remote communication through solute carriers and ATP binding cassette drug transporter pathways: An update on the Remote Sensing and Signaling Hypothesis. *Mol. Pharmacol.* **2011**, *79*, 795–805. [CrossRef]
14. Nigam, S.K.; Bush, K.T.; Martovetsky, G.; Ahn, S.Y.; Liu, H.C.; Richard, E.; Bhatnagar, V.; Wu, W. The organic anion transporter (OAT) family: A systems biology perspective. *Physiol. Rev.* **2015**, *95*, 83–123. [CrossRef]
15. Nigam, S.K. What do drug transporters really do? *Nat. Rev. Drug Discov.* **2014**, *14*, 29–44. [CrossRef]
16. Rosenthal, S.B.; Bush, K.T.; Nigam, S.K. A Network of SLC and ABC Transporter and DME Genes Involved in Remote Sensing and Signaling in the Gut-Liver-Kidney Axis. *Sci. Rep.* **2019**, *9*, 11879. [CrossRef]
17. Bhatnagar, V.; Richard, E.L.; Wu, W.; Nievergelt, C.M.; Lipkowitz, M.S.; Jeff, J.; Maihofer, A.X.; Nigam, S.K. Analysis of ABCG2 and other urate transporters in uric acid homeostasis in chronic kidney disease: Potential role of remote sensing and signaling. *Clin. Kidney J.* **2016**, *9*, 444–453. [CrossRef]

18. Yano, H.; Tamura, Y.; Kobayashi, K.; Tanemoto, M.; Uchida, S. Uric acid transporter ABCG2 is increased in the intestine of the 5/6 nephrectomy rat model of chronic kidney disease. *Clin. Exp. Nephrol.* **2014**, *18*, 50–55. [CrossRef]
19. Nigam, S.K.; Bhatnagar, V. The systems biology of uric acid transporters: The role of remote sensing and signaling. *Curr. Opin. Nephrol. Hypertens.* **2018**, *27*, 305–313. [CrossRef]
20. Langelueddecke, C.; Roussa, E.; Fenton, R.; Wolff, N.; Lee, W.K.; Thévenod, F. Lipocalin-2 (24p3/neutrophil gelatinase-associated lipocalin (NGAL)) receptor is expressed in distal nephron and mediates protein endocytosis. *J. Biol. Chem.* **2012**, *287*, 159–169. [CrossRef]
21. Kaler, G.; Truong, D.M.; Sweeney, D.E.; Logan, D.W.; Nagle, M.; Wu, W.; Eraly, S.A.; Nigam, S.K. Olfactory mucosa-expressed organic anion transporter, Oat6, manifests high affinity interactions with odorant organic anions. *Biochem. Biophys. Res. Commun.* **2006**, *351*, 872–876. [CrossRef]
22. Wishart, D.S.; Feunang, Y.D.; Guo, A.C.; Lo, E.J.; Marcu, A.; Grant, J.R.; Sajed, T.; Johnson, D.; Li, C.; Sayeeda, Z.; et al. DrugBank 5.0: A major update to the DrugBank database for 2018. *Nucleic Acids Res.* **2018**, *46*, D1074–D1082. [CrossRef]
23. Smoot, M.E.; Ono, K.; Ruscheinski, J.; Wang, P.L.; Ideker, T. Cytoscape 2.8: New features for data integration and network visualization. *Bioinformatics* **2011**, *27*, 431–432. [CrossRef]
24. Bremer, J. Carnitine. Metabolism and functions. *Physiol. Rev.* **1983**, *63*, 1420–1480. [CrossRef]
25. Blumberg, A.L.; Denny, S.E.; Marshall, G.E.; Needleman, P. Blood vessel hormone interactions: Angiotensin, bradykinin, and prostaglandins. *Am. J. Physiol.* **1977**, *232*, H305–H310. [CrossRef]
26. Wikoff, W.R.; Nagle, M.A.; Kouznetsova, V.L.; Tsigelny, I.F.; Nigam, S.K. Untargeted metabolomics identifies enterobiome metabolites and putative uremic toxins as substrates of organic anion transporter 1 (Oat1). *J. Proteome Res.* **2011**, *10*, 2842–2851. [CrossRef]
27. Vallon, V.; Eraly, S.A.; Rao, S.R.; Gerasimova, M.; Rose, M.; Nagle, M.; Anzai, N.; Smith, T.; Sharma, K.; Nigam, S.K.; et al. A role for the organic anion transporter OAT3 in renal creatinine secretion in mice. *Am. J. Physiol. Ren. Physiol.* **2012**, *302*, F1293–F1299. [CrossRef]
28. Wu, W.; Bush, K.T.; Nigam, S.K. Key Role for the Organic Anion Transporters, OAT1 and OAT3, in the in vivo Handling of Uremic Toxins and Solutes. *Sci. Rep.* **2017**, *7*, 1–9. [CrossRef]
29. Kimura, H.; Takeda, M.; Narikawa, S.; Enomoto, A.; Ichida, K.; Endou, H. Human organic anion transporters and human organic cation transporters mediate renal transport of prostaglandins. *J. Pharmacol. Exp. Ther.* **2002**, *301*, 293–298. [CrossRef]
30. Bush, K.T.; Wu, W.; Lun, C.; Nigam, S.K. The drug transporter OAT3 (SLC22A8) and endogenous metabolite communication via the gut–liver–kidney axis. *J. Biol. Chem.* **2017**, *292*, 15789–15803. [CrossRef]
31. Wu, W.; Bush, K.T.; Liu, H.C.; Zhu, C.; Abagyan, R.; Nigam, S.K. Shared ligands between organic anion transporters (OAT1 and OAT6) and odorant receptors. *Drug Metab. Dispos.* **2015**, *43*, 1855–1863. [CrossRef]
32. Monte, J.C.; Nagle, M.A.; Eraly, S.A.; Nigam, S.K. Identification of a novel murine organic anion transporter family member, OAT6, expressed in olfactory mucosa. *Biochem. Biophys. Res. Commun.* **2004**, *323*, 429–436. [CrossRef]
33. Bien, S.A.; Su, Y.R.; Conti, D.V.; Harrison, T.A.; Qu, C.; Guo, X.; Lu, Y.; Albanes, D.; Auer, P.L.; Banbury, B.L.; et al. Genetic variant predictors of gene expression provide new insight into risk of colorectal cancer. *Hum. Genet.* **2019**, *138*, 307–326. [CrossRef]
34. Wu, X.; Kekuda, R.; Huang, W.; Fei, Y.J.; Leibach, F.H.; Chen, J.; Conway, S.J.; Ganapathy, V. Identity of the organic cation transporter OCT3 as the extraneuronal monoamine transporter (uptake2) and evidence for the expression of the transporter in the brain. *J. Biol. Chem.* **1998**, *273*, 32776–32786. [CrossRef]
35. Shen, H.; Liu, T.; Morse, B.L.; Zhao, Y.; Zhang, Y.; Qiu, X.; Chen, C.; Lewin, A.C.; Wang, X.T.; Liu, G.; et al. Characterization of Organic Anion Transporter 2 (SLC22A7): A Highly Efficient Transporter for Creatinine and Species-Dependent Renal Tubular Expression. *Drug Metab. Dispos.* **2015**, *43*, 984–993. [CrossRef]
36. Köttgen, A.; Albrecht, E.; Teumer, A.; Vitart, V.; Krumsiek, J.; Hundertmark, C.; Pistis, G.; Ruggiero, D.; O'Seaghdha, C.M.; Haller, T.; et al. Genome-wide association analyses identify 18 new loci associated with serum urate concentrations. *Nat. Genet.* **2013**, *45*, 145–154. [CrossRef]
37. Shin, S.Y.; Fauman, E.B.; Petersen, A.K.; Krumsiek, J.; Santos, R.; Huang, J.; Arnold, M.; Erte, I.; Forgetta, V.; Yang, T.P. An atlas of genetic influences on human blood metabolites. *Nat. Genet.* **2014**, *46*, 543–550. [CrossRef]

38. Sun, W.; Wu, R.R.; Van Poelje, P.D.; Erion, M.D. Isolation of a family of organic anion transporters from human liver and kidney. *Biochem. Biophys. Res. Commun.* **2001**, *283*, 417–422. [CrossRef]
39. Eraly, S.A.; Vallon, V.; Rieg, T.; Gangoiti, J.A.; Wikoff, W.R.; Siuzdak, G.; Barshop, B.A.; Nigam, S.K. Multiple organic anion transporters contribute to net renal excretion of uric acid. *Physiol. Genom.* **2008**, *33*, 180–192. [CrossRef]
40. Hagos, Y.; Stein, D.; Ugele, B.; Burckhardt, G.; Bahn, A. Human renal organic anion transporter 4 operates as an asymmetric urate transporter. *J. Am. Soc. Nephrol.* **2007**, *18*, 430–439. [CrossRef]
41. Maxwell, S.R.; Thomason, H.; Sandler, D.; Leguen, C.; Baxter, M.A.; Thorpe, G.H.; Jones, A.F.; Barnett, A.H. Antioxidant status in patients with uncomplicated insulin-dependent and non-insulin-dependent diabetes mellitus. *Eur. J. Clin. Investig.* **1997**, *27*, 484–490. [CrossRef]
42. Sakiyama, M.; Matsuo, H.; Shimizu, S.; Nakashima, H.; Nakayama, A.; Chiba, T.; Naito, M.; Takada, T.; Suzuki, H.; Hamajima, N.; et al. A common variant of organic anion transporter 4 (OAT4/SLC22A11) gene is associated with renal underexcretion type gout. *Drug Metab. Pharmacokinet.* **2014**, *29*, 208–210. [CrossRef]
43. Cha, S.H.; Sekine, T.; Kusuhara, H.; Yu, E.; Kim, J.Y.; Kim, D.K.; Sugiyama, Y.; Kanai, Y.; Endou, H. Molecular cloning and characterization of multispecific organic anion transporter 4 expressed in the placenta. *J. Biol. Chem.* **2000**, *275*, 4507–4512. [CrossRef]
44. Tomi, M.; Eguchi, H.; Ozaki, M.; Tawara, T.; Nishimura, S.; Higuchi, K.; Maruyama, T.; Nishimura, T.; Nakashima, E. Role of OAT4 in uptake of estriol precursor 16α-hydroxydehydroepiandrosterone sulfate into human placental syncytiotrophoblasts from fetus. *Endocrinology* **2015**, *156*, 2704–2712. [CrossRef]
45. Skwara, P.; Schömig, E.; Gründemann, D. A novel mode of operation of SLC22A11: Membrane insertion of estrone sulfate versus translocation of uric acid and glutamate. *Biochem. Pharmacol.* **2017**, *128*, 74–82. [CrossRef]
46. Shiraya, K.; Hirata, T.; Hatano, R.; Nagamori, S.; Wiriyasermkul, P.; Jutabha, P.; Matsubara, M.; Muto, S.; Tanaka, H.; Asano, S.; et al. A novel transporter of SLC22 family specifically transports prostaglandins and co-localizes with 15-hydroxyprostaglandin dehydrogenase in renal proximal tubules. *J. Biol. Chem.* **2010**, *285*, 22141–22151. [CrossRef]
47. Long, T.; Hicks, M.; Yu, H.C.; Biggs, W.H.; Kirkness, E.F.; Menni, C.; Zierer, J.; Small, K.S.; Mangino, M.; Messier, H.; et al. Whole-genome sequencing identifies common-to-rare variants associated with human blood metabolites. *Nat. Genet.* **2017**, *49*, 568–578. [CrossRef]
48. Yee, S.W.; Stecula, A.; Chien, H.C.; Zou, L.; Feofanova, E.V.; Van Borselen, M.; Cheung, K.W.K.; Yousri, N.A.; Suhre, K.; Kinchen, J.M.; et al. Unraveling the functional role of the orphan solute carrier, SLC22A24 in the transport of 2 steroid conjugates through metabolomic and genome-wide association studies. *PLoS Genet.* **2019**, *15*, e1008208. [CrossRef]
49. Shin, H.J.; Anzai, N.; Enomoto, A.; He, X.; Kim, D.K.; Endou, H.; Kanai, Y. Novel liver-specific organic anion transporter OAT7 that operates the exchange of sulfate conjugates for short chain fatty acid butyrate. *Hepatology* **2007**, *45*, 1046–1055. [CrossRef]
50. Sardiello, M.; Annunziata, I.; Roma, G.; Ballabio, A. Sulfatases and sulfatase modifying factors: An exclusive and promiscuous relationship. *Hum. Mol. Genet.* **2005**, *14*, 3203–3217. [CrossRef]
51. Papatheodorou, I.; Fonseca, N.A.; Keays, M.; Tang, Y.A.; Barrera, E.; Bazant, W.; Burke, M.; Füllgrabe, A.; Fuentes, A.M.P.; George, N.; et al. Expression Atlas: Gene and protein expression across multiple studies and organisms. *Nucleic Acids Res.* **2018**, *46*, D246–D251. [CrossRef]
52. Bahn, A.; Hagos, Y.; Reuter, S.; Balen, D.; Brzica, H.; Krick, W.; Burckhardt, B.C.; Sabolić, I.; Burckhardt, G. Identification of a new urate and high affinity nicotinate transporter - human organic anion transporter 10 (hOAT10, SLC22A13). *J. Biol. Chem.* **2008**, *283*, 16332–16341. [CrossRef]
53. Uhl, G.R.; Liu, Q.R.; Drgon, T.; Johnson, C.; Walther, D.; Rose, J.E.; David, S.P.; Niaura, R.; Lerman, C. Molecular genetics of successful smoking cessation: Convergent genome-wide association study results. *Arch. Gen. Psychiatry* **2008**, *65*, 683–693. [CrossRef]
54. Uhl, G.R.; Drgon, T.; Li, C.Y.; Johnson, C.; Liu, Q.R. Smoking and smoking cessation in disadvantaged women: Assessing genetic contributions. *Drug Alcohol Depend.* **2009**, *104*, S58–S63. [CrossRef]
55. Maruyama, S.Y.; Ito, M.; Ikami, Y.; Okitsu, Y.; Ito, C.; Toshimori, K.; Fujii, W.; Yogo, K. A critical role of solute carrier 22a14 in sperm motility and male fertility in mice. *Sci. Rep.* **2016**, *6*, 36468. [CrossRef]
56. Bennett, K.M.; Liu, J.; Hoelting, C.; Stoll, J. Expression and analysis of two novel rat organic cation transporter homologs, SLC22A17 and SLC22A23. *Mol. Cell. Biochem.* **2011**, *352*, 143–154. [CrossRef]

57. Wan-Jie, C.; Wei-Yi, O.; Gavin, D. Lipocalin 2 and lipocalin 2 receptor in neuron-glia interactions following injury. *Front. Cell. Neurosci.* **2016**, *10*. [CrossRef]
58. Zhao, Z.Z.; Croft, L.; Nyholt, D.R.; Chapman, B.; Treloar, S.A.; Hull, M.L.; Montgomery, G.W. Evaluation of polymorphisms in predicted target sites for micro RNAs differentially expressed in endometriosis. *Mol. Hum. Reprod.* **2011**, *17*, 92–103. [CrossRef]
59. Serrano León, A.; Amir Shaghaghi, M.; Yurkova, N.; Bernstein, C.N.; El-Gabalawy, H.; Eck, P. Single-nucleotide polymorphisms in SLC22A23 are associated with ulcerative colitis in a Canadian white cohort. *Am. J. Clin. Nutr.* **2014**, *100*, 289–294. [CrossRef]
60. Aberg, K.; Adkins, D.E.; Liu, Y.; McClay, J.L.; Bukszár, J.; Jia, P.; Zhao, Z.; Perkins, D.; Stroup, T.S.; Lieberman, J.A.; et al. Genome-wide association study of antipsychotic-induced QTc interval prolongation. *Pharmacogenomics J.* **2012**, *12*, 165–172. [CrossRef]
61. Nigam, A.K.; Li, J.G.; Lall, K.; Shi, D.; Bush, K.T.; Bhatnagar, V.; Abagyan, R.; Nigam, S.K. Unique metabolite preferences of the drug transporters OAT1 and OAT3 analyzed by machine learning. *J. Biol. Chem.* **2020**, *RA119*, 010729. [CrossRef]
62. Busch, A.E.; Quester, S.; Ulzheimer, J.C.; Gorboulev, V.; Akhoundova, A.; Waldegger, S.; Lang, F.; Koepsell, H. Monoamine neurotransmitter transport mediated by the polyspecific cation transport rOCT1. *FEBS Lett.* **1996**, *395*, 153–156. [CrossRef]
63. Gründemann, D.; Liebich, G.; Kiefer, N.; Köster, S.; Schömig, E. Selective substrates for non-neuronal monoamine transporters. *Mol. Pharmacol.* **1999**, *56*, 1–10. [CrossRef]
64. Urakami, Y.; Kimura, N.; Okuda, M.; Inui, K.I. Creatinine transport by basolateral organic cation transporter hOCT2 in the human kidney. *Pharm. Res.* **2004**, *21*, 976–981. [CrossRef]
65. Enomoto, A.; Wempe, M.F.; Tsuchida, H.; Shin, H.J.; Cha, S.H.; Anzai, N.; Goto, A.; Sakamoto, A.; Niwa, T.; Kanai, Y.; et al. Molecular identification of a novel carnitine transporter specific to human testis: Insights into the mechanism of carnitine recognition. *J. Biol. Chem.* **2002**, *277*, 36262–36271. [CrossRef]
66. Ohashi, R.; Tamai, I.; Yabuuchi, H.; Nezu, J.I.; Oku, A.; Sai, Y.; Shimane, M.; Tsuji, A. Na+-dependent carnitine transport by organic cation transporter (OCTN2): Its pharmacological and toxicological relevance. *J. Pharmacol. Exp. Ther.* **1999**, *291*, 778–784.
67. Gründemann, D.; Harlfinger, S.; Golz, S.; Geerts, A.; Lazar, A.; Berkels, R.; Jung, N.; Rubbert, A.; Schömig, E. Discovery of the ergothioneine transporter. *Proc. Natl. Acad. Sci. USA* **2005**, *102*, 5256–5261. [CrossRef]
68. Cheah, I.K.; Halliwell, B. Ergothioneine; antioxidant potential, physiological function and role in disease. *Biochim. et Biophys. Acta Mol. Basis Dis.* **2012**, *1822*, 784–793. [CrossRef]
69. Ogden, T.H.; Rosenberg, M.S. Multiple sequence alignment accuracy and phylogenetic inference. *Syst. Biol.* **2006**, *55*, 314–328. [CrossRef]
70. Wu, W.; Baker, M.E.; Eraly, S.A.; Bush, K.T.; Nigam, S.K. Analysis of a large cluster of SLC22 transporter genes, including novel USTs, reveals species-specific amplification of subsets of family members. *Physiol. Genom.* **2009**, *38*, 116–124. [CrossRef]
71. Yokoyama, H.; Anzai, N.; Ljubojevic, M.; Ohtsu, N.; Sakata, T.; Miyazaki, H.; Nonoguchi, H.; Islam, R.; Onozato, M.; Tojo, A.; et al. Functional and immunochemical characterization of a novel organic anion transporter Oat8 (Slc22a9) in rat renal collecting duct. *Cell. Physiol. Biochem.* **2008**, *21*, 269–278. [CrossRef]
72. Eraly, S.A.; Monte, J.C.; Nigam, S.K. Novel slc22 transporter homologs in fly, worm, and human clarify the phylogeny of organic anion and cation transporters. *Physiol. Genom.* **2004**, *18*, 12–24. [CrossRef]
73. Eraly, S.A.; Nigam, S.K. Novel human cDNAs homologous to Drosophila Orct and mammalian carnitine transporters. *Biochem. Biophys. Res. Commun.* **2002**, *297*, 1159–1166. [CrossRef]
74. Quistgaard, E.M.; Löw, C.; Guettou, F.; Nordlund, P. Understanding transport by the major facilitator superfamily (MFS): Structures pave the way. *Nat. Rev. Mol. Cell Biol.* **2016**, *17*, 123–132. [CrossRef]
75. Inana, G.; Piatigorsky, J.; Norman, B.; Slingsby, C.; Blundell, T. Gene and protein structure of a β-crystallin polypeptide in murine lens: Relationship of exons and structural motifs. *Nature* **1983**, *302*, 310–315. [CrossRef]
76. Casper, J.; Zweig, A.S.; Villarreal, C.; Tyner, C.; Speir, M.L.; Rosenbloom, K.R.; Raney, B.J.; Lee, C.M.; Lee, B.T.; Karolchik, D.; et al. The UCSC Genome Browser database: 2018 update. *Nucleic Acids Res.* **2018**, *46*, D762–D769.
77. Altschul, S.F.; Gish, W.; Miller, W.; Myers, E.W.; Lipman, D.J. Basic local alignment search tool. *J. Mol. Biol.* **1990**, *215*, 403–410. [CrossRef]

78. Madeira, F.; Park, Y.M.; Lee, J.; Buso, N.; Gur, T.; Madhusoodanan, N.; Basutkar, P.; Tivey, A.R.; Potter, S.C.; Finn, R.D. The EMBL-EBI search and sequence analysis tools APIs in 2019. *Nucleic Acids Res.* **2019**, *47*, W636–W641. [CrossRef]
79. Sievers, F.; Higgins, D.G. Clustal Omega for making accurate alignments of many protein sequences. *Protein Sci.* **2018**, *27*, 135–145. [CrossRef]
80. Sievers, F.; Wilm, A.; Dineen, D.; Gibson, T.J.; Karplus, K.; Li, W.; Lopez, R.; McWilliam, H.; Remmert, M.; Söding, J.; et al. Fast, scalable generation of high-quality protein multiple sequence alignments using Clustal Omega. *Mol. Syst. Biol.* **2011**, *7*. [CrossRef]
81. Katoh, K.; Standley, D.M. MAFFT multiple sequence alignment software version 7: Improvements in performance and usability. *Mol. Biol. Evol.* **2013**, *30*, 772–780. [CrossRef] [PubMed]
82. Abagyan, R.; Totrov, M.; Kuznetsov, D. ICM—A new method for protein modeling and design: Applications to docking and structure prediction from the distorted native conformation. *J. Comput. Chem.* **1994**, *15*, 488–506. [CrossRef]
83. Letunic, I.; Bork, P. Interactive Tree Of Life (iTOL) v4: Recent updates and new developments. *Nucleic Acids Res.* **2019**, *47*, W256–W259. [CrossRef] [PubMed]
84. Saitou, N.; Nei, M. The neighbor-joining method: A new method for reconstructing phylogenetic trees. *Mol. Biol. Evol.* **1987**, *4*, 406–425. [PubMed]
85. Reddy, V.S.; Saier, M.H. BioV Suite—A collection of programs for the study of transport protein evolution. *FEBS J.* **2012**, *279*, 2036–2046. [CrossRef] [PubMed]
86. Smith, T.F.; Waterman, M.S. Identification of common molecular subsequences. *J. Mol. Biol.* **1981**, *147*, 195–197. [CrossRef]
87. Bailey, T.L.; Elkan, C. Fitting a mixture model by expectation maximization to discover motifs in biopolymers. *Proc. Int. Conf. Intell. Syst. Mol. Biol.* **1994**, *2*, 28–36.
88. Dobson, L.; Reményi, I.; Tusnády, G.E. CCTOP: A Consensus Constrained TOPology prediction web server. *Nucleic Acids Res.* **2015**, *43*, W408–W412. [CrossRef]
89. Johns, S.J. TOPO2, Transmembrane Protein Display Software. Available online: http://www.sacs.ucsf.edu/TOPO2/ (accessed on 3 March 2020).
90. Suhre, K.; Shin, S.Y.; Petersen, A.K.; Mohney, R.P.; Meredith, D.; Wägele, B.; Altmaier, E.; Deloukas, P.; Erdmann, J.; Grundberg, E.; et al. Human metabolic individuality in biomedical and pharmaceutical research. *Nature* **2011**, *477*, 54–62. [CrossRef]
91. Kastenmüller, G.; Raffler, J.; Gieger, C.; Suhre, K. Genetics of human metabolism: An update. *Human Mol. Genet.* **2015**, *24*, R93–R101. [CrossRef]

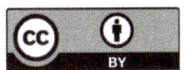

© 2020 by the authors. Licensee MDPI, Basel, Switzerland. This article is an open access article distributed under the terms and conditions of the Creative Commons Attribution (CC BY) license (http://creativecommons.org/licenses/by/4.0/).

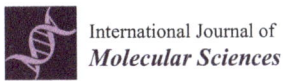

Review

Organic Cation Transporters in the Lung—Current and Emerging (Patho)Physiological and Pharmacological Concepts

Mohammed Ali Selo [1,2,*], Johannes A. Sake [1], Carsten Ehrhardt [1] and Johanna J. Salomon [3,*]

1. School of Pharmacy and Pharmaceutical Sciences and Trinity Biomedical Sciences Institute (TBSI), Trinity College Dublin, Dublin 2, Ireland; jsake@tcd.ie (J.A.S.); ehrhardc@tcd.ie (C.E.)
2. Faculty of Pharmacy, University of Kufa, 540011 Al-Najaf, Iraq
3. Translational Lung Research Center Heidelberg (TLRC), German Center for Lung Research (DZL), Department of Translational Pulmonology, University of Heidelberg, 69120 Heidelberg, Germany
* Correspondence: selom@tcd.ie (M.A.S.); Johanna.Salomon@med.uni-heidelberg.de (J.J.S.)

Received: 30 October 2020; Accepted: 27 November 2020; Published: 1 December 2020

Abstract: Organic cation transporters (OCT) 1, 2 and 3 and novel organic cation transporters (OCTN) 1 and 2 of the solute carrier 22 (SLC22) family are involved in the cellular transport of endogenous compounds such as neurotransmitters, L-carnitine and ergothioneine. OCT/Ns have also been implicated in the transport of xenobiotics across various biological barriers, for example biguanides and histamine receptor antagonists. In addition, several drugs used in the treatment of respiratory disorders are cations at physiological pH and potential substrates of OCT/Ns. OCT/Ns may also be associated with the development of chronic lung diseases such as allergic asthma and chronic obstructive pulmonary disease (COPD) and, thus, are possible new drug targets. As part of the Special Issue "Physiology, Biochemistry and Pharmacology of Transporters for Organic Cations", this review provides an overview of recent findings on the (patho)physiological and pharmacological functions of organic cation transporters in the lung.

Keywords: pulmonary drug delivery; SLC22A1–5; lung epithelium; drug uptake; β2-agonists; chronic lung diseases; anticholinergics

---

1. Introduction

Organic cation transmembrane transporters belonging to the solute carrier family 22 (i.e., SLC22A1–A5) are increasingly recognised as "impactors" of drug disposition in the respiratory tract [1–3]. SLC22A1–A5 transporters can be further divided according to the driving force of cation transport into membrane-potential-sensitive organic cation transporters (OCTs) or Na$^+$ and pH-dependent novel organic cation transporters (OCTNs) [4,5]. The human OCT subclass consists of OCT1 (SLC22A1), OCT2 (SLC22A2) and OCT3 (SLC22A3), whereas the OCTN subclass includes OCTN1 (SLC22A4) and OCTN2 (SLC22A5). According to the human protein atlas, hOCT1 is a 61 kDa protein exhibiting a broad tissue distribution with high expression levels in the liver [6,7]. hOCT2, with a less ubiquitous expression pattern than hOCT1 and hOCT3, is most strongly expressed in the kidneys with an approximate molecular size of 63 kDa [6,8]. The tissue expression pattern of OCT3 (61 kDa) is very broad, with high levels being observed in the liver, skeletal muscle, placenta and heart [8,9]. OCTN1 and OCTN2 also exhibit broad tissue distribution, and both are approximately 62 kDa proteins [8,9]. OCT/N transporters participate in the cellular transport of a broad spectrum of endogenous and exogenous organic cations and zwitterions such as neurotransmitters and xenobiotics. Thus, they are involved in clinical drug–transporter interactions and at the same time, they perform important physiological functions [9,10]. OCT1, for example mediates thiamine uptake, modulates hepatic glucose and lipid metabolism and thereby plays a role in hepatic steatosis [11,12]. In the brain, OCT2 and OCT3 are involved in the regulation of a variety of normal central nervous system functions related to mood as well as salt-intake behaviour and osmoregulation [13–15]. Detailed information on OCTs' expression and function in organs (except for the lung) was recently reviewed and can be found in this Special Issue of International Journal of Molecular Sciences [16]. With a focus on the lung, reviews by Salomon et al. [2] and Nickel et al. [3] have provided comprehensive overviews of pulmonary OCT/Ns' expression and function to the reader. Generally, OCTs in airway epithelial and smooth muscle cells accept physiological substrates such as dopamine, histamine, serotonin and acetylcholine. OCTN1 and OCTN2 mediate the uptake of ergothioneine (ESH) and L-carnitine, respectively. The exact roles of OCT/N transporters in lung (patho)physiology and pharmacology, however, are still not fully understood, and these topics are discussed in this review.

2. Expression and Subcellular Localisation of OCT/Ns in Lung-Derived Cell Lines, Pulmonary Cell Cultures and Lung Tissues in Health and Disease

The expression of OCT/Ns in the lung has been studied in several cell lines of human respiratory epithelial origin (e.g., A549, NCI-H441, BEAS-2B, Calu-3 and 16HBE14o-), in primary airway epithelial cells and in lung tissues on the mRNA and protein level [17–23], and has been reviewed comprehensively in our pervious publication [3]. There is some consensus that OCT1, OCT3, OCTN1 and OCTN2 are found ubiquitously throughout the lung epithelium. OCT2 expression is more controversial. The transporter was absent in many of lung-derived cell lines [17,18,23–26], except for NCI-H441 [20,27]. In the case of primary cultures of human tracheal, bronchial and alveolar epithelial cells and in human whole-lung tissue, a lot of conflicting data have been published [17,19,21,23,25,28,29].

The regional expression and subcellular localisation of OCT/Ns in the airways remains, to some extent, elusive. Immunohistochemistry (IHC) studies carried out in human bronchi revealed positive OCT1 and OCT2 staining in the apical membrane of ciliated epithelial cells, intracellular OCT1 staining in ciliated epithelial cells, and OCT3 staining in the basolateral membrane of intermediate cells and the entire plasma membrane of basal cells [28]. OCT3 transcript and protein expression were confirmed in primary human bronchial and vascular smooth muscle cells [30]. Positive OCTN1 and OCTN2 stainings were observed on the apical and the lateral membranes of human primary bronchial epithelial cells [31]. OCTN1 showed the strongest expression of all OCT/Ns in bronchi but was found to be expressed at a lower degree in peripheral lung tissue [32]. Data are still scarce on cell-type-specific expression of OCT/Ns, and hence it is rather difficult to identify the physiological function of each transporter protein. We highlighted this issue in another review in 2016 [3], however, the field has not advanced significantly since then.

A limited number of studies have been published connecting OCT/N expression to lung diseases. Genome-wide association studies (GWAS) have identified *SLC22A5* variants being linked to primary systemic carnitine deficiency and asthma [33,34]. Furthermore, due to its potential role in histamine release and clearance in the airways, an association between *SLC22A3* gene polymorphisms and the severity of asthma has been proposed [35,36]. No differences in mRNA expression levels of OCT1, OCT3, OCTN1 and OCTN2 between ex-smokers with a severe stage of COPD and healthy subjects were reported in a study by Berg and colleagues [32]. Subsequently, the same group's IHC analysis confirmed OCTN1 and OCTN2 expression in the epithelial cells of the bronchi, bronchioles and alveolar type II epithelial cells as well as in alveolar macrophages. However, no differences between COPD and healthy subjects were visible in IHC [31]. It should be noted that neither was immunoblot analysis carried out nor were IHC signal intensities measured in order to quantify potential differences in protein expression between the two groups. In another study, Calu-3 cells were grown for 21 days under air-interfaced culture (AIC) conditions and exposed to pro-inflammatory lipopolysaccharide (LPS) or house dust mite extract (HDM) to simulate asthmatic-like conditions at the epithelium in vitro [37]. The LPS challenge significantly upregulated the expression of OCT1, OCT3, OCTN1 and OCTN2 on mRNA and protein levels. HDM had similar effects on OCT1, OCT3 and OCTN2 mRNA and protein expression. However, when Calu-3 cells grown for the same duration and under similar conditions were exposed to LPS for shorter periods of time, other researchers did not observe any change in mRNA levels of OCT1, OCT3 [24] or OCTN2 [38]. Stimulation with tumour necrosis factor-α (TNF-α) and the Th2-cytokine, IL-4 also did not result in any change in OCT1, OCT3 [24] and OCTN2 mRNA levels [38]. Regretfully, in neither study, were mRNA expression data supported by protein expression analysis. In contrast, when alveolar A549 cells were exposed to similar LPS concentrations, mRNA and protein levels of OCTN1 and OCTN2 were downregulated, which was accompanied by a significant reduction in the uptake of the model substrate 4-[4-(dimethylamino)-styryl]-N-methylpyridinium (ASP$^+$) [39]. Likewise, challenging A549 cells with cigarette smoke extract (CSE), LPS or both caused a significant reduction in OCTN1 and OCTN2 mRNA expression levels [40]. It has been demonstrated that A549 and BEAS-2B cells respond distinctly, in terms of cytokine release, to LPS stimulation [41]. The latter may suggest different pathways involved in alveolar and bronchial epithelial cells upon LPS challenge and, together with different LPS exposure times used in the above-mentioned studies, may explain the discrepancies in OCT/N expression regulation observed in response to LPS stimulation in Calu-3 and A549 cells. Overall, some promising first results suggest that there indeed could be differences in OCT/N expression (and function) in healthy vs. diseased lungs, which needs to be further investigated using appropriate in vitro and experimental animal models as well as lung tissue specimens from patients with respiratory diseases.

OCT/N expression and subcellular localisation in the lungs need to be conclusively studied. For example, cell surface protein biotinylation should be performed to obtain clear-cut subcellular localisation data for OCT/Ns. However, it is essential to use high-quality antibodies, which might have to be generated first. Proteomics profiling will help not only to quantify expression levels of OCT/Ns but also to look into the association between molecular pathways of OCT/Ns in the lung, in health and disease [42]. Lastly, single-cell analysis approaches will allow to sort cell populations of the lung and to determine the expression of OCT/Ns in individual cells (i.e., epithelial vs. immune cells). In this context, first evidence was given that alveolar macrophages also express OCTN1 and OCTN2 [31].

3. OCT/Ns (SLC22A1–A5) Transporter Function in Lung Physiology and Pathophysiology

Despite being involved in the transport of essential endogenous substrates (Figure 1), little information is available about the role of OCT/Ns in physiological functions and under pathological conditions in the lung. Uncovering (patho)physiological functions of OCT/Ns in the lung is a key step in developing new drug therapies for respiratory disorders [10,43]. Molecular investigations are necessary to further identify and validate potential endogenous substrates of OCT/Ns. Transport studies of substrate candidates are traditionally performed utilising radioactive isotopes or liquid chromatography–mass spectrometry. Potentially, a novel assay that detects shifts in thermostability of the transporter protein in the presence of specific substrates may be employed to detect transporter–substrate interactions of lung OCT/Ns [44]. The main advantage of this assay is that it allows large-scale screening to identify candidate substrates from libraries of unlabelled compounds. However, the assay cannot discriminate between substrates, inhibitors or competitors and requires purified proteins. Novel approaches such as transporter tandems might also help to assess the influence of gene polymorphisms on OCT/Ns functional activity and to determine their (patho)physiological consequences in the lung [45] (see Section 3.5 for further details).

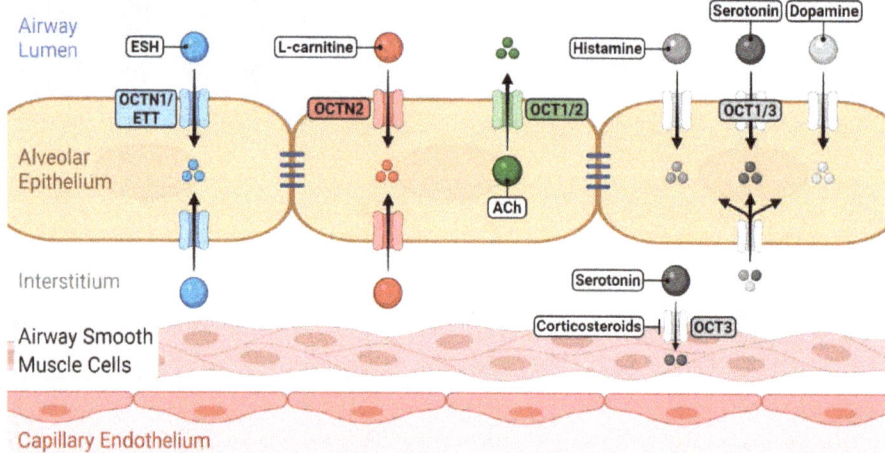

Figure 1. Role of novel/organic cation transporters (OCT/Ns) in pulmonary disposition of endogenous substrates. OCTN1/ergothioneine (ESH) transporter (ETT) mediates the uptake of ESH, which possesses antioxidant and anti-inflammatory properties. OCTN2 mediates L-carnitine uptake, which is essential for cellular energy production. OCTs may participate in the uptake/release of a number of neurotransmitters into/from airway epithelial and smooth muscle cells. Many of these induce bronchoconstriction, regulate mucus secretion and clearance and are linked to the pathophysiology of asthma. The localisation of OCT/Ns, whether apical or basolateral in airway epithelium, is still elusive.

3.1. OCT1, 2 and 3

OCTs transport a wide range of physiologically important endogenous substrates, including hormones such as prostaglandin E_2 and neurotransmitters such as acetylcholine (ACh), dopamine, serotonin, epinephrine, norepinephrine and histamine [3,6,46,47]. In the lung, the current knowledge of OCTs in these molecular interplays is primarily limited to non-neuronal ACh and serotonin transport. OCT1/Oct1 and OCT2/Oct2 have been demonstrated to be involved in the luminal release of non-neuronal ACh in human airway epithelial cells in vitro [28] and in mice in vivo [48]. ACh has various physiological functions in the airway. It regulates mucus secretion and clearance, bronchoconstriction, histamine release from mast cells [49–53] and promotes airway remodelling, particularly during inflammatory lung diseases such as asthma and COPD [51,54]. ACh has also been reported to have a negative impact on the progression of human lung cancer by acting as a growth factor [55]. In the case of serotonin, suppression of OCT3 by corticosterone has been reported to block serotonin-induced bronchoconstriction in mice [48].

Recent insights underline the importance of the above-mentioned neurotransmitters in pulmonary (patho)physiology. A study carried out in mice linked dopamine to a higher susceptibility of children to asthma compared to that of adults [56]. The study showed that sympathetic nerves innervating young mice lungs primarily produce dopamine, which triggers inflammatory reactions related to asthma [56]. Similarly, histamine is a bronchoconstrictor and plays a role in the pathogenesis of asthma and a number of other allergic disorders [36,57,58]. In addition to its bronchoconstricting action, higher plasma levels of serotonin have been observed in asthmatic [59] and COPD patients [60]. Despite having their own high-affinity physiological transporters (e.g., SLC6A3), alteration in OCT activity has been reported to influence the homoeostasis of these neurotransmitters and may result in pathophysiological consequences in the lungs. For example, knocking out of OCT2 and OCT3 in mice resulted in mood abnormality by interfering with monoamine neurotransmitters' clearance in the brain [13,61].

OCTs are also involved in interactions between therapeutic drugs with endogenous substrates. In this context, a number of commonly prescribed drugs have been shown to interfere with the uptake of histamine and monoamine neurotransmitters (i.e., serotonin, epinephrine, norepinephrine and dopamine) into OCT1-overexpressing HEK-293 cells and primary human hepatocytes [46,62]. However, such potential interactions have not yet been investigated in cells of lung origin. Answering further questions on physiological function, therefore, remains challenging. As mentioned previously, OCT2 is either absent or expressed at low levels in human airway epithelium. Thus, the focus shall be on OCT1 (>OCT3) to assess whether alterations in the expression and/or activity of these transporters result in pathophysiological consequences due to changes in the pulmonary disposition of the above-mentioned endogenous substrates. In particular, increased OCT1 and/or OCT3 activity can enhance dopamine uptake into respiratory epithelial cells, which is subsequently metabolised intracellularly by histamine N-methyltransferase [36,63], resulting in reduced neurotransmitter concentration in the extracellular airways space, which may have a positive impact on childhood asthma and/or vice versa.

3.2. OCTN1

OCTN1 facilitates the cellular uptake of its physiological substrate, ESH [64]. Gründemann and colleagues have demonstrated that the transporter is highly specific for ESH and hence the name "ergothioneine transporter" (ETT) has been proposed instead of OCTN1 [65,66]. Expression of OCTN1 in distinct tissues can, therefore, serve as a specific molecular indicator of intracellular ESH activity [65,66]. According to a number of in vitro and in vivo studies, ESH acts as a powerful free-radical scavenger and can modulate inflammation [67–70]. Polymorphisms in the *SLC22A4* gene have been linked with susceptibility to many chronic inflammatory diseases such as ulcerative colitis and Crohn's disease [71–73] as well as to tooth loss and adiposity in women [74]. In the lung, a protective role for ESH against inflammatory and oxidative-stress-induced damage has been demonstrated. For instance, pre-treatment of alveolar epithelial A549 cells with ESH inhibited TNF-α and H_2O_2-mediated IL-8 release and activation of nuclear factor kappa B (NF-κB) [75]. ESH was, therefore, proposed as a potential therapeutic intervention for chronic inflammatory pulmonary disorders such as COPD [76,77]. In a rat model of acute respiratory distress syndrome, intravenous ESH treatment before and after cytokine insufflation attenuated acute lung injury and inflammation [78]. The authors, however, did not carry out detailed histopathological studies to support their results. The physiologic transporter of ESH (i.e., OCTN1) itself was not considered in these studies. For drawing conclusions on the clinical impact, it is not only essential to investigate the substrate itself but also potential links between these respiratory disorders and reduced OCTN1 activity, e.g., through genetic polymorphisms or drug–drug interactions.

3.3. OCTN2

OCTN2 mediates the uptake of L-carnitine [6,79] and hence controls its homoeostasis, which is achieved by endogenous biosynthesis (mainly in the liver and kidney), intake from the diet and renal reabsorption [80]. L-carnitine is a highly polar zwitterionic and naturally occurring compound that plays a key physiological role in the mitochondrial β-oxidation of fatty acids and, consequently, in cellular energy production [80,81]. The process of fatty acid oxidation involves the consumption of large amounts of oxygen, which are reduced to H_2O, resulting in reduction in intracellular reactive oxygen species formation. L-carnitine also regulates the activity of several enzymes involved in protection against oxidative-stress-induced damage [82]. Based on in vitro and in vivo studies, L-carnitine can scavenge free radicals and counteract oxidants such as peroxyl radicals, hydrogen peroxide and peroxynitrite [83–87]. Reduced intracellular L-carnitine levels in turn impair cellular energy generation and result in deterioration of the function of several organs [80].

The clinical relevance of the substrate L-carnitine in lung (patho)physiology is well investigated. Studies have demonstrated that reduction in oxidative stress levels and increased activities of many antioxidant enzymes following administration of L-carnitine supplements are seen in healthy volunteers [88], suggesting a protective role against oxidative-stress-induced damage [89]. Moreover, lower serum L-carnitine levels were found in children with moderate persistent asthma compared to those in healthy volunteers, and six months of L-carnitine supplementation to the asthmatic children improved childhood-asthma control test and pulmonary function test parameters [90]. A significant reduction in serum L-carnitine level was observed in asthmatic children during acute exacerbations and shortly thereafter. The difference in L-carnitine levels between the groups of healthy and asthmatic children, however, was not significant [91]. These data should be carefully considered due to low numbers of patients and healthy controls included in the above-mentioned studies. L-carnitine also plays a role in pulmonary surfactant synthesis. In murine alveolar epithelium, it was proposed that when fatty acid oxidation is impaired, pulmonary surfactant levels and lung function are decreased [92]. Acylcarnitines, which are catabolised from carnitine, directly inhibit the activity of alveolar surfactant [92]. Furthermore, L-carnitine has been proposed to play a role in respiratory distress syndrome (RDS). Treatment of new-borns with RDS with L-carnitine has been demonstrated to reduce surfactant requirement, to shorten the duration of mechanical ventilation needed and to reduce the incidence of bronchopulmonary dysplasia [93]. These clinical findings, however, were not yet linked to the expression and function of OCTN2. In the future, these data could permit an identification of a clinically relevant dysregulation or dysfunction of the physiological transporter in these respiratory disorders. Lately, OCTN2-mediated L-carnitine uptake, via maintaining energy supply, was discussed to play a role in sustaining respiratory ciliary beating and consequently, airway mucociliary clearance, by which excess mucus and potentially harmful foreign particles are removed from the airways [94].

Due to the physiological importance of OCTN2 in regulating L-carnitine homoeostasis, data on expression and function in different preclinical models is steadily increasing. In vitro studies confirmed a cellular OCTN2-mediated accumulation of L-carnitine and acetyl-L-carnitine in human respiratory epithelial cell models [22,95,96]. However, when acetyl-L-carnitine uptake into a number of respiratory epithelial cell lines (i.e., NCl-H441, A549 and Calu-3 cells) was compared to that in primary alveolar epithelial cells, the kinetics and inhibitor specificities were significantly different, similar to the functions of OCTs (see Section 3.4) [22]. In vivo studies revealed an active accumulation of L-carnitine in mice trachea without a systemic absorption [97]. This was supported by studies in an intact isolated, perfused rat-lung model, where data revealed no carnitine-sensitive pulmonary absorption [95].

3.4. Functional Studies Using Exogenous OCT/N Substrates

The uptake and transport of xenobiotics has been reviewed before [98]. To measure OCT/Ns' function, the fluorescent dye ASP$^+$ [19,27,98,99] has often been used. ASP$^+$, however, lacks selectivity as an OCT substrate as it is also a substrate for a number of plasma membrane neurotransmitter transporters [100,101]. Tetraethylammonium (TEA), 1-methyl-4-phenylpyridinium (MPP$^+$) and decynium-22 [6] have been used mainly in in vitro studies and are more specific for OCTs but lack selectivity for the individual OCT subtypes [18,102]. Distinct TEA uptake kinetics and patterns of OCT inhibitory effects were observed in NCl-H441, A549 and Calu-3 cell lines when compared to those in primary alveolar epithelial cells [102]. These results point out the relevance of a physiological epithelial cell model. When MPP$^+$ uptake was studied, only the above-mentioned respiratory epithelial cell lines were used [18]. The authors suggested differential contributions of OCTs to the MPP$^+$ uptake [18]. Thus, these results have to be carefully discussed in terms of physiological propagation. To our knowledge, no other data on pulmonary OCT/N-mediated drug transport was published since our last review in 2016 [3]. It is still a rather difficult assignment to conclusively determine the regional OCT/N transporter activity in the lung. The affinities of OCTs for exogenous and endogenous substrates have been comprehensively summarised in several reviews [6,9,103] with a focus on the liver and the kidneys. Studies of clinically relevant OCT-involving drug–drug interactions have recently been reviewed by Koepsell [103,104]. In the lung, very few pharmacokinetic studies have been performed [18,102,105]. Interactions of beta-agonists, corticosteroids and anticholinergics may occur in the lung, and we have focussed on recent data in Section 4; however these studies are mainly based on interaction of drugs and model substrates.

3.5. Relation of OCT/N Expression, Subcellular Localisation and Function

Some of the reported discrepancies in OCT/N expression levels mentioned in Section 2 are likely due to inconsistencies in passage numbers, time in culture, culture conditions (i.e., AIC vs. liquid-covered conditions (LCC)) and medium supplements. For example, OCT3 transcripts were detected in Calu-3 cells grown for 21, but not for 14, days [25]. Higher OCTN1 and OCTN2 mRNA levels were observed in 16HBE14o- cells cultured for 18 days than in those grown for 11 days [17]. Culturing Caco-2 cells in media supplemented with high glucose concentrations has been shown to reduce OCT3 activity and mRNA and protein expression levels [106]. Likewise, cell culture conditions and time in culture have been demonstrated to have a significant impact on the mRNA expression levels of a number of SLC transporters in Calu-3 [107] and primary human nasal epithelial cells [108]. Method standardisation is, therefore, crucial for future studies in order to validate epithelial cell models and freshly isolated human lung epithelial cells as surrogates for in vivo studies. Furthermore, a lack of high-quality antibodies has been a major challenge in OCT/N research. In particular, when using commercially available antibodies for protein detection via confocal laser scanning microscopy, the localisation of the observed signals was not always unambiguous (see below). This also constrains investigations in novel in vitro cell systems, such as 3D epithelial cell models, to evaluate their suitability as models for OCT/N research. For further reading on pulmonary epithelial cell models, please refer to the following reviews and publications [109–112].

Investigating the activity of a transporter protein can be more challenging than studying variations in its mRNA or gene product expression. Much of lung OCT/N research is solely based on expression analysis [17,23,113,114] and hence presents a strongly unilateral view on OCT/Ns. Expression studies using immunoblotting or liquid chromatography–tandem mass spectrometry (LC-MS/MS) may not precisely foretell a transporter's activity due to the detection of inactive intracellular transporter protein. LC-MS/MS has been used to study the expression levels of a number of transporters, including OCT/Ns, in the plasma membranes fractions isolated, via gradient centrifugation, from human whole-lung tissues, primary cells and a number of lung-derived cell lines [20,21,29]. The purity of plasma membrane fractions, however, could not be confirmed. Transporter tandems has been recently proposed as a precise tool to determine a transporter's activity in the plasma membrane [45]. In short, a link is created between two transporters by joining their cDNAs in a single open reading frame, resulting in a 1:1 stoichiometry and, thereby, enabling to measure the activity of one transporter by the activity of the second one. For example, OCTN1–OCT2 tandems were used to assess the activity of OCTN1 [45]. Moreover, linking OCTN1 as a reference transporter with a number of SLC and SLCO transporters (i.e., OCT1, OCT2, OAT1, OAT3, OATP1B1 and OATP1B3), has demonstrated that transporter tandems can be a useful tool to assess the activity of transporters belonging to other families [45]. However, there must be no functional overlap between the reference and the test transporter of the tandem, which must be verified by uptake experiments with the individual unconnected transporters. In addition, suitable linker peptides should be used between the two transporters. The sequence and the length of the linkers as well as the order of transporters in the tandems may have a strong impact on transporters' expression and activity and, therefore, must be carefully validated [45].

Activity studies using ASP^+ suggested OCT/N localisation on the apical side of Calu-3 cell monolayers grown under AIC conditions for 21 days [25]. IHC analysis, which confirmed the expression of OCT1, OCT3 and OCTN2, however, was inconclusive regarding the subcellular localisation of the transporters [25]. In contrast, bidirectional MPP^+ transport across Calu-3 monolayers grown under similar conditions and for similar duration was proposed to be mediated by both OCT1 and OCT3 at the apical and OCT3 at the basolateral side of the polarised monolayers [18]. In the same study, transport studies carried out in NCI-H441 and A549 cells suggested apical expression of OCT1 and OCT3 [18]. The authors, however, could not support their data with proper subcellular localisation experiments. More recently, MPP$^+$ uptake studies, indicated that OCT1 and OCT3 are active on the basolateral membrane of the 3D cell model composed of normal human bronchial epithelial cells [24]. L-carnitine transport studies suggested OCTN2 to be active on the basolateral side of Calu-3 cells and the 3D cell model [38]. IHC analysis was suggestive of a basolateral localisation of the transporter in Calu-3 monolayers, but the signals were inconclusive in the 3D cell model [38].

Taken together, these data suggest that functional activity studies may fail to accurately predict the subcellular localisation and/or expression of OCT/Ns and vice versa. Thus, monitoring expression and function of OCT/Ns simultaneously is necessary to define active transporter proteins and to determine the source of published discrepancies in either expression or functional analysis.

4. Pharmacological Aspects of OCT/N Transporters in the Lung

4.1. Interaction of OCT/N Transporters with Inhaled Drugs

Inhaled bronchodilator drugs must pass through the airway epithelial barrier to reach their target receptors in the underlying airway smooth muscle cells. Many of these drugs belonging to the muscarinic receptor antagonists and β_2-agonists are cations and are positively charged at physiological pH-values of the lung lining fluid. Thus, OCT/Ns may play a potential role in their pulmonary disposition, pharmacokinetics, safety and efficacy profile. The involvement of OCT/N transporters in interactions with inhaled drugs has been intensively discussed in previous reviews [2,3].

The role of OCT/Ns in the pulmonary disposition of inhaled drugs is an ongoing research topic; however, data are mainly limited to in vitro studies. Despite being essential for initial screenings of inhaled drugs' interactions with membrane transporters, in vitro studies are insufficient to confirm the clinical significances of such interactions, and a number of challenges and disadvantages are associated with them. First, an ideal in vitro lung epithelial model for drug disposition studies still does not exist. Second, the different cell composition of proximal and distal lung epithelium may result in different OCT/N expression and activity profiles [17,98]. Third, determination of inhaled drug concentrations in the epithelial lining fluid following drug inhalation is extremely difficult because of the complex anatomical nature of the lung [25,115]. Thus, the concentrations of inhaled drugs applied in in vitro studies to assess their interaction with OCT/N transporters may be clinically irrelevant. The concentration of drugs used in in vitro studies is of particular importance because it influences the ratio of passive membrane diffusion and transporter-mediated uptake [9]. Generally, when high concentrations are used, passive membrane permeation predominates resulting in an underestimation of the transporter impact [9]. In vitro data may, therefore, not predict the in vivo airway-to-blood absorption process accurately and should be carefully considered. Validation can be achieved by ex vivo, in vivo and clinical studies [10]. Recent reviews have covered preclinical models (in vitro, ex vivo and in vivo) that are currently implemented in pulmonary drug delivery studies [111,112]. Moreover, new experimental in silico models such as Mimetikos Preludium™ (Emmace Consulting) and SimCyp Simulator™ (Certara) can be used to estimate the regional absorption of inhaled drugs [116,117]. It is necessary to point out that such in silico models may fail to precisely describe the pulmonary pharmacokinetics of drugs because the validity of the simulation depends on the quality (and quantity) of data used to inform the model. These data, however, are scarce and were generated under different experimental conditions. Moreover, none of these models has been specifically designed for use in pulmonary drug delivery. Nonetheless, in silico models might prove useful to assess the impact of OCT/Ns in pulmonary disposition of inhaled drugs, once sufficient and reliable in vitro and in vivo data have been generated to inform them.

Many questions related to the pharmacological roles of OCT/Ns in the lung have been raised and remain open. Which member of the family is of particular importance? Are OCT/N–drug interactions clinically relevant, and do they influence drug efficacy and toxicity?

4.1.1. Interaction with β_2-Agonists

Ehrhardt et al. were the first to propose the involvement OCT/Ns in the active transport of salbutamol across monolayers of human bronchial epithelial cell lines in vitro [118]. In another study, salbutamol was suggested to be a specific substrate and inhibitor of OCT1 in human distal respiratory epithelial cells [105]. Horvath and colleagues observed that OCTN2 function can be inhibited by salbutamol and formoterol in normal human bronchial epithelial (NHBE) cells in vitro [19]. Whilst they found no role for OCT/Ns in the transepithelial transport of salbutamol across the cell monolayers, paracellular diffusion was suggested to be the predominant mediator of the inhaled drug translocation across lung mucosa [119]. Salbutamol, formoterol and ipratropium bromide have also been demonstrated to inhibit OCT1, OCT3, OCTN1 and OCTN2 in bronchial epithelial Calu-3 cells [25]. A number of nonsteroidal anti-inflammatory drugs interfered with salbutamol uptake into Calu-3 cells via a mechanism involving the inhibition of OCT transporters [120]. In a more recent study, data showed that epithelial asthmatic-like challenges can enhance the transepithelial permeability of salbutamol through OCT transporters' overexpression in vitro [37]. A delay in the pulmonary absorption of salbutamol and GW597901, a long-acting β_2-agonist, was observed in isolated human lung reperfusion model after nebulisation of L-carnitine via a mechanism involving competition with the OCTN2 transporter [121]. However, the authors could not determine the duration of delay due to the limited viability time of the model.

Fenoterol, a short-acting β_2-agonist, has been identified as a substrate of OCT1 [122,123]. When a number of heritable OCT1 variants were overexpressed in HEK-293 cells, the uptake of this drug was completely abolished or substantially reduced [123]. Clinically, following intravenous administration of fenoterol to healthy individuals with heritable non-functional hOCT1 alleles, the systemic exposure was approximately two-folds higher than in individuals with functional hOCT alleles due to reduced hepatic clearance. Consequently, the drug caused more pronounced undesirable effects such as increased heart rate and blood glucose levels in OCT1-deficient individuals [123]. Further, OCT3 was proposed to mediate the uptake of cationic β_2-agonists into their site of action (i.e., bronchial smooth muscle cells) [124]. In another study, it was demonstrated that inhibition of OCT3 in vascular smooth muscle cells, via corticosteroids, could reduce the vascular clearance of cationic β_2-agonists and, therefore, increase their airway retention time. The authors, therefore, suggested that combining inhaled corticosteroids with β_2-agonists may improve the pharmacologic response to the latter [30]. However, they did not discuss whether the inhibition of OCT3 in airway smooth muscle cells may instead have a negative impact on β_2-agonists' action by reducing their uptake into their target site.

Taken together, OCT1 and OCTN2 seem to be the main members involved in interaction with β_2-agonists in airway epithelial cells; whereas, OCT3 is mainly involved in the uptake and clearance of β_2-agonists into/from airway smooth muscle cells (Figure 2). By now, studies provide evidence that cationic β_2-agonists are substrates as well as inhibitors of OCT/Ns. Based on the available data, the clinical significance of such interactions remains to be investigated.

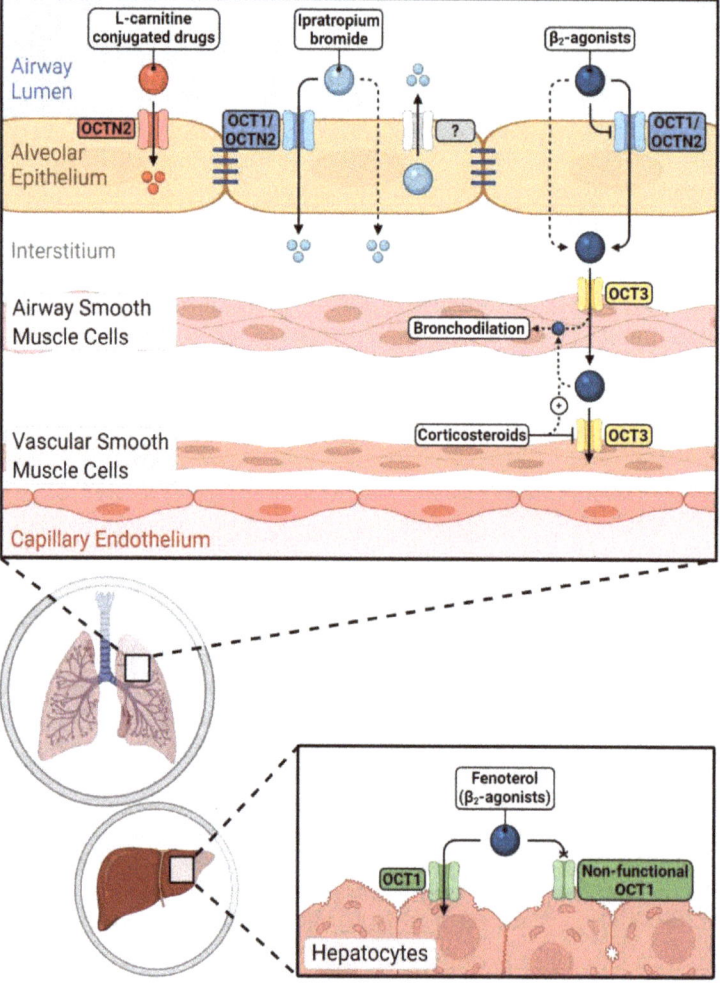

Figure 2. Impacts of novel/organic cation transporters (OCT/Ns) on pulmonary and systemic disposition of inhaled drugs. Inhaled cationic β_2-agonists' epithelial transport is mediated either by OCT/Ns (mainly OCT1 and OCTN2) or passive diffusion. Corticosteroids can increase the airway retention of β_2-agonists by inhibiting OCT3 in vascular smooth muscle cells. Hepatic clearance of fenoterol is reduced in carriers of non-functional OCT1 alleles. Ipratropium bromide uptake via airway epithelium is more complex and OCT/Ns, unidentified efflux transporters and passive diffusion are participating. OCTN2 mediates the uptake of L-carnitine-conjugated prodrugs and nanoparticles into pulmonary epithelial cells improving pulmonary delivery of the parent drugs.

4.1.2. Interaction with Anticholinergic Drugs

Short-acting ipratropium bromide and long-acting tiotropium bromide and glycopyrronium anticholinergic drugs have been shown to be substrates of OCTs and OCTN2 [97,122,125]. OCTN2 was reported to be the predominant mediator of ipratropium bromide uptake into BEAS-2B bronchial epithelial cells [126]. In contrast, ipratropium bromide transport studies across Calu-3 monolayers revealed a net secretion sensitive to inhibition by MPP$^+$ and TEA but not L-carnitine, suggesting the involvement of OCTs and ruling out any role for OCTN2 in drug flux across cell monolayers [127].

Moreover, the study revealed the presence of an active efflux mechanism that extrudes the bronchodilator to the apical chamber, which could be inhibited by MPP$^+$, TEA and probenecid. The latter has been reported to inhibit multidrug-resistance-associated proteins (MRPs) [128] and organic anion transporters (OATs) [129]. However, there is no report, to our knowledge, that indicates ipratropium bromide as a substate of MRPs. OATs were undetectable in Calu-3 monolayers grown under similar condition [130]. Anions, including probenecid, have been proposed to inhibit OCTs [6] and thus might be involved in the interaction between probenecid and ipratropium bromide. However, the authors were unable to confirm this hypothesis and suggested that an apically localised OCT1 and other unidentified efflux transporters may be involved in the luminal recycling of the inhaled drug [127]. In this context, ipratropium bromide has been recognised as a substate of multidrug and toxin extrusion (MATE) transporters [131], which are reported to mediate cationic drugs' efflux across the apical membrane of tubular renal cells and hepatocytes [132]. The authors of the above-mentioned study concluded that ipratropium absorption across respiratory epithelium is a complex process in which both passive diffusion and carrier-mediated uptake and efflux processes play a role [127]. Recently, the involvement of the amino acid transporter B$^{0,+}$ (ATB$^{0,+}$), which can also mediate cellular uptake of organic cations [98] and L-carnitine was discussed [133]. The transporter was taken into consideration in two recent studies in which ipratropium bromide, but not tiotropium bromide nor glycopyrrolate, was shown to inhibit OCTN2-mediated basolateral uptake of L-carnitine [38] and OCT-mediated MPP$^+$ uptake [24] into 3D human bronchial epithelial cell model and Calu-3 cells. It remains to be validated whether ATB$^{0,+}$ plays such an important role in drug disposition.

Not many ex vivo studies have been carried out to assess the interaction of anticholinergic drugs with OCT/N transporters. The uptake of ipratropium bromide, but not tiotropium bromide, was shown to be carrier mediated in lung slices obtained from drug-naïve rats [134]. In contrast, a study carried out in an isolated and perfused rat lung model suggested passive diffusion to be the main driving force for the overall absorption of ipratropium bromide across the lung epithelial barrier and that OCT/Ns play no role in the process [95]. Meanwhile, in vitro uptake experiments showed a significant role for OCTs in the uptake of ipratropium bromide into primary rat alveolar epithelial cells and into three human pulmonary epithelial cell lines (i.e., A549, BEAS-2B, 16HBE14o-).

Overall, the importance of OCT/Ns in the pulmonary disposition of anticholinergic drugs remains to some extent contradictory between in vitro and ex vivo studies. Data point towards an involvement of OCT1 and OCTN2 in the interaction with ipratropium bromide (Figure 2).

4.2. OCTN2 as a Target to Enhance Pulmonary Drug Delivery

Conjugation of drugs or nanodrug delivery systems with a specific transporter's substrate to promote drug transfer across biological barriers has emerged as a strategy to improve drug delivery [135,136]. OCTN2-targeted nanodrug delivery systems have been successfully used to enhance the oral bioavailability of nanoparticles [137]. As far as the pulmonary drug delivery is concerned, Mo and colleagues synthesised a carnitine ester prodrug of prednisolone (i.e., prednisolone succinate-L-carnitine (PDSC)). The uptake of the prodrugs into BEAS-2B cells was enhanced and could be inhibited by L-carnitine, indicating it was an OCTN2-mediated process. The prodrug displayed improved duration of action with the free prednisolone being slowly released inside the cells resulting in longer suppression of LPS-induced release of IL-6 by BEAS-2B cells in vitro [138]. In a follow-up study, the asthmatic guinea pig model was treated with the prodrug and showed less severe vascular pathologies, restricted asthma induced airway thickenings and lower inflammatory cell count in bronchoalveolar fluid when compared to animals treated with unconjugated prednisolone [139]. However, a link to alterations in OCTN2 expression levels was not investigated in this model.

OCTN2 may be a potential target to enhance the pulmonary delivery of inhaled drugs to achieve a better therapeutic outcome. As mentioned before, L-carnitine itself has antioxidant properties and may confer additional beneficial effects when conjugated with inhaled drugs used for the treatment of respiratory disorders such as asthma and COPD (Figure 2).

5. Conclusions and Future Perspectives

Reliable epithelial cell models most closely reflecting the situation in vivo are necessary to assess the role of OCT/Ns in pulmonary (patho)physiology and drug disposition. Recent in vitro studies discussed in this review are mainly based on continuously growing cell lines such as Calu-3 [24,37,38] or A549 [40]. Comparison of OCTN2 and OCT function in respiratory epithelial cell models (i.e., Calu-3, A549 and NCl-H441) to that in human alveolar primary epithelial cells showed vast differences in kinetics and inhibitor profiles, underlining the importance of this topic [22,102]. MatTek's EpiAirway model has been proposed as a phenotypic 3D model in which OCT/Ns were found to be functionally active at the basolateral membrane only [24,38]. These data show that an "ideal" in vitro epithelial cell model for OCTN/-based research is still elusive. To overcome some of the challenges, much effort has been undertaken to establish isolated and perfused lung models to predict in vivo drug absorption [140,141]. Furthermore, a porcine isolated and perfused lung model for pulmonary pathophysiological studies was established [142]. Porcine lungs are very similar to their human counterparts in term of size, anatomy and physiological characteristics, and this model may therefore be a promising ex vivo surrogate for inhalation biopharmaceutical investigations. When using other species, the consideration of any potential species differences in OCT/Ns' activity between laboratory animals and human is of crucial importance. In this Special Issue, Floerl and colleagues demonstrate a good functional correlation between rat, mouse and human OCT1 in terms of interactions between a number of investigated drugs [143]. Other OCT/Ns expression and activity profiles, however, still need to be thoroughly investigated in these models.

Studies have only started considering the airway microenvironment of lung diseases on inhaled drug disposition by, e.g., modelling asthma-like conditions in vitro [37] or utilising tissue from patients [31]. The presence of mucus and airway inflammation is a crucial factor for the absorption of β_2-agonists, e.g., salbutamol [37,144,145]. An in vitro model was developed to study mucus interaction with aerosolised drugs by applying a thin layer of porcine tracheal mucus. Results showed that mucus delayed the absorption of all inhaled tested drugs (i.e., salbutamol, formoterol and indacaterol, ipratropium bromide and glycopyrronium) but to a varying extent [145]. The thickness of the mucus layer in the model, however, was about 10-fold higher than that of the mucus film covering the airways in vivo, and thus, the observed influences are very likely overestimated. These studies considering the impact of the mucus are still in their infancy and need further technical and methodological refinement.

Following recent achievements in proteomics and microbiome analysis, which has been highly "boosted" in the last years [146,147], insights into the pathology of airway diseases become increasingly available. Several studies have shown that the airway microbiome is disturbed in patients with COPD [148,149], likely contributing to the pathology of diseases. It is yet unknown but necessary to investigate any potential change in OCT/Ns' functions in such specific pathologic airway environments. These studies will rely on patient-derived material. By implementing, e.g., cultures of human primary 2D airway epithelial cell cultures or 3D airway spheroids [150,151], screenings of OCT/N substrates and inhibitors will greatly advance insights into responses of pulmonary drug disposition. Furthermore, this avenue of research will facilitate the analysis of effects of gene polymorphisms and gender on OCT/Ns' expression and function (towards "individualised pharmaceutics"). Gender-related differences in the expression and activity of a number of SLC and ATP-binding cassette transporters have been observed in hepatic [152–154] and renal tissue [155]. Sakamoto et al. showed first evidences in their pulmonary expression profiles that females had two-fold higher levels of OCT1 and OCTN1 compared to those in males [21].

To summarise, according to the current state of knowledge, OCT/Ns have a potential pharmacological impact in the lung. The understanding of their regulation is pivotal for the development of novel inhaled drug therapies.

Author Contributions: Conceptualisation of the review: M.A.S., J.A.S., C.E. and J.J.S.; writing: M.A.S. and J.J.S.; preparation of the figures: J.A.S.; critical reading: J.A.S. and C.E. All authors have read and agreed to the published version of the manuscript.

Funding: This work was financially supported by grants from the German Ministry for Education and Research (FKZ 82DZL004A1 to JJS), Enterprise Ireland (IP/2019/0797) and Niederösterreichische Forschungs- und Bildungsges.m.b.H. (NFB LSC17-009).

Acknowledgments: The figures were created with BioRender.com

Conflicts of Interest: The authors declare no conflict of interest.

Abbreviations

ACh	Acetylcholine
AIC	Air-interfaced culture
ASP$^+$	4-[4-(dimethylamino)-styryl]-N-methylpyridinium
ATB$^{0,+}$	Amino acid transporter B$^{0,+}$
COPD	Chronic obstructive pulmonary disease
CSE	Cigarette smoke extract
ESH	Ergothioneine
ETT	Ergothioneine transporter
HDM	House dust mite extract
IHC	Immunohistochemistry
LCC	Liquid-covered conditions
LC-MS/MS	Liquid chromatography–tandem mass spectrometry
LPS	Lipopolysaccharide
MATE	Multidrug and toxin extrusion
MPP$^+$	1-methyl-4-phenylpyridinium
MRPs	Multidrug-resistance-associated proteins
NF-κB	Nuclear factor kappa B
NHBE	Normal human bronchial epithelial
OATs	Organic anion transporters
OCT	Organic cation transporter
OCTN	Novel organic cation transporter
PDSC	Prednisolone succinate-L-carnitine
RDS	Respiratory distress syndrome
SLC	Solute carrier
TEA	Tetraethylammonium
TNF-α	Tumour necrosis factor α

References

1. Bosquillon, C. Drug transporters in the lung—Do they play a role in the biopharmaceutics of inhaled drugs? *J. Pharm. Sci.* **2010**, *99*, 2240–2255. [CrossRef] [PubMed]
2. Salomon, J.J.; Ehrhardt, C. Organic cation transporters in the blood–air barrier: Expression and implications for pulmonary drug delivery. *Ther. Deliv.* **2012**, *3*, 735–747. [CrossRef] [PubMed]
3. Nickel, S.; Clerkin, C.G.; Selo, M.A.; Ehrhardt, C. Transport mechanisms at the pulmonary mucosa: Implications for drug delivery. *Expert Opin. Drug Deliv.* **2016**, *13*, 667–690. [CrossRef] [PubMed]
4. Engelhart, D.; Granados, J.C.; Shi, D.; Saier, M.H.; Baker, M.E.; Abagyan, R.; Nigam, S.K.; Saier, M.H. Systems Biology Analysis Reveals Eight SLC22 Transporter Subgroups, Including OATs, OCTs, and OCTNs. *Int. J. Mol. Sci.* **2020**, *21*, 1791. [CrossRef] [PubMed]
5. Selo, M.A.; Al-Alak, H.H.; Ehrhardt, C. Lung transporters and absorption mechanisms in the lungs. In *Inhalation Aerosols: Physical and Biological Basis for Therapy*, 3rd ed.; Hickey, A.J., Mansour, H.M., Eds.; CRC Press: New York, NY, USA, 2019; Volume 1, pp. 57–70.
6. Koepsell, H.; Lips, K.; Volk, C. Polyspecific Organic Cation Transporters: Structure, Function, Physiological Roles, and Biopharmaceutical Implications. *Pharm. Res.* **2007**, *24*, 1227–1251. [CrossRef] [PubMed]

7. Uhlen, M.; Oksvold, P.; Fagerberg, L.; Lundberg, E.; Jonasson, K.; Forsberg, M.; Zwahlen, M.; Kampf, C.; Wester, K.; Hober, S.; et al. Towards a knowledge-based Human Protein Atlas. *Nat. Biotechnol.* **2010**, *28*, 1248–1250. [CrossRef]
8. The Human Protein Atlas 19 November 2020. Available online: https://www.proteinatlas.org/ (accessed on 23 November 2020).
9. Koepsell, H. Organic Cation Transporters in Health and Disease. *Pharmacol. Rev.* **2020**, *72*, 253–319. [CrossRef]
10. The International Transporter Consortium; International Transporter Consortium; Giacomini, K.M.; Huang, S.; Tweedie, D.J.; Benet, L.Z.; Brouwer, K.L.R.; Chu, X.; Dahlin, A.; Evers, R.; et al. Membrane transporters in drug development. *Nat. Rev. Drug Discov.* **2010**, *9*, 215–236. [CrossRef]
11. Chen, L.; Yee, S.W.; Giacomini, K.M. OCT1 in hepatic steatosis and thiamine disposition. *Cell Cycle* **2015**, *14*, 283–284. [CrossRef]
12. Chen, L.; Shu, Y.; Liang, X.; Chen, E.C.; Yee, S.W.; Zur, A.A.; Li, S.; Xu, L.; Keshari, K.R.; Lin, M.J.; et al. OCT1 is a high-capacity thiamine transporter that regulates hepatic steatosis and is a target of metformin. *Proc. Natl. Acad. Sci. USA* **2014**, *111*, 9983–9988. [CrossRef]
13. Bacq, A.; Balasse, L.; Biala, G.; Guiard, B.P.; Gardier, A.; Schinkel, A.; Louis, F.; Vialou, V.; Martres, M.-P.; Chevarin, C.; et al. Organic cation transporter 2 controls brain norepinephrine and serotonin clearance and antidepressant response. *Mol. Psychiatry* **2012**, *17*, 926–939. [CrossRef]
14. Couroussé, T.; Gautron, S. Role of organic cation transporters (OCTs) in the brain. *Pharmacol. Ther.* **2015**, *146*, 94–103. [CrossRef]
15. Vialou, V.V.; Amphoux, A.; Zwart, R.; Giros, B.; Gautron, S. Organic Cation Transporter 3 (Slc22a3) Is Implicated in Salt-Intake Regulation. *J. Neurosci.* **2004**, *24*, 2846–2851. [CrossRef]
16. Samodelov, S.L.; Kullak-Ublick, G.A.; Gai, Z.; Visentin, M. Organic Cation Transporters in Human Physiology, Pharmacology, and Toxicology. *Int. J. Mol. Sci.* **2020**, *21*, 7890. [CrossRef]
17. Endter, S.; Francombe, D.; Gumbleton, M.; Ehrhardt, C. RT-PCR analysis of ABC, SLC and SLCO drug transporters in human lung epithelial cell models. *J. Pharm. Pharmacol.* **2009**, *61*, 583–591. [CrossRef]
18. Ingoglia, F.; Visigalli, R.; Rotoli, B.M.; Barilli, A.; Riccardi, B.; Puccini, P.; Dall'Asta, V. Functional characterization of the organic cation transporters (OCTs) in human airway pulmonary epithelial cells. *Biochim. Biophys. Acta* **2015**, *1848*, 1563–1572. [CrossRef]
19. Horvath, G.; Schmid, N.; Fragoso, M.A.; Schmid, A.; Conner, G.E.; Salathe, M.; Wanner, A. Epithelial Organic Cation Transporters Ensure pH-Dependent Drug Absorption in the Airway. *Am. J. Respir. Cell Mol. Biol.* **2007**, *36*, 53–60. [CrossRef]
20. Sakamoto, A.; Matsumaru, T.; Yamamura, N.; Suzuki, S.; Uchida, Y.; Tachikawa, M.; Terasaki, T. Drug Transporter Protein Quantification of Immortalized Human Lung Cell Lines Derived from Tracheobronchial Epithelial Cells (Calu-3 and BEAS2-B), Bronchiolar–Alveolar Cells (NCI-H292 and NCI-H441), and Alveolar Type II-like Cells (A549) by Liquid Chromatography–Tandem Mass Spectrometry. *J. Pharm. Sci.* **2015**, *104*, 3029–3038. [CrossRef]
21. Sakamoto, A.; Matsumaru, T.; Yamamura, N.; Uchida, Y.; Tachikawa, M.; Ohtsuki, S.; Terasaki, T. Quantitative expression of human drug transporter proteins in lung tissues: Analysis of regional, gender, and interindividual differences by liquid chromatography–tandem mass spectrometry. *J. Pharm. Sci.* **2013**, *102*, 3395–3406. [CrossRef]
22. Salomon, J.J.; Gausterer, J.C.; Selo, M.A.; Hosoya, K.-I.; Huwer, H.; Schneider-Daum, N.; Lehr, C.-M.; Ehrhardt, C. OCTN2-Mediated Acetyl-l-Carnitine Transport in Human Pulmonary Epithelial Cells In Vitro. *J. Pharm. Sci.* **2019**, *11*, 396. [CrossRef]
23. Courcot, E.; Leclerc, J.; Lafitte, J.-J.; Mensier, E.; Jaillard, S.; Gosset, P.; Shirali, P.; Pottier, N.; Broly, F.; Lo-Guidice, J.-M. Xenobiotic Metabolism and Disposition in Human Lung Cell Models: Comparison with In Vivo Expression Profiles. *Drug Metab. Dispos.* **2012**, *40*, 1953–1965. [CrossRef] [PubMed]
24. Barilli, A.; Visigalli, R.; Ferrari, F.; Di Lascia, M.; Riccardi, B.; Puccini, P.; Dall'Asta, V.; Rotoli, B.M. Organic Cation Transporters (OCTs) in EpiAirway™, a Cellular Model of Normal Human Bronchial Epithelium. *Biomedicines* **2020**, *8*, 127. [CrossRef] [PubMed]
25. Mukherjee, M.; Pritchard, D.; Bosquillon, C. Evaluation of air-interfaced Calu-3 cell layers for investigation of inhaled drug interactions with organic cation transporters in vitro. *Int. J. Pharm.* **2012**, *426*, 7–14. [CrossRef] [PubMed]

26. Mukherjee, M.; Latif, M.; Pritchard, D.; Bosquillon, C. In-cell Western™ detection of organic cation transporters in bronchial epithelial cell layers cultured at an air–liquid interface on Transwell ® inserts. *J. Pharmacol. Toxicol. Methods* **2013**, *68*, 184–189. [CrossRef]
27. Salomon, J.J.; Muchitsch, V.E.; Gausterer, J.C.; Schwagerus, E.; Huwer, H.; Daum, N.; Lehr, C.-M.; Ehrhardt, C. The Cell Line NCl-H441 Is a Usefulin VitroModel for Transport Studies of Human Distal Lung Epithelial Barrier. *Mol. Pharm.* **2014**, *11*, 995–1006. [CrossRef]
28. Lips, K.S.; Volk, C.; Schmitt, B.M.; Pfeil, U.; Arndt, P.; Miska, D.; Ermert, L.; Kummer, W.; Koepsell, H. Polyspecific Cation Transporters Mediate Luminal Release of Acetylcholine from Bronchial Epithelium. *Am. J. Respir. Cell Mol. Biol.* **2005**, *33*, 79–88. [CrossRef]
29. Fallon, J.K.; Houvig, N.; Booth-Genthe, C.L.; Smith, P.C. Quantification of membrane transporter proteins in human lung and immortalized cell lines using targeted quantitative proteomic analysis by isotope dilution nanoLC–MS/MS. *J. Pharm. Biomed. Anal.* **2018**, *154*, 150–157. [CrossRef]
30. Horvath, G.; Mendes, E.S.; Schmid, N.; Schmid, A.; Conner, G.E.; Salathe, M.; Wanner, A. The effect of corticosteroids on the disposal of long-acting β2-agonists by airway smooth muscle cells. *J. Allergy Clin. Immunol.* **2007**, *120*, 1103–1109. [CrossRef]
31. Berg, T.; Hegelund-Myrbäck, T.; Öckinger, J.; Zhou, X.; Brännström, M.; Hagemann-Jensen, M.; Werkstrom, V.; Seidegård, J.; Grunewald, J.; Nord, M.; et al. Expression of MATE1, P-gp, OCTN1 and OCTN2, in epithelial and immune cells in the lung of COPD and healthy individuals. *Respir. Res.* **2018**, *19*, 68. [CrossRef]
32. Berg, T.; Myrbäck, T.H.; Olsson, M.; Seidegård, J.; Werkström, V.; Zhou, X.; Grunewald, J.; Gustavsson, L.; Nord, M. Gene expression analysis of membrane transporters and drug-metabolizing enzymes in the lung of healthy and COPD subjects. *Pharmacol. Res. Perspect.* **2014**, *2*, e00054. [CrossRef]
33. Shrine, N.; Portelli, M.A.; John, C.; Artigas, M.S.; Bennett, N.; Hall, R.; Lewis, J.; Henry, A.P.; Billington, C.K.; Ahmad, A.; et al. Moderate-to-severe asthma in individuals of European ancestry: A genome-wide association study. *Lancet Respir. Med.* **2019**, *7*, 20–34. [CrossRef]
34. Moffatt, M.F.; Gut, I.G.; Demenais, F.; Strachan, D.P.; Bouzigon, E.; Heath, S.; Von Mutius, E.; Farrall, M.; Lathrop, M.; Cookson, W.O. A Large-Scale, Consortium-Based Genomewide Association Study of Asthma. *N. Engl. J. Med.* **2010**, *363*, 1211–1221. [CrossRef] [PubMed]
35. Yamauchi, K.; Shikanai, T.; Nakamura, Y.; Kobayashi, H.; Ogasawara, M.; Maeyama, K. Roles of Histamine in the Pathogenesis of Bronchial Asthma and Reevaluation of the Clinical Usefulness of Antihistamines. *Yakugaku Zasshi* **2011**, *131*, 185–191. [CrossRef] [PubMed]
36. Yamauchi, K.; Ogasawara, M. The Role of Histamine in the Pathophysiology of Asthma and the Clinical Efficacy of Antihistamines in Asthma Therapy. *Int. J. Mol. Sci.* **2019**, *20*, 1733. [CrossRef]
37. Mukherjee, M.; Cingolani, E.; Pritchard, D.; Bosquillon, C. Enhanced expression of Organic Cation Transporters in bronchial epithelial cell layers following insults associated with asthma—Impact on salbutamol transport. *Eur. J. Pharm. Sci.* **2017**, *106*, 62–70. [CrossRef] [PubMed]
38. Rotoli, B.M.; Visigalli, R.; Barilli, A.; Ferrari, F.; Bianchi, M.G.; Di Lascia, M.; Riccardi, B.; Puccini, P.; Dall'Asta, V. Functional analysis of OCTN2 and ATB$^{0,+}$ in normal human airway epithelial cells. *PLoS ONE* **2020**, *15*, e0228568. [CrossRef]
39. Li, D.; Qi, C.; Zhou, J.; Wen, Z.; Zhu, X.; Xia, H.; Song, J. LPS-induced inflammation delays the transportation of ASP+ due to down-regulation of OCTN1/2 in alveolar epithelial cells. *J. Drug Target.* **2019**, *28*, 437–447. [CrossRef]
40. Qi, C.; Zhou, J.; Wang, Z.; Fang, X.; Li, D.; Jin, Y.; Song, J. Cigarette smoke extract combined with lipopolysaccharide reduces OCTN1/2 expression in human alveolar epithelial cells in vitro and rat lung in vivo under inflammatory conditions. *Int. Immunopharmacol.* **2020**, *87*, 106812. [CrossRef]
41. Schulz, C.; Farkas, L.; Wolf, K.; Krätzel, K.; Eissner, G.; Pfeifer, M. Differences in LPS-Induced Activation of Bronchial Epithelial Cells (BEAS-2B) and Type II-Like Pneumocytes (A-549). *Scand. J. Immunol.* **2002**, *56*, 294–302. [CrossRef]
42. Al-Majdoub, Z.M.; Al Feteisi, H.; Achour, B.; Warwood, S.; Neuhoff, S.; Rostami-Hodjegan, A.; Barber, J. Proteomic Quantification of Human Blood–Brain Barrier SLC and ABC Transporters in Healthy Individuals and Dementia Patients. *Mol. Pharm.* **2019**, *16*, 1220–1233. [CrossRef]
43. Liang, Y.; Ligong, C.; Chen, L. The physiological role of drug transporters. *Protein Cell* **2015**, *6*, 334–350. [CrossRef]

44. Majd, H.; King, M.S.; Palmer, S.M.; Smith, A.C.; Elbourne, L.D.; Paulsen, I.T.; Sharples, D.; Henderson, P.J.; Kunji, E.R. Screening of candidate substrates and coupling ions of transporters by thermostability shift assays. *eLife* **2018**, *7*. [CrossRef]
45. Tschirka, J.; Bach, M.; Kisis, I.; Lemmen, J.; Gnoth, M.J.; Gründemann, D. Transporter tandems—Precise tools for normalizing active transporter in the plasma membrane. *Biochem. J.* **2020**, *477*, 4191–4206. [CrossRef] [PubMed]
46. Boxberger, K.H.; Hagenbuch, B.; Lampe, J.N. Common drugs inhibit human organic cation transporter 1 (OCT1)-mediated neurotransmitter uptake. *Drug Metab. Dispos.* **2014**, *42*, 990–995. [CrossRef] [PubMed]
47. Yoshikawa, T.; Yanai, K. Histamine Clearance Through Polyspecific Transporters in the Brain. *Muscarinic Recept.* **2016**, *241*, 173–187. [CrossRef]
48. Kummer, W.; Wiegand, S.; Akinci, S.; Wessler, I.; Schinkel, A.H.; Wess, J.; Koepsell, H.; Haberberger, R.V.; Lips, K. Role of acetylcholine and polyspecific cation transporters in serotonin-induced bronchoconstriction in the mouse. *Respir. Res.* **2006**, *7*, 65. [CrossRef]
49. Kummer, W.; Krasteva, G. Non-neuronal cholinergic airway epithelium biology. *Curr. Opin. Pharmacol.* **2014**, *16*, 43–49. [CrossRef]
50. Wessler, I.; Kirkpatrick, C.J.; Racké, K. Non-neuronal acetylcholine, a locally acting molecule, widely distributed in biological systems: Expression and function in humans. *Pharmacol. Ther.* **1998**, *77*, 59–79. [CrossRef]
51. Kolahian, S.; Gosens, R. Cholinergic Regulation of Airway Inflammation and Remodelling. *J. Allergy* **2012**, *2012*, 1–9. [CrossRef]
52. Belmonte, K.E. Cholinergic Pathways in the Lungs and Anticholinergic Therapy for Chronic Obstructive Pulmonary Disease. *Proc. Am. Thorac. Soc.* **2005**, *2*, 297–304. [CrossRef]
53. Reinheimer, T.; Baumgärtner, D.; Höhle, K.-D.; Racké, K.; Wessler, I. Acetylcholine via Muscarinic Receptors Inhibits Histamine Release from Human Isolated Bronchi. *Am. J. Respir. Crit. Care Med.* **1997**, *156*, 389–395. [CrossRef] [PubMed]
54. Gosens, R.; Zaagsma, J.; Meurs, H.; Halayko, A.J. Muscarinic receptor signaling in the pathophysiology of asthma and COPD. *Respir. Res.* **2006**, *7*, 73. [CrossRef] [PubMed]
55. Friedman, J.R.; Richbart, S.D.; Merritt, J.C.; Brown, K.C.; Nolan, N.A.; Akers, A.T.; Lau, J.K.; Robateau, Z.R.; Miles, S.L.; Dasgupta, P. Acetylcholine signaling system in progression of lung cancers. *Pharmacol. Ther.* **2019**, *194*, 222–254. [CrossRef] [PubMed]
56. Wang, W.; Cohen, J.A.; Wallrapp, A.; Trieu, K.G.; Barrios, J.; Shao, F.; Krishnamoorthy, N.; Kuchroo, V.K.; Jones, M.R.; Fine, A.; et al. Age-Related Dopaminergic Innervation Augments T Helper 2-Type Allergic Inflammation in the Postnatal Lung. *Immunity* **2019**, *51*, 1102–1118.e7. [CrossRef] [PubMed]
57. Thangam, E.B.; Jemima, E.A.; Singh, H.; Baig, M.S.; Khan, M.; Mathias, C.B.; Church, M.K.; Saluja, R. The Role of Histamine and Histamine Receptors in Mast Cell-Mediated Allergy and Inflammation: The Hunt for New Therapeutic Targets. *Front. Immunol.* **2018**, *9*, 1873. [CrossRef]
58. Gelfand, E.W. Role of histamine in the pathophysiology of asthma: Immunomodulatory and anti-inflammatory activities of H1-receptor antagonists. *Am. J. Med.* **2002**, *113*, 2–7. [CrossRef]
59. Cazzola, M.; Matera, M.G. 5-HT modifiers as a potential treatment of asthma. *Trends Pharmacol. Sci.* **2000**, *21*, 13–16. [CrossRef]
60. Pirina, P.; Zinellu, E.; Paliogiannis, P.; Fois, A.G.; Marras, V.; Sotgia, S.; Carru, C.; Zinellu, A. Circulating serotonin levels in COPD patients: A pilot study. *BMC Pulm. Med.* **2018**, *18*, 167. [CrossRef]
61. Wultsch, T.; Grimberg, G.; Schmitt, A.; Painsipp, E.; Wetzstein, H.; Breitenkamp, A.F.S.; Gründemann, D.; Schömig, E.; Lesch, K.P.; Gerlach, M.; et al. Decreased anxiety in mice lacking the organic cation transporter 3. *J. Neural Transm.* **2009**, *116*, 689–697. [CrossRef]
62. Yee, S.W.; Lin, L.; Merski, M.; Keiser, L.G.M.J.; Gupta, A.; Zhang, Y.; Chien, H.-C.; Shoichet, B.K.; Giacomini, K.M. Prediction and validation of enzyme and transporter off-targets for metformin. *J. Pharmacokinet. Pharmacodyn.* **2015**, *42*, 463–475. [CrossRef]
63. Sekizawa, K.; Nakazawa, H.; Morikawa, M.; Yamauchi, K.; Maeyama, K.; Watanabe, T.; Sasaki, H. Histamine N-methyltransferase inhibitor potentiates histamine- and antigen-induced airway microvascular leakage in guinea pigs. *J. Allergy Clin. Immunol.* **1995**, *96*, 910–916. [CrossRef]
64. Gründemann, D.; Harlfinger, S.; Golz, S.; Geerts, A.; Lazar, A.; Berkels, R.; Jung, N.; Rubbert, A.; Schömig, E. Discovery of the ergothioneine transporter. *Proc. Natl. Acad. Sci. USA* **2005**, *102*, 5256–5261. [CrossRef] [PubMed]

65. Tschirka, J.; Kreisor, M.; Betz, J.; Gründemann, D. Substrate Selectivity Check of the Ergothioneine Transporter. *Drug Metab. Dispos.* **2018**, *46*, 779–785. [CrossRef] [PubMed]
66. Grigat, S.; Harlfinger, S.; Pal, S.; Striebinger, R.; Golz, S.; Geerts, A.; Lazar, A.; Schömig, E.; Gründemann, D. Probing the substrate specificity of the ergothioneine transporter with methimazole, hercynine, and organic cations. *Biochem. Pharmacol.* **2007**, *74*, 309–316. [CrossRef]
67. Cheah, I.K.; Tang, R.M.; Yew, T.S.; Lim, K.H.; Halliwell, B. Administration of Pure Ergothioneine to Healthy Human Subjects: Uptake, Metabolism, and Effects on Biomarkers of Oxidative Damage and Inflammation. *Antioxid. Redox Signal.* **2017**, *26*, 193–206. [CrossRef]
68. Halliwell, B.; Cheah, I.K.; Tang, R.M.Y. Ergothioneine—A diet-derived antioxidant with therapeutic potential. *FEBS Lett.* **2018**, *592*, 3357–3366. [CrossRef]
69. Cheah, I.; Halliwell, B. Could Ergothioneine Aid in the Treatment of Coronavirus Patients? *Antioxidants* **2020**, *9*, 595. [CrossRef]
70. Asahi, T.; Wu, X.; Shimoda, H.; Hisaka, S.; Harada, E.; Kanno, T.; Nakamura, Y.; Kato, Y.; Osawa, T. A mushroom-derived amino acid, ergothioneine, is a potential inhibitor of inflammation-related DNA halogenation. *Biosci. Biotechnol. Biochem.* **2015**, *80*, 313–317. [CrossRef]
71. Waller, S.; Tremelling, M.; Bredin, F.; Godfrey, L.; Howson, J.; Parkes, M. Evidence for association of OCTN genes and IBD5 with ulcerative colitis. *Gut* **2006**, *55*, 809–814. [CrossRef]
72. Lin, Z.; Nelson, L.; Franke, A.; Poritz, L.; Li, T.Y.; Wu, R.; Wang, Y.; MacNeill, C.; Thomas, N.J.; Schreiber, S.; et al. OCTN1 variant L503F is associated with familial and sporadic inflammatory bowel disease. *J. Crohns Colitis* **2010**, *4*, 132–138. [CrossRef]
73. Peltekova, V.D.; Wintle, R.F.; Rubin, L.A.; Amos, C.I.; Huang, Q.; Gu, X.; Newman, B.; Van Oene, M.; Cescon, D.; Greenberg, G.; et al. Functional variants of OCTN cation transporter genes are associated with Crohn disease. *Nat. Genet.* **2004**, *36*, 471–475. [CrossRef] [PubMed]
74. Meisel, P.; Pagels, S.; Grube, M.; Jedlitschky, G.; Völzke, H.; Kocher, T. Tooth loss and adiposity: Possible role of carnitine transporter (OCTN1/2) polymorphisms in women but not in men. *Clin. Oral Investig.* **2020**, 1–9. [CrossRef] [PubMed]
75. Rahman, I.; Gilmour, P.S.; Jimenez, L.A.; Biswas, S.K.; Antonicelli, F.; Aruoma, O.I. Ergothioneine inhibits oxidative stress- and TNF-α-induced NF-κB activation and interleukin-8 release in alveolar epithelial cells. *Biochem. Biophys. Res. Commun.* **2003**, *302*, 860–864. [CrossRef]
76. Biswas, S.; Hwang, J.W.; Kirkham, P.A.; Rahman, I. Pharmacological and Dietary Antioxidant Therapies for Chronic Obstructive Pulmonary Disease. *Curr. Med. Chem.* **2013**, *20*, 1496–1530. [CrossRef]
77. Rahman, I.; Kilty, I. Antioxidant Therapeutic Targets in COPD. *Curr. Drug Targets* **2006**, *7*, 707–720. [CrossRef]
78. Repine, J.E.; Elkins, N.D. Effect of ergothioneine on acute lung injury and inflammation in cytokine insufflated rats. *Prev. Med.* **2012**, *54*, S79–S82. [CrossRef]
79. Ohashi, R.; Tamai, I.; Yabuuchi, H.; Nezu, J.I.; Oku, A.; Sai, Y.; Shimane, M.; Tsuji, A. Na(+)-dependent carnitine transport by organic cation transporter (OCTN2): Its pharmacological and toxicological relevance. *J. Pharmacol. Exp. Ther.* **1999**, *291*, 778–784.
80. Longo, N.; Frigeni, M.; Pasquali, M. Carnitine transport and fatty acid oxidation. *Biochim. Biophys. Acta (BBA) Bioenerg.* **2016**, *1863*, 2422–2435. [CrossRef]
81. Tamai, I.; Ohashi, R.; Nezu, J.-I.; Yabuuchi, H.; Oku, A.; Shimane, M.; Sai, Y.; Tsuji, A. Molecular and Functional Identification of Sodium Ion-dependent, High Affinity Human Carnitine Transporter OCTN2. *J. Biol. Chem.* **1998**, *273*, 20378–20382. [CrossRef]
82. Kremser, K.; Stangl, H.; Pahan, K.; Singh, I. Nitric Oxide Regulates Peroxisomal Enzyme Activities. *Clin. Chem. Lab. Med.* **1995**, *33*, 763–774. [CrossRef]
83. Ferreira, G.C.; McKenna, M.C. l-Carnitine and Acetyl-l-carnitine Roles and Neuroprotection in Developing Brain. *Neurochem. Res.* **2017**, *42*, 1661–1675. [CrossRef]
84. Gülçin, I. Antioxidant and antiradical activities of l-carnitine. *Life Sci.* **2006**, *78*, 803–811. [CrossRef]
85. Solarska, K.; Lewinska, A.; Karowicz-Bilińska, A.; Bartosz, G. The antioxidant properties of carnitine in vitro. *Cell. Mol. Biol. Lett.* **2010**, *15*, 90–97. [CrossRef]
86. Şener, G.; Paskaloğlu, K.; Şatiroglu, H.; Alican, I.; Kaçmaz, A.; Sakarcan, A. L-Carnitine Ameliorates Oxidative Damage due to Chronic Renal Failure in Rats. *J. Cardiovasc. Pharmacol.* **2004**, *43*, 698–705. [CrossRef]
87. Le Borgne, F.; Ravaut, G.; Bernard, A.; Demarquoy, J. L-carnitine protects C2C12 cells against mitochondrial superoxide overproduction and cell death. *World J. Biol. Chem.* **2017**, *8*, 86–94. [CrossRef]

88. Cao, Y.; Qu, H.-J.; Li, P.; Wang, C.-B.; Wang, L.-X.; Han, Z.-W. Single dose administration of L-carnitine improves antioxidant activities in healthy subjects. *Tohoku J. Exp. Med.* **2011**, *224*, 209–213. [CrossRef]
89. Lee, B.-J.; Lin, J.-S.; Lin, Y.-C.; Lin, P.-T. Effects of L-carnitine supplementation on oxidative stress and antioxidant enzymes activities in patients with coronary artery disease: A randomized, placebo-controlled trial. *Nutr. J.* **2014**, *13*, 79. [CrossRef]
90. Al-Biltagi, M.; Isa, M.; Bediwy, A.S.; Helaly, N.; El Lebedy, D.D. L-Carnitine Improves the Asthma Control in Children with Moderate Persistent Asthma. *J. Allergy 2012*, **2012**, 1–7. [CrossRef]
91. Asilsoy, S.; Soylu, O.B.; Karaman, O.; Uzuner, N.; Kavukçu, S. Serum total and free carnitine levels in children with asthma. *World J. Pediatr.* **2009**, *5*, 60–62. [CrossRef]
92. Otsubo, C.; Bharathi, S.; Uppala, R.; Ilkayeva, O.R.; Wang, N.; McHugh, K.; Zou, Y.; Wang, J.; Alcorn, J.F.; Zuo, Y.Y.; et al. Long-chain Acylcarnitines Reduce Lung Function by Inhibiting Pulmonary Surfactant. *J. Biol. Chem.* **2015**, *290*, 23897–23904. [CrossRef]
93. Öztürk, M.A.; Kardas, Z.; Kardas, F.; Güneş, T.; Kurtoglu, S. Effects of L-carnitine supplementation on respiratory distress syndrome development and prognosis in premature infants: A single blind randomized controlled trial. *Exp. Ther. Med.* **2016**, *11*, 1123–1127. [CrossRef]
94. Gustavsson, L.; Bosquillon, C.; Gumbleton, M.; Hegelund-Myrbäck, T.; Nakanishi, T.; Price, D.; Tamai, I.; Zhou, X.-H. *Drug Transporters in the Lung: Expression and Potential Impact on Pulmonary Drug Disposition*; Royal Society of Chemistry (RSC): Cambridge, UK, 2016; Chapter 6; Volume 1, pp. 184–228.
95. Al-Jayyoussi, G.; Price, D.F.; Kreitmeyr, K.; Keogh, J.P.; Smith, M.W.; Gumbleton, M.; Morris, C.J. Absorption of ipratropium and l-carnitine into the pulmonary circulation of the ex-vivo rat lung is driven by passive processes rather than active uptake by OCT/OCTN transporters. *Int. J. Pharm.* **2015**, *496*, 834–841. [CrossRef]
96. Ohashi, R.; Tamai, I.; Nezu, J.-I.; Nikaido, H.; Hashimoto, N.; Oku, A.; Sai, Y.; Shimane, M.; Tsuji, A. Molecular and Physiological Evidence for Multifunctionality of Carnitine/Organic Cation Transporter OCTN2. *Mol. Pharmacol.* **2001**, *59*, 358–366. [CrossRef]
97. Nakanishi, T.; Hasegawa, Y.; Haruta, T.; Wakayama, T.; Tamai, I. In Vivo Evidence of Organic Cation Transporter-Mediated Tracheal Accumulation of the Anticholinergic Agent Ipratropium in Mice. *J. Pharm. Sci.* **2013**, *102*, 3373–3381. [CrossRef]
98. Salomon, J.J.; Endter, S.; Tachon, G.; Falson, F.; Buckley, S.T.; Ehrhardt, C. Transport of the fluorescent organic cation 4-(4-(dimethylamino)styryl)-N-methylpyridinium iodide (ASP+) in human respiratory epithelial cells. *Eur. J. Pharm. Biopharm.* **2012**, *81*, 351–359. [CrossRef]
99. Macdonald, C.; Shao, D.; Oli, A.; Agu, R.U. Characterization of Calu-3 cell monolayers as a model of bronchial epithelial transport: Organic cation interaction studies. *J. Drug Target.* **2013**, *21*, 97–106. [CrossRef]
100. Solis, E.; Zdravkovic, I.; Tomlinson, I.D.; Noskov, S.Y.; Rosenthal, S.J.; DeFelice, L.J. 4-(4-(Dimethylamino) phenyl)-1-methylpyridinium (APP+) Is a Fluorescent Substrate for the Human Serotonin Transporter. *J. Biol. Chem.* **2012**, *287*, 8852–8863. [CrossRef]
101. Schwartz, J.W.; Blakely, R.D.; DeFelice, L.J. Binding and Transport in Norepinephrine Transporters. *J. Biol. Chem.* **2003**, *278*, 9768–9777. [CrossRef]
102. Salomon, J.J.; Gausterer, J.C.; Yahara, T.; Hosoya, K.-I.; Huwer, H.; Hittinger, M.; Schneider-Daum, N.; Lehr, C.-M.; Ehrhardt, C. Organic cation transporter function in different in vitro models of human lung epithelium. *Eur. J. Pharm. Sci.* **2015**, *80*, 82–88. [CrossRef]
103. Koepsell, H. Multiple binding sites in organic cation transporters require sophisticated procedures to identify interactions of novel drugs. *Biol. Chem.* **2019**, *400*, 195–207. [CrossRef]
104. Koepsell, H. Role of organic cation transporters in drug–drug interaction. *Expert Opin. Drug Metab. Toxicol.* **2015**, *11*, 1619–1633. [CrossRef] [PubMed]
105. Salomon, J.J.; Hagos, Y.; Petzke, S.; Kühne, A.; Gausterer, J.C.; Hosoya, K.-I.; Ehrhardt, C. Beta-2 Adrenergic Agonists Are Substrates and Inhibitors of Human Organic Cation Transporter 1. *Mol. Pharm.* **2015**, *12*, 2633–2641. [CrossRef] [PubMed]
106. Faria, A.; Monteiro, R.; Pestana, D.; Martel, F.; De Freitas, V.; Mateus, N.; Calhau, C. Impact of culture media glucose levels on the intestinal uptake of organic cations. *Cytotechnology* **2010**, *62*, 23–29. [CrossRef] [PubMed]
107. Kreft, M.E.; Jerman, U.D.; Lasič, E.; Hevir-Kene, N.; Rižner, T.L.; Peternel, L.; Kristan, K. The characterization of the human cell line Calu-3 under different culture conditions and its use as an optimized in vitro model to investigate bronchial epithelial function. *Eur. J. Pharm. Sci.* **2015**, *69*, 1–9. [CrossRef]

108. Kreft, M.E.; Tratnjek, L.; Lasič, E.; Hevir, N.; Rižner, T.L.; Kristan, K. Different Culture Conditions Affect Drug Transporter Gene Expression, Ultrastructure, and Permeability of Primary Human Nasal Epithelial Cells. *Pharm. Res.* **2020**, *37*, 170. [CrossRef]
109. Forbes, B.; Ehrhardt, C. Human respiratory epithelial cell culture for drug delivery applications. *Eur. J. Pharm. Biopharm.* **2005**, *60*, 193–205. [CrossRef]
110. Sporty, J.L.; Horálková, L.; Ehrhardt, C. In vitrocell culture models for the assessment of pulmonary drug disposition. *Expert Opin. Drug Metab. Toxicol.* **2008**, *4*, 333–345. [CrossRef]
111. Sakagami, M. In vitro, ex vivo and in vivo methods of lung absorption for inhaled drugs. *Adv. Drug Deliv. Rev.* **2020**. [CrossRef]
112. Bosquillon, C.; Madlova, M.; Patel, N.; Clear, N.; Forbes, B. A Comparison of Drug Transport in Pulmonary Absorption Models: Isolated Perfused rat Lungs, Respiratory Epithelial Cell Lines and Primary Cell Culture. *Pharm. Res.* **2017**, *34*, 2532–2540. [CrossRef]
113. Bleasby, K.; Castle, J.C.; Roberts, C.J.; Cheng, C.; Bailey, W.J.; Sina, J.F.; Kulkarni, A.V.; Hafey, M.J.; Evers, R.; Johnson, J.M.; et al. Expression profiles of 50 xenobiotic transporter genes in humans and pre-clinical species: A resource for investigations into drug disposition. *Xenobiotica* **2006**, *36*, 963–988. [CrossRef]
114. Leclerc, J.; Ngangue, E.C.-N.; Cauffiez, C.; Allorge, D.; Pottier, N.; Lafitte, J.-J.; Debaert, M.; Jaillard, S.; Broly, F.; Lo-Guidice, J.-M. Xenobiotic metabolism and disposition in human lung: Transcript profiling in non-tumoral and tumoral tissues. *Biochimie* **2011**, *93*, 1012–1027. [CrossRef] [PubMed]
115. Selo, M.A.; Delmas, A.-S.; Springer, L.; Zoufal, V.; Sake, J.A.; Clerkin, C.G.; Huwer, H.; Schneider-Daum, N.; Lehr, C.-M.; Nickel, S.; et al. Tobacco Smoke and Inhaled Drugs Alter Expression and Activity of Multidrug Resistance-Associated Protein-1 (MRP1) in Human Distal Lung Epithelial Cells in vitro. *Front. Bioeng. Biotechnol.* **2020**, *8*, 1030. [CrossRef] [PubMed]
116. Kolli, A.R.; Kuczaj, A.K.; Martin, F.; Hayes, A.W.; Peitsch, M.C.; Hoeng, J. Bridging inhaled aerosol dosimetry to physiologically based pharmacokinetic modeling for toxicological assessment: Nicotine delivery systems and beyond. *Crit. Rev. Toxicol.* **2019**, *49*, 725–741. [CrossRef]
117. Bäckman, P.; Arora, S.; Couet, W.; Forbes, B.; De Kruijf, W.; Paudel, A. Advances in experimental and mechanistic computational models to understand pulmonary exposure to inhaled drugs. *Eur. J. Pharm. Sci.* **2018**, *113*, 41–52. [CrossRef]
118. Ehrhardt, C.; Kneuer, C.; Bies, C.; Lehr, C.-M.; Kim, K.-J.; Bakowsky, U. Salbutamol is actively absorbed across human bronchial epithelial cell layers. *Pulm. Pharmacol. Ther.* **2005**, *18*, 165–170. [CrossRef]
119. Unwalla, H.J.; Horvath, G.; Roth, F.D.; Conner, G.E.; Salathe, M. Albuterol Modulates Its Own Transepithelial Flux via Changes in Paracellular Permeability. *Am. J. Respir. Cell Mol. Biol.* **2012**, *46*, 551–558. [CrossRef]
120. Mamlouk, M.; Young, P.M.; Bebawy, M.; Haghi, M.; Mamlouk, S.; Mulay, V.; Traini, D. Salbutamol Sulfate Absorption across Calu-3 Bronchial Epithelia Cell Monolayer is Inhibited in the Presence of Common Anionic NSAIDs. *J. Asthma* **2013**, *50*, 334–341. [CrossRef]
121. Gnadt, M.; Trammer, B.; Freiwald, M.; Kardziev, B.; Bayliss, M.K.; Edwards, C.D.; Schmidt, M.; Friedel, G.; Högger, P. Methacholine delays pulmonary absorption of inhaled β2-agonists due to competition for organic cation/carnitine transporters. *Pulm. Pharmacol. Ther.* **2012**, *25*, 124–134. [CrossRef]
122. Hendrickx, R.; Johansson, J.G.; Lohmann, C.; Jenvert, R.-M.; Blomgren, A.; Börjesson, L.; Gustavsson, L. Identification of Novel Substrates and Structure–Activity Relationship of Cellular Uptake Mediated by Human Organic Cation Transporters 1 and 2. *J. Med. Chem.* **2013**, *56*, 7232–7242. [CrossRef]
123. Tzvetkov, M.V.; Matthaei, J.; Pojar, S.; Faltraco, F.; Vogler, S.; Prukop, T.; Seitz, T.; Brockmöller, J. Increased Systemic Exposure and Stronger Cardiovascular and Metabolic Adverse Reactions to Fenoterol in Individuals with HeritableOCT1Deficiency. *Clin. Pharmacol. Ther.* **2018**, *103*, 868–878. [CrossRef]
124. Horvath, G.; Mendes, E.S.; Schmid, N.; Schmid, A.; Conner, G.E.; Fregien, N.L.; Salathe, M.; Wanner, A. Rapid nongenomic actions of inhaled corticosteroids on long-acting β2-agonist transport in the airway. *Pulm. Pharmacol. Ther.* **2011**, *24*, 654–659. [CrossRef] [PubMed]
125. Nakanishi, T.; Haruta, T.; Shirasaka, Y.; Tamai, I. Organic Cation Transporter-Mediated Renal Secretion of Ipratropium and Tiotropium in Rats and Humans. *Drug Metab. Dispos.* **2010**, *39*, 117–122. [CrossRef]
126. Nakamura, T.; Nakanishi, T.; Haruta, T.; Shirasaka, Y.; Keogh, J.P.; Tamai, I. Transport of Ipratropium, an Anti-Chronic Obstructive Pulmonary Disease Drug, Is Mediated by Organic Cation/Carnitine Transporters in Human Bronchial Epithelial Cells: Implications for Carrier-Mediated Pulmonary Absorption. *Mol. Pharm.* **2010**, *7*, 187–195. [CrossRef]

127. Panduga, V.; Stocks, M.J.; Bosquillon, C. Ipratropium is 'luminally recycled' by an inter-play between apical uptake and efflux transporters in Calu-3 bronchial epithelial cell layers. *Int. J. Pharm.* **2017**, *532*, 328–336. [CrossRef]
128. Zhou, S.-F.; Wang, L.-L.; Di, Y.M.; Xue, C.C.; Duan, W.; Li, C.G.; Li, Y. Substrates and inhibitors of human multidrug resistance associated proteins and the implications in drug development. *Curr. Med. Chem.* **2008**, *15*, 1981–2039. [CrossRef]
129. Shitara, Y.; Sato, H.; Sugiyama, Y. EVALUATION OF DRUG-DRUG INTERACTION IN THE HEPATOBILIARY AND RENAL TRANSPORT OF DRUGS. *Annu. Rev. Pharmacol. Toxicol.* **2005**, *45*, 689–723. [CrossRef]
130. Hutter, V.; Chau, D.Y.; Hilgendorf, C.; Brown, A.; Cooper, A.; Zann, V.; Pritchard, D.I.; Bosquillon, C. Digoxin net secretory transport in bronchial epithelial cell layers is not exclusively mediated by P-glycoprotein/MDR1. *Eur. J. Pharm. Biopharm.* **2014**, *86*, 74–82. [CrossRef]
131. Chen, J.; Brockmöller, J.; Seitz, T.; König, J.; Tzvetkov, M.V.; Chen, X. Tropane alkaloids as substrates and inhibitors of human organic cation transporters of the SLC22 (OCT) and the SLC47 (MATE) families. *Biol. Chem.* **2017**, *398*, 237–249. [CrossRef]
132. Müller, F.; König, J.; Hoier, E.; Mandery, K.; Fromm, M.F. Role of organic cation transporter OCT2 and multidrug and toxin extrusion proteins MATE1 and MATE2-K for transport and drug interactions of the antiviral lamivudine. *Biochem. Pharmacol.* **2013**, *86*, 808–815. [CrossRef]
133. Ingoglia, F.; Visigalli, R.; Rotoli, B.M.; Barilli, A.; Riccardi, B.; Puccini, P.; Dall'Asta, V. Functional activity of L-carnitine transporters in human airway epithelial cells. *Biochim. Biophys. Acta (BBA) Biomembr.* **2016**, *1858*, 210–219. [CrossRef]
134. Bäckström, E.; Lundqvist, A.; Boger, E.; Svanberg, P.; Ewing, P.; Hammarlund-Udenaes, M.; Fridén, M. Development of a Novel Lung Slice Methodology for Profiling of Inhaled Compounds. *J. Pharm. Sci.* **2016**, *105*, 838–845. [CrossRef]
135. Su, H.; Wang, Y.; Liu, S.; Wang, Y.; Liu, Q.; Liu, G.; Chen, Q. Emerging transporter-targeted nanoparticulate drug delivery systems. *Acta Pharm. Sin. B* **2019**, *9*, 49–58. [CrossRef]
136. Kou, L.; Bhutia, Y.D.; Yao, Q.; He, Z.; Sun, J.; Ganapathy, V. Transporter-Guided Delivery of Nanoparticles to Improve Drug Permeation across Cellular Barriers and Drug Exposure to Selective Cell Types. *Front. Pharmacol.* **2018**, *9*, 27. [CrossRef]
137. Kou, L.; Yao, Q.; Sun, M.; Wu, C.; Wang, J.; Luo, Q.; Wang, G.; Du, Y.; Fu, Q.; He, Z.; et al. Cotransporting Ion is a Trigger for Cellular Endocytosis of Transporter-Targeting Nanoparticles: A Case Study of High-Efficiency SLC22A5 (OCTN2)-Mediated Carnitine-Conjugated Nanoparticles for Oral Delivery of Therapeutic Drugs. *Adv. Health Mater.* **2017**, *6*. [CrossRef]
138. Mo, J.; Shi, S.; Zhang, Q.; Gong, T.; Sun, X.; Zhang, Z.-R. Synthesis, Transport and Mechanism of a Type I Prodrug: L-Carnitine Ester of Prednisolone. *Mol. Pharm.* **2011**, *8*, 1629–1640. [CrossRef]
139. Mo, J.; Lim, L.Y.; Zhang, Z.-R. l-Carnitine ester of prednisolone: Pharmacokinetic and pharmacodynamic evaluation of a type I prodrug. *Int. J. Pharm.* **2014**, *475*, 123–129. [CrossRef]
140. Eriksson, J.; Sjögren, E.; Lennernäs, H.; Thörn, H. Drug Absorption Parameters Obtained Using the Isolated Perfused Rat Lung Model Are Predictive of Rat In Vivo Lung Absorption. *AAPS J.* **2020**, *22*, 71. [CrossRef]
141. Eriksson, J.; Thörn, H.; Sjögren, E.; Holmstén, L.; Rubin, K.; Lennernäs, H. Pulmonary Dissolution of Poorly Soluble Compounds Studied in an ex Vivo Rat Lung Model. *Mol. Pharm.* **2019**, *16*, 3053–3064. [CrossRef]
142. Kamusella, P.C.; Wissgott, C.; Grosse-Siestrup, C.; Dittrich, S.; Hegemann, O.; Koios, D.; Von Massenbach, J.; Meissler, M.; Unger, V.; Groneberg, D.A.; et al. A model of isolated, autologously hemoperfused porcine slaughterhouse lungs. *ALTEX* **2009**, *26*, 279–284. [CrossRef]
143. Floerl, S.; Kuehne, A.; Hagos, Y. Functional and Pharmacological Comparison of Human, Mouse, and Rat Organic Cation Transporter 1 toward Drug and Pesticide Interaction. *Int. J. Mol. Sci.* **2020**, *21*, 6871. [CrossRef]
144. Cingolani, E.; Alqahtani, S.; Sadler, R.C.; Prime, D.; Stolnik, S.; Bosquillon, C. In vitro investigation on the impact of airway mucus on drug dissolution and absorption at the air-epithelium interface in the lungs. *Eur. J. Pharm. Biopharm.* **2019**, *141*, 210–220. [CrossRef]
145. Alqahtani, S.; Roberts, C.J.; Stolnik, S.; Bosquillon, C. Development of an In Vitro System to Study the Interactions of Aerosolized Drugs with Pulmonary Mucus. *Pharmaceutics* **2020**, *12*, 145. [CrossRef]
146. Faner, R.; Agustí, À. COPD: Algorithms and clinical management. *Eur. Respir. J.* **2017**, *50*, 1701733. [CrossRef]
147. Aebersold, R.; Mann, M. Mass-spectrometric exploration of proteome structure and function. *Nat. Cell Biol.* **2016**, *537*, 347–355. [CrossRef]

148. Erb-Downward, J.R.; Thompson, D.L.; Han, M.K.; Freeman, C.M.; McCloskey, L.; Schmidt, L.A.; Young, V.B.; Toews, G.B.; Curtis, J.L.; Sundaram, B.; et al. Analysis of the Lung Microbiome in the "Healthy" Smoker and in COPD. *PLoS ONE* **2011**, *6*, e16384. [CrossRef]
149. Garcia-Nuñez, M.; Millares, L.; Pomares, X.; Ferrari, R.; Pérez-Brocal, V.; Gallego, M.; Espasa, M.; Moya, A.; Monsó, E. Severity-Related Changes of Bronchial Microbiome in Chronic Obstructive Pulmonary Disease. *J. Clin. Microbiol.* **2014**, *52*, 4217–4223. [CrossRef]
150. Brewington, J.J.; Filbrandt, E.T.; LaRosa, F.; Ostmann, A.J.; Strecker, L.M.; Szczesniak, R.D.; Clancy, J.P. Detection of CFTR function and modulation in primary human nasal cell spheroids. *J. Cyst. Fibros.* **2018**, *17*, 26–33. [CrossRef]
151. Sachs, N.; Papaspyropoulos, A.; Ommen, D.D.Z.; Heo, I.; Böttinger, L.; Klay, D.; Weeber, F.; Huelsz-Prince, G.; Iakobachvili, N.; Amatngalim, G.D.; et al. Long-term expanding human airway organoids for disease modeling. *EMBO J.* **2019**, *38*. [CrossRef]
152. Yang, L.; Li, Y. Sex Differences in the Expression of Drug-Metabolizing and Transporter Genes in Human Liver. *J. Drug Metab. Toxicol.* **2012**, *3*, 1000119. [CrossRef]
153. Lyn-Cook, B.; Starlard-Davenport, A.; Word, B.; Green, B.; Wise, C.; Ning, B.; Huang, Y. Gender differences in expression of drug transporter genes in human livers: Microarray and real-time PCR analysis. *AACR* **2008**, *14*, B34.
154. Schuetz, E.G.; Furuya, K.N.; Schuetz, J.D. Interindividual variation in expression of P-glycoprotein in normal human liver and secondary hepatic neoplasms. *J. Pharmacol. Exp. Ther.* **1995**, *275*, 1011–1018.
155. Joseph, S.; Nicolson, T.J.; Hammons, G.; Word, B.; Green-Knox, B.; Lyn-Cook, B. Expression of drug transporters in human kidney: Impact of sex, age, and ethnicity. *Biol. Sex Differ.* **2015**, *6*, 4. [CrossRef]

Publisher's Note: MDPI stays neutral with regard to jurisdictional claims in published maps and institutional affiliations.

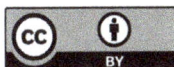

© 2020 by the authors. Licensee MDPI, Basel, Switzerland. This article is an open access article distributed under the terms and conditions of the Creative Commons Attribution (CC BY) license (http://creativecommons.org/licenses/by/4.0/).

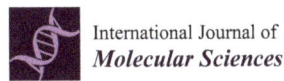

Review

Organic Cation Transporters in Human Physiology, Pharmacology, and Toxicology

Sophia L. Samodelov [1], Gerd A. Kullak-Ublick [1,2], Zhibo Gai [1,3,*] and Michele Visentin [1,*]

1. Department of Clinical Pharmacology and Toxicology, University Hospital Zurich, University of Zurich, 8006 Zurich, Switzerland; sophia.samodelov@usz.ch (S.L.S.); gerd.kullak@usz.ch (G.A.K.-U.)
2. Mechanistic Safety, CMO & Patient Safety, Global Drug Development, Novartis Pharma, 4056 Basel, Switzerland
3. Experimental Center, Shandong University of Traditional Chinese Medicine, Jinan 250355, China
* Correspondence: zhibo.gai@usz.ch (Z.G.); michele.visentin@usz.ch (M.V.); Tel.: +86-177-6358-1814 (Z.G.); +41-44-556-31-48 (M.V.)

Received: 4 September 2020; Accepted: 21 October 2020; Published: 24 October 2020

Abstract: Individual cells and epithelia control the chemical exchange with the surrounding environment by the fine-tuned expression, localization, and function of an array of transmembrane proteins that dictate the selective permeability of the lipid bilayer to small molecules, as actual gatekeepers to the interface with the extracellular space. Among the variety of channels, transporters, and pumps that localize to cell membrane, organic cation transporters (OCTs) are considered to be extremely relevant in the transport across the plasma membrane of the majority of the endogenous substances and drugs that are positively charged near or at physiological pH. In humans, the following six organic cation transporters have been characterized in regards to their respective substrates, all belonging to the solute carrier 22 (SLC22) family: the organic cation transporters 1, 2, and 3 (OCT1–3); the organic cation/carnitine transporter novel 1 and 2 (OCTN1 and N2); and the organic cation transporter 6 (OCT6). OCTs are highly expressed on the plasma membrane of polarized epithelia, thus, playing a key role in intestinal absorption and renal reabsorption of nutrients (e.g., choline and carnitine), in the elimination of waste products (e.g., trimethylamine and trimethylamine N-oxide), and in the kinetic profile and therapeutic index of several drugs (e.g., metformin and platinum derivatives). As part of the Special Issue Physiology, Biochemistry, and Pharmacology of Transporters for Organic Cations, this article critically presents the physio-pathological, pharmacological, and toxicological roles of OCTs in the tissues in which they are primarily expressed.

Keywords: hepatotoxicity; nephrotoxicity; organic cation transporter; solute carrier

1. Introduction

The organic cation transporters are primarily members of the solute carrier 22 (SLC22) family, which itself belongs to the solute carrier (SLC) superfamily, the largest group of membrane transporters comprising 65 SLC families (SLC1–65) with more than 400 identified genes thus far (for details on the SLC classification, we refer to the curated BioParadigms.org online SLC table) [1]. SLCs regulate the transport of most of the molecules essential for cell life across biomembranes and they have been linked to more than a hundred monogenic disorders [2]. In the human SLC22 family, six organic cation transporters have been characterized in regard to their respective substrates. The organic cation transporters 1, 2, and 3 (OCT1–3) are encoded by the genes *SLC22A1*, -*2*, and -*3*. The organic cation/carnitine transporter novel 1 and 2 (OCTN1 and N2) and the organic cation transporter 6 (OCT6) are encoded by the *SLC22A4*, -*5*, and -*16*, respectively [3]. Other members of the human SLC22 family comprise eight anion transporters (OATs), one urate transporter (URAT1), and fourteen orphan proteins, as no substrate thereof has yet been identified (Figure 1) [1]. Phylogenetic analyses suggest that SLC22 transporters may have evolved over 450 million years ago, with putative SLC22 orthologues found in worms, sea urchins, flies, and ciona [4]. The transporters discussed in this review are the highly related members OCT1–3 and OCTN1–2, as well as the more recently characterized OCT6, encoded by *SLC22A16* and cloned alongside with *SLC22A15* in 2002. Because no substrate of the latter has yet been identified, it will not be discussed in this review (see [5] Eraly et al., [6] Okada et al., [7] Zhu et al., and [8] Drake et al. for the current status of information on human SLC22A15).

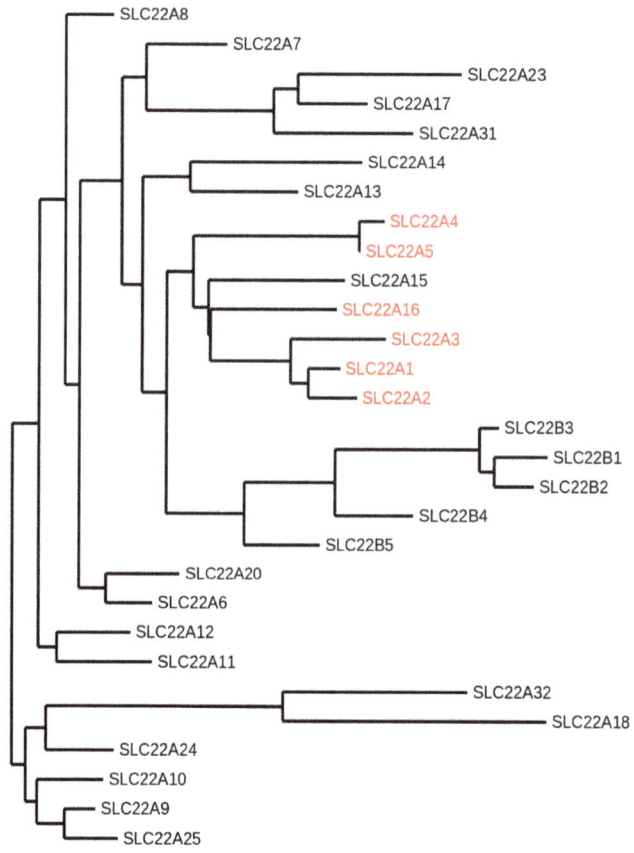

Figure 1. Phylogram of the human solute carrier 22 (SLC22) family members. The following protein sequence were used: SLC22A1 (O15245.2), SLC22A2 (O15244.2), SLC22A3 (O75751.1), SLC22A4 (Q9H015.3), SLC22A5 (O76082.1), SLC22A6 (Q4U2R8.1), SLC22A7 (Q9Y694.1), SLC22A8 (Q8TCC7.1), SLC22A9 (Q8IVM8.1), SLC22A10 (Q63ZE4.2), SLC22A11 (Q9NSA0.1), SLC22A12 (Q96S37.1), SLC22A13 (Q9Y226.2), SLC22A14 (Q9Y267.4), SLC22A15 (Q8IZD6.1), SLC22A16 (Q86VW1.1), SLC22A17 (Q8WUG5.1), SLC22A18 (Q96BI1.3), SLC22A20 (A6NK97.1), SLC22A23 (A1A5C7.2), SLC22A24 (Q8N4F4.2), SLC22A25 (Q6T423.2), SLC22A31 (A6NKX4.4), SLC22A32 (Q14728.1), SLC22B1 (Q7L0J3.1), SLC22B2 (Q7L1I2.1), SLC22B3 (Q496J9.1), SLC22B4 (Q8N4V2.1), and SLC22B5 (Q8N434.2). The organic cation transporters are highlighted in red. The SLC22A15 transporter that clusters with the other organic cation transporters has not been functionally characterized yet. This phylogeny was generated using the open access software Phylogeny.fr [9–11].

The putative human OCT proteins consist of 12 transmembrane domains (TMDs), intracellular N- and C-termini, one extracellular loop between the first and the second TMD, and one intracellular loop between the sixth and the seventh TMD (Figure 2). Currently, no crystal structure of OCTs has been resolved; hence, the topology and the mode of transport of OCTs are largely based on computational modeling with *E. coli* LacY permease and structure-function characterization. In this model, the binding pocket within the outward-open binding cleft is likely to have overlapping binding sites. The binding of the substrate leads to a series of conformational changes for the release of the substrate into the cytosol. Thereafter, the transporter, empty or loaded with a substrate bound in the inward conformation, can switch back to the outward-open conformation [12,13]. Although most of these studies have been performed on rat Oct1 and Oct2, this mechanistic model is considered to also be valid for the human OCTs. However, the differences between human and rodents concerning substrate selectivity warrant direct structure-function studies on the human OCTs to better understand how these transporters work in humans [14].

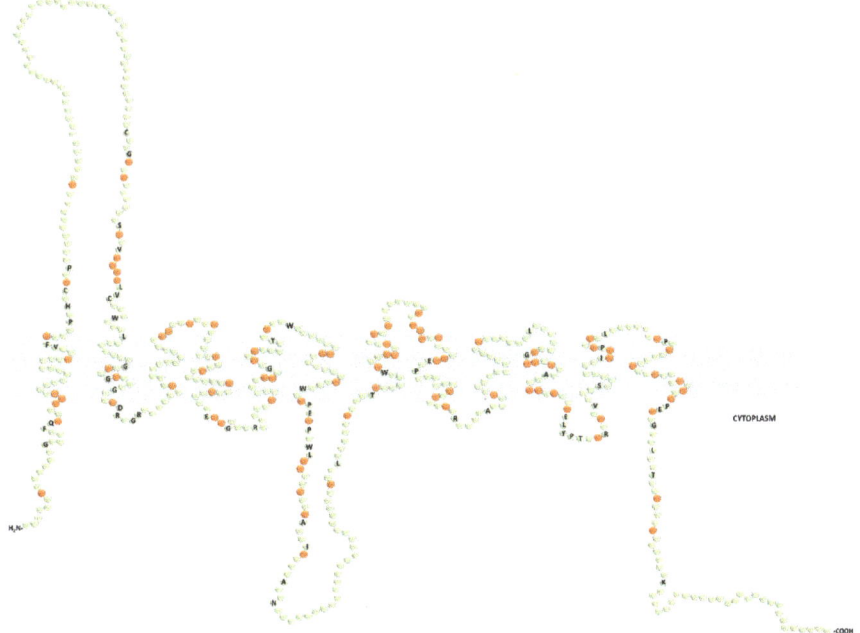

Figure 2. Predicted secondary structure of the functionally characterized human organic cation transporters (OCTs). Prediction was generated with the Protter open access software from the input protein sequence Q86VW1.1 (OCT6) and aligned by CLUSTALW open access software with the following protein sequences: SLC22A1 (O15245.2), SLC22A2 (O15244.2), SLC22A3 (O75751.1), SLC22A4 (Q9H015.3), and SLC22A5 (O76082.1). The labeled and non-labeled residues in green color represent the fully conserved and the non-conserved amino acids, respectively. The orange color indicates the semiconserved residues.

OCTs are known as polyspecific transporters because they recognize and transport a broad range of molecules, typically positively charged or zwitterions at physiological pH, such as the organic amines choline and carnitine, the neurotransmitters dopamine and serotonin, the microbiota products trimethylamine (TMA) and trimethylamine N-oxide (TMAO), and the vitamin B1 thiamine [15,16]. OCTs also facilitate the transport of a variety of drugs, including the anticancer platinum derivatives and ifosfamide, the antibiotics gentamicin, cephaloridine and colistin, and the antidiabetic metformin [3,15,17,18]. Ever since their identification, the thermodynamics, kinetics, and substrate specificities of OCTs have been characterized in different overexpressing systems, using prototypical substrates such as radiolabeled tetraethylammonium (TEA) and 1-methyl-4-phenylpyridinium (MPP$^+$), and the fluorescent compound 4-[4-(dimthylamino)-styryl]-N-methylpyridinium (ASP$^+$). In most cases, OCTs are Na$^+$-independent electrogenic transporters, whose activity is driven by the membrane potential across the plasma membrane. Thus, according to the electrochemical gradient of the substrate, OCTs can act as either influx or efflux systems. An exception is represented by OCTN2, which displays a bifunctional mode of transport. OCTN2 transports carnitine and its precursor γ-butyrobetaine in a Na$^+$-dependent manner, and other organic cations in a Na$^+$-independent manner [19]. OCTs are characterized by different influx kinetics. The OCTN2-mediated L-carnitine uptake seems to follow Michaelis–Menten kinetics [20]. OCT1 and OCT2 appear to have allosteric properties. Koepsell's group elegantly demonstrated that the rat Oct1 monomer functioned in an allosteric mode [21]. Likewise, our group has shown that the transport of structurally different substrates mediated by the human OCT2 likely involved two cooperative binding sites, suggesting that human OCT2 also had allosteric features [18,22,23].

Expression and localization studies in different species have revealed that OCT1, OCT2, and OCT6 displayed relatively narrow patterns of expression limited to individual organs or tissues. In humans, OCT1 is primarily expressed on the basolateral membrane of enterocytes and hepatocytes (intestines and liver) [24,25], and OCT2 is expressed on the basolateral membrane of proximal tubular cells (kidney) [26]. Initially, OCT6 was considered to be testis specific, as it had been detected only on the luminal membrane of the epididymal epithelium and in the Sertoli cells [27]. Lately, it has also been detected in endometria and in several cancers, suggesting a possible role of OCT6 in cancer resistance [28–39]. Noteworthy, in rodents, Oct1 has also been shown to be highly expressed on the basolateral membrane of proximal tubular cells and Oct2 in the brain and inner ear [40,41]. High expression levels in the intestine, liver, and kidneys of OCT1 and OCT2 advocates a cardinal role of these transporters in the intestinal absorption, tissue distribution, and hepatic and renal elimination of several widely prescribed drugs [42]. OCT3, OCTN1, and OCTN2 are more broadly expressed throughout the body [14,20,43–46]. In polarized epithelia, OCT1, -2, and -3 are restricted to the basolateral membrane. Through a mating-based split-ubiquitin system screening, it has been found that tetraspanin CD63, a four transmembrane domains protein that facilitates cell adhesion and motility, was a protein partner of OCT1, -2 and -3 [47,48]. It has also been demonstrated that CD63 was critical for the correct basolateral localization of OCT2 in proximal tubular cells [47]. The motif sequence that might be involved in the basolateral sorting of OCT1, -2 and -3 is not known. Still, it is noteworthy to highlight the presence of a fully conserved di-leucine sequence, a well-characterized basolateral sorting sequence, in the cytoplasmic tail of these transporters (Figure 2) [49]. Conversely, OCTN1, OCTN2, and OCT6 cellular localization may be tissue dependent. For instance, OCTN2 is expressed on the brush border membrane of enterocytes and proximal tubular cells, and on the sinusoidal membrane of hepatocytes [20,44–46,50–53]. The delivery of proteins to the apical surface most likely depends on multiple coordinated mechanisms, including N-glycosylation pattern, interacting protein partners, and membrane lipid content [49].

As part of the Special Issue Physiology, Biochemistry, and Pharmacology of Transporters for Organic Cations, this article provides a critical overview of the physiological, pharmacological, and toxicological impact and function of organic cation transporters in the key organ systems in which they are expressed. Sources for this review were obtained through extensive literature searches of publications browsing PubMed. Only papers published in the English language were considered.

2. Organic Cation Transporters (OCTs) in the Liver

There is a good deal of evidence that OCT1 and OCT3 are expressed in rodent, as well as human liver, whereas OCTN1 and OCTN2 may be expressed in rodent but not in the human hepatocytes. OCT1 represents the most studied hepatic OCT [15]. In this section, we discuss OCT1 primarily and mention some valuable, although not necessarily translatable, animal studies on liver Oct3 and Octn transporters. Oct1 was cloned from the rat in 1994 and found to be highly expressed in the liver and kidney [54]. The human OCT1 was cloned shortly after that and was found in the liver, at the sinusoidal side of hepatocytes, but only marginally expressed in the kidney [24,25]. The *SLC22A1* gene is under the control of the hepatic nuclear transcription factor HNF-4a. When it binds to the promoter region of the *SLC22A1* gene, HNF-4a activates the transcription of the OCT1 mRNA. The HNF-4a-mediated transcriptional activation of the *SLC22A1* gene is inhibited by the bile acid chenodeoxycholic acid, which is the most potent endogenous ligand of the nuclear receptor farnesoid X receptor (FXR) [55]. Indeed, the hepatic expression of OCT1 is lower in patients and animals with cholestasis, a condition in which bile acids accumulate in the liver because of an inefficient elimination in the bile [24,56–58]. A number of independent studies have shown that OCT1 expression was also reduced in liver tumors. Although the role of OCT1 in liver carcinogenesis has not been elucidated, it is conceivable that the expression level of OCT1 is likely to determine the pattern of fluorocholine hepatic accumulation, a positron emission tomography (PET) tracer, a substrate of OCT1 that shows promising results in the differential diagnosis of intrahepatic lesions [59–61]. At the protein level, OCT1 can be regulated by protein kinase A (PKA) and Ca^{++}/calmodulin [62]. Recently, by using rat Oct1 reconstituted in nanodiscs, it has been found that the allosteric binding of rat Oct1 was regulated through interactions with the surrounding lipid microenvironment [63].

Thus far, OCT1 has been primarily characterized from a pharmacological perspective, and its physiological role has only been partially defined. Recently, it has been shown that the total Oct1 knockout mouse, viable with no apparent deficiencies or phenotype, displayed an increased ratio of AMP to ATP, which activated the energy sensor AMP-activated kinase (AMPK), and substantially reduced triglyceride levels in the liver [64]. This phenotype seems to be due to the reduced uptake of thiamine in the Oct1-deficient animals. Thiamine (vitamin B1) is involved in energy transformation pathways as a cofactor of the pyruvate dehydrogenase complex, the α-ketoglutarate dehydrogenase, and the branched-chain α-ketoacid dehydrogenase [65]. Thiamine deficiency compromises the ability of the cell to synthesize ATP, resulting in a constitutive phosphorylation of AMPK, and increased catabolic rate and energy consumption [64,66]. When human OCT1 is expressed in the $Oct1^{-/-}$ mouse, the transgenic liver appears to become prone to steatosis, indicating a role of OCT1 in hepatic lipid and energy metabolism [66]. The pharmacological relevance of OCT1 has been facilitated by the flourishing of pharmacogenomics studies in the last two decades. There is extensive clinical evidence suggesting that the therapeutic effects and toxicity of drugs could be changed in subsets of individuals carrying a certain genetic variant of the *SLC22A1* gene encoding for OCT1. In the *SLC22A1* gene, many nonsynonymous single nucleotide polymorphisms (SNPs) have been identified, some affecting expression or transport activity and others altering substrate selectivity [67]. Genetic variants of the *SLC22A1* gene have been associated with altered pharmacokinetics and pharmacodynamics of several drugs including opioids, the $β_2$ agonist fenoterol, and metformin [68–72]. For instance, carriers of the p.Met420del (rs35191146) or p.Arg61Cys (rs12208357) variants, which are associated with decreased transport activity, experienced reduced therapeutic effects, assessed through a glucose tolerance test, as compared with individuals carrying OCT1 wild-type [64,69].

OCT3 colocalizes with OCT1 in the sinusoidal hepatocyte membrane [24]. The role of OCT3 in liver physiology is probably linked to the homeostasis of molecules that are not substrates of OCT1, such as the neurotransmitters adrenaline, noradrenaline, and histamine [14,73]. Studies have shown that the degree of hepatic fibrosis and ductular reaction induced by bile duct ligation or carbon tetrachloride (CCl_4) treatment was significantly higher in $Oct3^{-/-}$ than wild-type mice, because of an overproduction of TGFβ by stellate cells [74]. As adrenaline and histamine have been shown to promote fibrotic remodeling of the airways and the heart, respectively [75,76], it is possible that the different handling of these neurotransmitters concurs to the excessive hepatic remodeling observed in $Oct3^{-/-}$ mice. Similar to OCT1, the hepatic expression of OCT3 is significantly affected by cholestasis in both humans and rodents; however, the mechanism of transcription repression might be different [24].

OCTN2, encoded by the *SLC22A5* gene, is a high-affinity, Na^+-dependent, electrogenic carnitine carrier [20]. Carnitine is a vitamin-like compound, highly enriched in red meat or synthesized from γ-butyrobetaine in liver, kidney, and brain [77]. About 25% is synthesized in the body, while the rest is derived from dietary meats [78]. Carnitine is primarily involved in the translocation of mid- and long-chain fatty acids from the cytosol into the mitochondrial matrix, where fatty acid β-oxidation takes place [79]. An important experimental model for the comprehension of carnitine's physiological role is the juvenile visceral steatosis (jvs) mouse. Jvs mice are characterized by impaired intestinal absorption, tissue distribution, and reabsorption of carnitine, which leads to systemic carnitine deficiency resulting in hepatic steatosis, hypoglycemia, hyperammonaemia, and growth retardation [80]. Shortly after being cloned, Octn2/OCTN2 was found mutated in jvs mice, as well as in patients with systemic carnitine deficiency (OMIM212149) [81]. Notably, OCTN2 can also transport, in a Na^+-dependent manner, γ-butyrobetaine, the carnitine precursor (K_m~13 μM) [19]. The role of Ocnt2 in the hepatic uptake of carnitine has been demonstrated in primary cultured mouse hepatocytes, which showed a K_m of ~5 μM, consistent with a high-affinity system [52,53]. Carnitine deficiency in the liver, over loss of Octn2, leads to an accumulation of fatty acids in the cytoplasm of hepatocytes. In line with the pivotal role of carnitine in lipid metabolism, the Octn2 expression level is closely linked to lipid homeostasis. The nuclear receptor Pparα, activated by free fatty acids, has been shown to induce the mRNA expression of Octn2 in rodents and pigs in several tissues, including the liver [82–87]. Insulin, which positively correlates with fatty acids oxidation in human skeletal muscle [88] has been associated with an increase in carnitine uptake and expression of OCTN2 in skeletal muscle [89]. Taken together, these findings suggest that OCTN2 induction represents an adaptive protective mechanism against lipid metabolism dysfunction.

Mouse Octn1 was found to be expressed in non-parenchymal mouse liver cells, with reports showing functional expression in stellate cells. Upregulation of Octn1 and activation of stellate cells, after treatment with the liver toxin dimethylnitrosamine, were seen to lead to increased liver levels of the natural, nutrient-derived, OCTN1 substrate, antioxidant ergothioneine, which resulted in protection from inflammation, oxidative stress, and more severe liver fibrosis [90]. Although OCNT1 was originally cloned from fetal human liver tissue, neither OCTN1 nor OCTN2 seem to be expressed in adult human liver tissue, although low amounts of mRNA may be detected [91,92]. This highlights the historical difficulties of discerning the physiological and pharmacological relevance of each transporter in humans, in accordance with varying tissue expression patterns.

3. OCTs in the Kidney

OCT2 and OCTN2, and to a lesser extent, OCT3 and OCTN1 are expressed in the human kidney. OCT2 and OCT3 are considered to be expressed on the basolateral side of proximal tubule cells [26,93], while OCTN2 and OCTN1 are located (assumed for OCTN1) at the apical brush border membrane [15,94]. The expression pattern of Octs is different in rodents, where Oct1 colocalizes with Oct2 at the basolateral membrane of proximal tubule cells. Mice lacking $Oct2^{-/-}$ are normal, suggesting that the expression of Oct1 alone is sufficient to sustain normal renal function. Because of this functional redundancy, our understanding of the potential role of OCT2 primarily relies on studies that employ mice lacking both Oct1 and Oct2 ($Oct1/2^{-/-}$), which display an impaired tubular secretion of organic cations [95].

OCT2 has been well characterized for its relevance in creatinine tubular secretion, although creatinine has been shown to be a substrate of all the above listed transporters, at least in vitro [96]. Creatinine is largely cleared from the blood by glomerular filtration; however, 10–40% of creatinine is actively secreted into the collecting duct for excretion in proximal tubules [26,97]. OCT2 is deemed to be responsible for the majority of the uptake of creatinine, aided by OAT2 and most likely OCT3, into the tubule cells for subsequent active secretion into the collecting duct over apically (urine-facing)-located SLC47 family members (multidrug and toxin extrusion MATE transporters, MATE1 and MATE2-K) [98–100]. The most well-known drugs that lead to transient elevation of serum creatinine through interference at the transporter level with OATs, OCTs, or MATEs are cimetidine, isavuconazole, ranolazine, trimethoprim, vandetanib, probenecid, and pyrimethamine and several antivirals used in the treatment of HIV (dolutegravir, rilpivirine, and cobicistat) [96,101–103]. Elevations in serum creatinine under treatment with these compounds do not underlie pathological interruption of kidney function. As serum creatinine is widely used as a diagnostic marker in monitoring nephrotoxicity, drug development relies on the clear delineation between nephrotoxicity and non-pathological transient inhibition of creatinine secretion. Currently, guidance of drug regulatory agencies demands that each molecule in development be tested in vitro for inhibition of OCT2 transport activity in order to predict potential drug–drug interactions [104,105]. An example of a drug–transporter interaction leading to a drug–drug interaction is the reduction in renal metformin secretion by the combined inhibition of MATE and, to a lesser extent, OCT2 and possibly OCT3, by cimetidine [106–112].

Actual kidney injury mediated by substrates of OCT2 most notably includes anticancer platinum agents, of which cisplatin is the most studied [113]. Cisplatin is a substrate of OCT2, whose toxicity stems from the intracellular accumulation by OCT2-mediated cellular uptake, as seen in rodent models [114–118]. Oct1/2$^{-/-}$ mice are partially resistant to cisplatin-induced nephrotoxicity [40,118,119]. Some protective effects of cimetidine co-application under cisplatin treatment have also been demonstrated in mice [40,117] and humans [120,121], with supporting in vitro evidence [122]. Another very small human study using the OCT2 inhibitor pantoprazole (proton-pump inhibitor) could not ameliorate cisplatin-caused nephrotoxicity in pediatric and adolescent cancer patients [123]. In rodents, it has been indicated that the drug-induced kidney injury incurred by the aminoglycoside gentamicin [18], triptolide [124], and the plant toxin ochratoxin A [125] was dependent on Oct2 expression and function. In vitro data also suggest that the nephrotoxic effects of the antiviral agents defovir, cidofovir, and tenofovir [126], and the anticancer agent ifosfamide also underlie OCT2 uptake [127].

Genetic polymorphisms in OCT2 and OCTN1 have been identified to affect metformin renal excretion, leading to significantly increased peak concentrations and larger serum areas under the curve. On the one hand, patients carrying the OCT2 p.Ala270Ser (rs316019) variant or the OCTN1 p.Thr306Ile (rs272893) may require, similar to those with renal impairment, metformin-dosing reductions [128]. Therefore, it is possible that OCTN1 on the apical membrane is involved in the secretion of metformin into the collecting duct. On the other hand, individuals carrying the OCT2 variant p.Ala270Ser (rs316019), associated with a lower OCT2 activity, benefit from a lower risk of cisplatin-induced nephrotoxicity [115,116].

OCTN2 is physiologically most relevant for the reabsorption of carnitine, where loss or non-functionality of this transporter leads to primary systemic carnitine deficiency through carnitine wasting by renal excretion [78,81,129–131]. This has been discussed in the previous section in the context of the liver, because the liver, skeletal muscles, and the heart are tissues that largely rely on fatty acid β-oxidation for energy production, and thus are affected most by carnitine deficiency. However, the underlying cause of primary systemic carnitine deficiency and resulting clinical manifestations also underlies intestinal absorption, as most carnitine is derived from the diet, and, most relevantly, OCTN2-mediated renal reabsorption. Patients with primary systemic carnitine deficiency usually present within the first four years of life with lethargy, irritability, and poor feeding; elevated liver enzymes, hypoketotic hypoglycemia, hyperammonemia, frequently hepatomegaly, and most notably, cardio and skeletal myopathies are observed in these patients. It is further associated with sudden infant death [132]. However, interestingly, some affected persons remain completely asymptomatic into adulthood or present with clinical manifestations of carnitine deficiency only as high fatigability or muscle weakness after exertion or not until metabolically stressed, such as under fasting, diet, or recurrent illness [78,133,134]. Primary systemic carnitine deficiency due to autosomal recessive OCTN2 mutations is treated by oral carnitine supplementation and leads to reduction in clinical manifestations although tissue levels of carnitine seem to remain low [132,135]. Despite the heterogeneous clinical picture for primary systemic carnitine deficiency, it remains clear the OCTN2 in the kidney largely dictates carnitine homeostasis through renal reabsorption, with potentially far reaching clinical implications in energy metabolism throughout the body when dysregulated or lost. Drug-induced systemic carnitine deficiency (and nephrotoxicity) in animals has also been reported. Treatment with colistin (a polymyxin) or cephaloridine (a beta-lactam) is associated with urinary loss of carnitine and systemic carnitine deficiency in rats and rabbits, respectively [136–138]. Colistin is transported by human OCTN2 in a Na$^+$-independent manner, whereas cephaloridine interaction with OCTN2 is Na$^+$-dependent [17,139,140].

4. OCTs in the Intestines

OCT1, OCT3, OCTN1, and OCTN2 are expressed in the intestines, where OCT1 and -3 are located at the basolateral membrane of enterocytes and OCTN1 and -2 at the brush border membrane [15,141]. Physiologically, these transporters are likely to contribute, along with other higher affinity uptake transporters, to the intestinal absorption of several dietary substrates. OCT1 and OCT3 may be involved in thiamine uptake at high nutritional concentrations in the intestine [15]. OCT1 and OCT3 might play a role in choline intestinal absorption in rodents but perhaps not in humans, as choline does not seem to be a substrate of the human OCT1 and OCT3 in vitro [59,142–145]. OCTN2, as the primary carnitine transporter, is also involved in the uptake of dietary carnitine. OCTN1 transports carnitine, although cannot compensate for the loss of OCTN1 in primary carnitine deficiency (addressed in Section 3), and is physiologically more relevant in the uptake of ergothioneine, at least in mice [146,147]. Several OCTN1 and OCTN2 genetic variants, which result in reduced expression or function of the transport protein, have been associated with a susceptibility to inflammatory bowel diseases such as Crohn's disease, ulcerative colitis, and irritable bowel syndrome [141,148–154]. Pharmacologically, OCT1 and OCTN1 (and likely OCT3) seem to be involved in the absorption of metformin, with gastrointestinal side effects or intolerance being associated with both OCT1 and OCTN1 reduced or loss-of-function variants [155–158].

5. OCTs in Other Tissues

To briefly summarize the above sections, framed in the context of what is known in terms of pathophysiology and pharmacological relevance, OCT1 plays more significant roles in the liver, while OCT2 and OCTN2 have very important functions in the kidney. The following sections address additional tissues, which are selected based on current research trends. We discuss even less well known or described functions of OCTs in additional (human) tissues, where much of the existing work stems from animal studies. We critically assess current themes in animal studies on OCTs and detail the limited studies on humans for each respective tissue. For a comprehensive summary on the state of knowledge about OCTs in human and rodent models based on tissue expression, we suggest consulting the extensive review by H. Koepsell [15].

5.1. Central Nervous System

A rather quickly growing number of studies have addressed Oct2 and Oct3 in regard to their roles in the central nervous system and blood-brain barrier in rodents [159–164]. Both transporters transport biogenic amines such as dopamine, epinephrine, norepinephrine, serotonin, and histamine, as well as other neurotransmitters and neuromodulators cyclo(His-Pro), salsolinol, and the l-arginine metabolite agmatine [3]. Oct3 has been found to be massively expressed in circumventricular organs. In addition, while both Oct2 and Oct3 appeared principally expressed in central neurons, Oct3 has also been found in astrocytes, in restricted brain areas such as the dorsomedial hypothalamus nucleus and substantia nigra [161,163], where it has been shown to influence stress-mediated increase in extracellular serotonin levels [162] and neurotoxicity [163]. The roles of Octs in the brain have mainly been examined in Oct2- and Oct3-deficient mice. In vivo, Oct2 invalidation appeared to have preferential consequences on serotonin and norepinephrine uptake and clearance [164], and Oct3 invalidation had more impact on dopamine signaling [161]. Invalidation of Oct2 in mice resulted in abnormal anxiety-related behavior in several conflict paradigms [164]. As compared with wild-type mice, Oct2-deficient mice showed altered sensitivity to the dual serotonin/norepinephrine reuptake inhibitor venlafaxine and the serotonin transporter (SERT) and norepinephrine transporter (NET) inhibitors, citalopram and reboxetine, respectively. Oct2 was recently shown to be an essential modulator of the short- and long-term responses to stress in rodents [165]. Oct2-deficient mice and wild-type mice treated with cimetidine, an OCT2 substrate, were protected from oxaliplatin-induced neurotoxicity [166,167]. This transporter is highly expressed in the limbic and prefrontal cortical regions [164,165], known to control the autonomic and endocrine responses to stress or threats. However, recent expression analyses of OCTs in both mouse and human blood brain barrier samples have revealed negligent to no expression of these transporters at this site [168]. It seems that further studies on the role and expression of OCTs in both rodents and humans are needed to assess the physiological and pharmacological relevance of these transporters in the central nervous system.

5.2. Inner Ear

As mentioned in the kidney section of this review, aminoglycoside antibiotics and anticancer platinum agents, most notably gentamicin and cisplatin, respectively, are known for their nephrotoxicity and also to induce irreversible hearing loss. While it cannot be disputed that these agents lead to ototoxicity, since evidence for the relevance of OCT2 in these processes has been presented in both rodents and gineau pigs, literature on humans on this topic is not abundant [169]. Additionally, conflicting evidence has been presented as to the localization of OCT2 in the inner ear structures in the experimental models used [40,170]. A human study with pediatric patients identified the most common OCT2 p.Ala270Ser (rs316019) variant to be protective against ototoxicity under cisplatin treatment. Another very small human study using the OCT2 inhibitor pantoprazole (proton-pump inhibitor) could not ameliorate cisplatin-caused ototoxicity in pediatric and adolescent cancer patients [123].

Interestingly, in humans, mutations in OCTN1 that seemingly affect the correct trafficking of the protein to the apical membrane of stria vascularis endothelial cells, were identified as causative in the screening of consanguineous Tunisian families with autosomal recessive non-syndromic hearing loss. Although the reasons behind the hearing loss were not clear, it was postulated in the study that altered energy status via reduced carnitine uptake in the stria vascularis in such patients may have led to oxidative stress and consequent cell damage resulting in profound hearing loss [171]. It is interesting to note that OCTN1 transports the potent food-derived antioxidant ergothioeine with high affinity, which illicits antioxidant/anti-inflammatory effects [147,172]. It should be noted that the authors of this study emphasized that no other comorbidities (Crohn's disease or other digestive issues) were reported among the patients assessed. This study provided an example of a quite severe phenotype with the loss-of-function of OCTN1. It would be interesting to assess whether or not this is a population effect in an already challenged patient population and whether or not OCTN2, demonstrating a much higher affinity for carnitine than OCTN1, is expressed in these tissues in humans. The latter is not known and not to be assumed, in the context of this study, should carnitine deficiency in the inner ear, and not the lack of other substrates such as ergothioeine, be the underlying cause for deafness.

5.3. Cardiovascular System

Trimethylamine N-oxide (TMAO), which is produced from trimethylamine (TMA) stemming from OCT substrates choline and carnitine from protein and lipid nutrients converted by microbiota in the gut, is associated with cardiovascular disease, and thus considered to be a potential novel pro-atherosclerotic molecule [173,174]. In mice, Oct2 is the major uptake transporter of TMAO, as Oct1/2 knockout mice show highly elevated plasma TMAO levels with reduced renal retention [175,176]. Conversely, the relevance of OCT2 or other OCTs in TMAO handling in humans is still questioned, as TMAO is excreted at a similar rate as creatinine in the human kidney, regardless of age and kidney function, and OCT2 variants are not associated with increased TMAO levels [175,176]. TMAO plasma levels in humans may be indirectly modulated by OCTs, over the uptake in the intestines of dietary nutrients, or directly controlled, in part, over the uptake in the kidney; the contribution of both remain to be elucidated. Interestingly, a choline-TMA lyase small molecule inhibitor has proven to be effective as an anti-atherothrombotic agent by its regulation of host microbe, cholesterol, and bile acid metabolism [177], indicating that inhibition of the conversion of choline, of which OCT2 is the main transporter, to TMA positively impacts cardiac health. In the context of primary systemic carnitine deficiency, oral supplementation of carnitine leads to elevated plasma concentrations of TMAO [178–181], whereas little information is available on long-term effects on the heart in this patient subset [132]. Several studies have questioned the cardiotoxic effects of TMAO in humans in conjunction with carnitine supplementation [176,177,182,183] and this rather hot topic in cardiovascular health has been extensively reviewed and discussed in recent years [184–187]. Inducing atherosclerosis in mice usually requires an ApoE$^{-/-}$ or Ldlr$^{-/-}$ genotype, also with or without high-fat diet [188,189]. It might be interesting to assess the endothelial function by organ chamber assay of aortic rings freshly isolated from Oct1/2$^{-/-}$ mice, to further study the role of TMAO, as well as the effects of dietary choline and carnitine handling, on cardiovascular health. It seems clear that more studies in both mice and man are required to fully understand the processes involved in the development of atherosclerosis and the contribution of choline, carnitine, and TMAO transport.

5.4. Skeletal Muscle

Response to metformin treatment underlies intestinal (OCTN1 and OCT1), hepatic (OCT1), and renal (OCT2) handling, and also transports into peripheral tissues on the level of the effect on metabolism in both skeletal muscle and adipose tissue. Indeed, the more ubiquitously expressed OCT3 has been implicated, both in mice and man, in the metabolic response to metformin in muscle tissue [107,190]. In addition, in relation to in muscle metabolism, OCTN2 is essential to the distribution of carnitine in muscle tissues and has been shown to be upregulated in muscle tissue in response to insulin [89]. Lack of transport of fatty acids into mitochondria due to insufficient intracellular carnitine levels presents as cardiomyopathies, which are common features of primary systemic carnitine deficiency [81].

5.5. Reproductive Organs

OCT6 was cloned in 2002 and directly identified as a carnitine transporter specifically expressed in the human testis in Sertoli cells and epididymal epithelium [5,27], and shortly after in endometria [39]. However, research on this newly identified OCT is ongoing and the physiological relevance in carnitine uptake in reproductive organs over this transporter is unclear. Mentionable from a pharmacological perspective, OCT6 has been found to be differentially expressed in several cancers, several SNPs of which have been associated with pharmacologic implications under treatment with anticancer agents doxorubicin, bleomycin-A5, adriamycin, and cyclophosphamide [28–38].

6. Conclusions

The recognition of OCTs as low affinity transporters of frequently prescribed drugs, such as several antibiotics and metformin, the flourishing of pharmacogenetics, and the development of rigorous drug–drug interaction studies for marketing approval have decisively contributed to elucidating the impact of the organ-specific and interorgan functions of these transporters and, in conjunction, their high pharmacological impact. However, with the exception of OCTN2, the understanding of the physio-pathological roles played by OCTs in humans is not fully understood. Comprehension of the roles played by OCTs in physiology is hampered by the partially different substrate specificity and tissue expression between rodents and humans and the lack of obvious phenotypes associated with loss of, or gain of, function of any of these transporters. In general, the phenotype of an organism is not the mere product of its genetic constitution but rather the manifestation of the interaction of the genetic background with various environmental influences. In the study of the physio-pathological role of any gene, the best-case scenario is that the phenotype of a genetic variant is apparent under standard environmental conditions. This is the case of the jvs animals lacking Octn2. Alternatively, the phenotype develops only in specific circumstances that the investigator must understand and optimize.

For instance, the potential role of OCTs in the elimination of toxins whose chronic exposure is associated with several aging-related diseases such as Parkinson's and cardiovascular disease, might suggest that the phenotype of Oct-deficient animals does not manifest just because the animals are not examined in the proper environment, or under the correct challenge or insult, or in the right moment of their life. This seems to be the case for OCT1 in steatosis onset [66] and for OCTN1 and OCTN2 in inflammatory disorders [191,192]. Similarly, the evidence that OCT1 and OCT2 are markedly downregulated in liver and kidney cancer, respectively, may suggest that a chronic impaired function of these transporters might be part of the carcinogenic process [22,59–61]. In addition, because frequently prescribed drugs are handled by OCTs, we must be confident that the knowledge gained on these transporters will continue to be highly relevant to drug development and patient care in the future, and will, to some extent, contribute to the understanding of the physiology of the OCTs. To conclude, we summarize this work with the statement that, with the current state of knowledge, it is conceivable, though in part only inferred from tissue expression patterns and functionality in the uptake of endogenous and xenobiotic substrates in vitro, that human OCT1 is relevant in the liver and intestine, OCT2 in the kidney, OCT6 in the reproductive system, and OCTN1, OCTN2, and OCT3 in several tissues, whereby the bulk of knowledge on the latter four transporters is historically less abundant than on the former two.

Funding: This work was funded by the Swiss National Science Foundation (grant 310030_175639 to G.A.K.-U.).

Acknowledgments: We would like to thank Sebastien Santini for the management of the Phylogeny.fr online platform, which was used to generate Figure 1 of this manuscript.

Conflicts of Interest: The authors declare no conflict of interest.

Abbreviations

OCT	Organic cation transporter
OCTN	Organic cation transporter novel
SLC	Solute carrier
TMA	Trimethylamine
TMAO	Trimethylamine N-oxide

References

1. Bioparadigms SLC TABLES. Available online: http://slc.bioparadigms.org/ (accessed on 5 April 2020).
2. Cesar-Razquin, A.; Snijder, B.; Frappier-Brinton, T.; Isserlin, R.; Gyimesi, G.; Bai, X.; Reithmeier, R.A.; Hepworth, D.; Hediger, M.A.; Edwards, A.M.; et al. A Call for Systematic Research on Solute Carriers. *Cell* **2015**, *162*, 478–487. [CrossRef]
3. Koepsell, H. The SLC22 family with transporters of organic cations, anions and zwitterions. *Mol. Asp. Med.* **2013**, *34*, 413–435. [CrossRef] [PubMed]
4. Zhu, C.; Nigam, K.B.; Date, R.C.; Bush, K.T.; Springer, S.A.; Saier, M.H., Jr.; Wu, W.; Nigam, S.K. Evolutionary Analysis and Classification of OATs, OCTs, OCTNs, and Other SLC22 Transporters: Structure-Function Implications and Analysis of Sequence Motifs. *PLoS ONE* **2015**, *10*, e0140569. [CrossRef] [PubMed]
5. Eraly, S.A.; Nigam, S.K. Novel human cDNAs homologous to Drosophila Orct and mammalian carnitine transporters. *Biochem. Biophys. Res. Commun.* **2002**, *297*, 1159–1166. [CrossRef]
6. Okada, R.; Koshizuka, K.; Yamada, Y.; Moriya, S.; Kikkawa, N.; Kinoshita, T.; Hanazawa, T.; Seki, N. Regulation of Oncogenic Targets by miR-99a-3p (Passenger Strand of miR-99a-Duplex) in Head and Neck Squamous Cell Carcinoma. *Cells* **2019**, *8*, 1535. [CrossRef]
7. Zhu, G.; Qian, M.; Lu, L.; Chen, Y.; Zhang, X.; Wu, Q.; Liu, Y.; Bian, Z.; Yang, Y.; Guo, S.; et al. O-GlcNAcylation of YY1 stimulates tumorigenesis in colorectal cancer cells by targeting SLC22A15 and AANAT. *Carcinogenesis* **2019**, *40*, 1121–1131. [CrossRef]
8. Drake, K.A.; Torgerson, D.G.; Gignoux, C.R.; Galanter, J.M.; Roth, L.A.; Huntsman, S.; Eng, C.; Oh, S.S.; Yee, S.W.; Lin, L.; et al. A genome-wide association study of bronchodilator response in Latinos implicates rare variants. *J. Allergy Clin. Immunol.* **2014**, *133*, 370–378. [CrossRef]

9. Phylogeny.fr: Robust Phylogenetic Analysis for the Non-Specialist. Available online: www.phylogeny.fr/index.cgi (accessed on 3 March 2020).
10. Dereeper, A.; Guignon, V.; Blanc, G.; Audic, S.; Buffet, S.; Chevenet, F.; Dufayard, J.F.; Guindon, S.; Lefort, V.; Lescot, M.; et al. Phylogeny.fr: Robust phylogenetic analysis for the non-specialist. *Nucleic Acids Res.* **2008**, *36*, W465-9. [CrossRef]
11. Dereeper, A.; Audic, S.; Claverie, J.M.; Blanc, G. BLAST-EXPLORER helps you building datasets for phylogenetic analysis. *BMS Evol. Biol.* **2010**, *10*, 8. [CrossRef]
12. Koepsell, H. Substrate recognition and translocation by polyspecific organic cation transporters. *Biol. Chem.* **2011**, *392*, 95–101. [CrossRef]
13. Schmitt, B.M.; Gorbunov, D.; Schlachtbauer, P.; Egenberger, B.; Gorboulev, V.; Wischmeyer, E.; Muller, T.; Koepsell, H. Charge-to-substrate ratio during organic cation uptake by rat OCT2 is voltage dependent and altered by exchange of glutamate 448 with glutamine. *Am. J. Physiol. Ren. Physiol.* **2009**, *296*, F709–F722. [CrossRef] [PubMed]
14. Koepsell, H.; Lips, K.; Volk, C. Polyspecific organic cation transporters: Structure, function, physiological roles, and biopharmaceutical implications. *Pharm. Res.* **2007**, *24*, 1227–1251. [CrossRef]
15. Koepsell, H. Organic Cation Transporters in Health and Disease. *Pharm. Rev.* **2020**, *72*, 253–319. [CrossRef] [PubMed]
16. Pelis, R.M.; Wright, S.H. SLC22, SLC44, and SLC47 transporters–organic anion and cation transporters: Molecular and cellular properties. *Curr. Top. Membr.* **2014**, *73*, 233–261. [PubMed]
17. Visentin, M.; Gai, Z.; Torozi, A.; Hiller, C.; Kullak-Ublick, G.A. Colistin is substrate of the carnitine/organic cation transporter 2 (OCTN2, SLC22A5). *Drug Metab. Dispos.* **2017**, *45*, 1240–1244. [CrossRef] [PubMed]
18. Gai, Z.; Visentin, M.; Hiller, C.; Krajnc, E.; Li, T.; Zhen, J.; Kullak-Ublick, G.A. Organic Cation Transporter 2 Overexpression May Confer an Increased Risk of Gentamicin-Induced Nephrotoxicity. *Antimicrob. Agents Chemother.* **2016**, *60*, 5573–5580. [CrossRef] [PubMed]
19. Fujita, M.; Nakanishi, T.; Shibue, Y.; Kobayashi, D.; Moseley, R.H.; Shirasaka, Y.; Tamai, I. Hepatic uptake of gamma-butyrobetaine, a precursor of carnitine biosynthesis, in rats. *Am. J. Physiol. Gastrointest. Liver Physiol.* **2009**, *297*, G681–G686. [CrossRef] [PubMed]
20. Tamai, I.; Ohashi, R.; Nezu, J.; Yabuuchi, H.; Oku, A.; Shimane, M.; Sai, Y.; Tsuji, A. Molecular and functional identification of sodium ion-dependent, high affinity human carnitine transporter OCTN2. *J. Biol. Chem.* **1998**, *273*, 20378–20382. [CrossRef]
21. Koepsell, H. Multiple binding sites in organic cation transporters require sophisticated procedures to identify interactions of novel drugs. *Biol. Chem.* **2019**, *400*, 195–207. [CrossRef]
22. Visentin, M.; Torozi, A.; Gai, Z.; Hausler, S.; Li, C.; Hiller, C.; Schraml, P.H.; Moch, H.; Kullak-Ublick, G.A. Fluorocholine Transport Mediated by the Organic Cation Transporter 2 (OCT2, SLC22A2): Implication for Imaging of Kidney Tumors. *Drug Metab. Dispos. Biol. Fate Chem.* **2018**, *46*, 1129–1136. [CrossRef]
23. Hormann, S.; Gai, Z.; Kullak-Ublick, G.A.; Visentin, M. Plasma Membrane Cholesterol Regulates the Allosteric Binding of 1-Methyl-4-Phenylpyridinium to Organic Cation Transporter 2 (SLC22A2). *J. Pharmacol. Exp. Ther.* **2020**, *372*, 46–53. [CrossRef]
24. Nies, A.T.; Koepsell, H.; Winter, S.; Burk, O.; Klein, K.; Kerb, R.; Zanger, U.M.; Keppler, D.; Schwab, M.; Schaeffeler, E. Expression of organic cation transporters OCT1 (SLC22A1) and OCT3 (SLC22A3) is affected by genetic factors and cholestasis in human liver. *Hepatology* **2009**, *50*, 1227–1240. [CrossRef] [PubMed]
25. Zhang, L.; Dresser, M.J.; Gray, A.T.; Yost, S.C.; Terashita, S.; Giacomini, K.M. Cloning and functional expression of a human liver organic cation transporter. *Mol. Pharmacol.* **1997**, *51*, 913–921. [CrossRef] [PubMed]
26. Motohashi, H.; Sakurai, Y.; Saito, H.; Masuda, S.; Urakami, Y.; Goto, M.; Fukatsu, A.; Ogawa, O.; Inui, K. Gene expression levels and immunolocalization of organic ion transporters in the human kidney. *J. Am. Soc. Nephrol.* **2002**, *13*, 866–874. [PubMed]
27. Enomoto, A.; Wempe, M.F.; Tsuchida, H.; Shin, H.J.; Cha, S.H.; Anzai, N.; Goto, A.; Sakamoto, A.; Niwa, T.; Kanai, Y.; et al. Molecular identification of a novel carnitine transporter specific to human testis. Insights into the mechanism of carnitine recognition. *J. Biol. Chem.* **2002**, *277*, 36262–36271. [CrossRef]
28. Sagwal, S.K.; Pasqual-Melo, G.; Bodnar, Y.; Gandhirajan, R.K.; Bekeschus, S. Combination of chemotherapy and physical plasma elicits melanoma cell death via upregulation of SLC22A16. *Cell Death Dis.* **2018**, *9*, 1179. [CrossRef]

29. Zhao, W.; Wang, Y.; Yue, X. SLC22A16 upregulation is an independent unfavorable prognostic indicator in gastric cancer. *Future Oncol.* **2018**, *14*, 2139–2148. [CrossRef]
30. Tecza, K.; Pamula-Pilat, J.; Lanuszewska, J.; Butkiewicz, D.; Grzybowska, E. Pharmacogenetics of toxicity of 5-fluorouracil, doxorubicin and cyclophosphamide chemotherapy in breast cancer patients. *Oncotarget* **2018**, *9*, 9114–9136. [CrossRef]
31. Faraji, A.; Dehghan Manshadi, H.R.; Mobaraki, M.; Zare, M.; Houshmand, M. Association of ABCB1 and SLC22A16 Gene Polymorphisms with Incidence of Doxorubicin-Induced Febrile Neutropenia: A Survey of Iranian Breast Cancer Patients. *PLoS ONE* **2016**, *11*, e0168519. [CrossRef]
32. Wu, Y.; Hurren, R.; MacLean, N.; Gronda, M.; Jitkova, Y.; Sukhai, M.A.; Minden, M.D.; Schimmer, A.D. Carnitine transporter CT2 (SLC22A16) is over-expressed in acute myeloid leukemia (AML) and target knockdown reduces growth and viability of AML cells. *Apoptosis* **2015**, *20*, 1099–1108. [CrossRef]
33. Bray, J.; Sludden, J.; Griffin, M.J.; Cole, M.; Verrill, M.; Jamieson, D.; Boddy, A.V. Influence of pharmacogenetics on response and toxicity in breast cancer patients treated with doxorubicin and cyclophosphamide. *Br. J. Cancer* **2010**, *102*, 1003–1009. [CrossRef]
34. Aouida, M.; Poulin, R.; Ramotar, D. The human carnitine transporter SLC22A16 mediates high affinity uptake of the anticancer polyamine analogue bleomycin-A5. *J. Biol. Chem.* **2010**, *285*, 6275–6284. [CrossRef] [PubMed]
35. Ota, K.; Ito, K.; Akahira, J.; Sato, N.; Onogawa, T.; Moriya, T.; Unno, M.; Abe, T.; Niikura, H.; Takano, T.; et al. Expression of organic cation transporter SLC22A16 in human epithelial ovarian cancer: A possible role of the adriamycin importer. *Int. J. Gynecol. Pathol.* **2007**, *26*, 334–340. [CrossRef] [PubMed]
36. Lal, S.; Wong, Z.W.; Jada, S.R.; Xiang, X.; Chen Shu, X.; Ang, P.C.; Figg, W.D.; Lee, E.J.; Chowbay, B. Novel SLC22A16 polymorphisms and influence on doxorubicin pharmacokinetics in Asian breast cancer patients. *Pharmacogenomics* **2007**, *8*, 567–575. [CrossRef] [PubMed]
37. Okabe, M.; Unno, M.; Harigae, H.; Kaku, M.; Okitsu, Y.; Sasaki, T.; Mizoi, T.; Shiiba, K.; Takanaga, H.; Terasaki, T.; et al. Characterization of the organic cation transporter SLC22A16: A doxorubicin importer. *Biochem. Biophys. Res. Commun.* **2005**, *333*, 754–762. [CrossRef]
38. Gong, S.; Lu, X.; Xu, Y.; Swiderski, C.F.; Jordan, C.T.; Moscow, J.A. Identification of OCT6 as a novel organic cation transporter preferentially expressed in hematopoietic cells and leukemias. *Exp. Hematol.* **2002**, *30*, 1162–1169. [CrossRef]
39. Sato, N.; Ito, K.; Onogawa, T.; Akahira, J.; Unno, M.; Abe, T.; Niikura, H.; Yaegashi, N. Expression of organic cation transporter SLC22A16 in human endometria. *Int. J. Gynecol. Pathol.* **2007**, *26*, 53–60. [CrossRef]
40. Ciarimboli, G.; Deuster, D.; Knief, A.; Sperling, M.; Holtkamp, M.; Edemir, B.; Pavenstadt, H.; Lanvers-Kaminsky, C.; am Zehnhoff-Dinnesen, A.; Schinkel, A.H.; et al. Organic cation transporter 2 mediates cisplatin-induced oto- and nephrotoxicity and is a target for protective interventions. *Am. J. Pathol.* **2010**, *176*, 1169–1180. [CrossRef]
41. Koepsell, H.; Schmitt, B.M.; Gorboulev, V. Organic cation transporters. *Rev. Physiol. Biochem. Pharmacol.* **2003**, *150*, 36–90.
42. Neuhoff, S.; Ungell, A.L.; Zamora, I.; Artursson, P. pH-dependent bidirectional transport of weakly basic drugs across Caco-2 monolayers: Implications for drug-drug interactions. *Pharm. Res.* **2003**, *20*, 1141–1148. [CrossRef]
43. Tamai, I.; China, K.; Sai, Y.; Kobayashi, D.; Nezu, J.; Kawahara, E.; Tsuji, A. Na(+)-coupled transport of L-carnitine via high-affinity carnitine transporter OCTN2 and its subcellular localization in kidney. *Biochim. et Biophys. Acta* **2001**, *1512*, 273–284. [CrossRef]
44. Meier, Y.; Eloranta, J.J.; Darimont, J.; Ismair, M.G.; Hiller, C.; Fried, M.; Kullak-Ublick, G.A.; Vavricka, S.R. Regional distribution of solute carrier mRNA expression along the human intestinal tract. *Drug Metab. Dispos. Biol. Fate Chem.* **2007**, *35*, 590–594. [CrossRef]
45. Sugiura, T.; Kato, Y.; Wakayama, T.; Silver, D.L.; Kubo, Y.; Iseki, S.; Tsuji, A. PDZK1 regulates two intestinal solute carriers (Slc15a1 and Slc22a5) in mice. *Drug Metab. Dispos. Biol. Fate Chem.* **2008**, *36*, 1181–1188. [CrossRef]
46. McCloud, E.; Ma, T.Y.; Grant, K.E.; Mathis, R.K.; Said, H.M. Uptake of L-carnitine by a human intestinal epithelial cell line, Caco-2. *Gastroenterology* **1996**, *111*, 1534–1540. [CrossRef]
47. Schulze, U.; Brast, S.; Grabner, A.; Albiker, C.; Snieder, B.; Holle, S.; Schlatter, E.; Schroter, R.; Pavenstadt, H.; Herrmann, E.; et al. Tetraspanin CD63 controls basolateral sorting of organic cation transporter 2 in renal proximal tubules. *Faseb. J. Off. Publ. Fed. Am. Soc. Exp. Biol.* **2017**, *31*, 1421–1433. [CrossRef]

48. Pols, M.S.; Klumperman, J. Trafficking and function of the tetraspanin CD63. *Exp. Cell Res.* **2009**, *315*, 1584–1592. [CrossRef]
49. Muth, T.R.; Caplan, M.J. Transport protein trafficking in polarized cells. *Annu. Rev. Cell Dev. Biol.* **2003**, *19*, 333–366. [CrossRef]
50. Koizumi, T.; Nikaido, H.; Hayakawa, J.; Nonomura, A.; Yoneda, T. Infantile disease with microvesicular fatty infiltration of viscera spontaneously occurring in the C3H-H-2(0) strain of mouse with similarities to Reye's syndrome. *Lab Anim.* **1988**, *22*, 83–87. [CrossRef] [PubMed]
51. Kato, Y.; Sugiura, M.; Sugiura, T.; Wakayama, T.; Kubo, Y.; Kobayashi, D.; Sai, Y.; Tamai, I.; Iseki, S.; Tsuji, A. Organic cation/carnitine transporter OCTN2 (Slc22a5) is responsible for carnitine transport across apical membranes of small intestinal epithelial cells in mouse. *Mol. Pharmacol.* **2006**, *70*, 829–837. [CrossRef]
52. Bohmer, T.; Eiklid, K.; Jonsen, J. Carnitine uptake into human heart cells in culture. *Biochim. et Biophys. Acta* **1977**, *465*, 627–633. [CrossRef]
53. Yokogawa, K.; Yonekawa, M.; Tamai, I.; Ohashi, R.; Tatsumi, Y.; Higashi, Y.; Nomura, M.; Hashimoto, N.; Nikaido, H.; Hayakawa, J.; et al. Loss of wild-type carrier-mediated L-carnitine transport activity in hepatocytes of juvenile visceral steatosis mice. *Hepatology* **1999**, *30*, 997–1001. [CrossRef]
54. Grundemann, D.; Gorboulev, V.; Gambaryan, S.; Veyhl, M.; Koepsell, H. Drug excretion mediated by a new prototype of polyspecific transporter. *Nature* **1994**, *372*, 549–552. [CrossRef] [PubMed]
55. Saborowski, M.; Kullak-Ublick, G.A.; Eloranta, J.J. The human organic cation transporter-1 gene is transactivated by hepatocyte nuclear factor-4alpha. *J. Pharmacol. Exp. Ther.* **2006**, *317*, 778–785. [CrossRef] [PubMed]
56. Ogawa, K.; Suzuki, H.; Hirohashi, T.; Ishikawa, T.; Meier, P.J.; Hirose, K.; Akizawa, T.; Yoshioka, M.; Sugiyama, Y. Characterization of inducible nature of MRP3 in rat liver. *Am. J. Physiol. Gastrointest. Liver Physiol.* **2000**, *278*, G438–G446. [CrossRef]
57. Denk, G.U.; Soroka, C.J.; Mennone, A.; Koepsell, H.; Beuers, U.; Boyer, J.L. Down-regulation of the organic cation transporter 1 of rat liver in obstructive cholestasis. *Hepatology* **2004**, *39*, 1382–1389. [CrossRef] [PubMed]
58. Jin, H.E.; Hong, S.S.; Choi, M.K.; Maeng, H.J.; Kim, D.D.; Chung, S.J.; Shim, C.K. Reduced antidiabetic effect of metformin and down-regulation of hepatic Oct1 in rats with ethynylestradiol-induced cholestasis. *Pharm. Res.* **2009**, *26*, 549–559. [CrossRef]
59. Visentin, M.; van Rosmalen, B.V.; Hiller, C.; Bieze, M.; Hofstetter, L.; Verheij, J.; Kullak-Ublick, G.A.; Koepsell, H.; Phoa, S.S.; Tamai, I.; et al. Impact of Organic Cation Transporters (OCT-SLC22A) on Differential Diagnosis of Intrahepatic Lesions. *Drug Metab. Dispos.* **2017**, *45*, 166–173. [CrossRef]
60. Heise, M.; Lautem, A.; Knapstein, J.; Schattenberg, J.M.; Hoppe-Lotichius, M.; Foltys, D.; Weiler, N.; Zimmermann, A.; Schad, A.; Grundemann, D.; et al. Downregulation of organic cation transporters OCT1 (SLC22A1) and OCT3 (SLC22A3) in human hepatocellular carcinoma and their prognostic significance. *BMC Cancer* **2012**, *12*, 109. [CrossRef]
61. Schaeffeler, E.; Hellerbrand, C.; Nies, A.T.; Winter, S.; Kruck, S.; Hofmann, U.; van der Kuip, H.; Zanger, U.M.; Koepsell, H.; Schwab, M. DNA methylation is associated with downregulation of the organic cation transporter OCT1 (SLC22A1) in human hepatocellular carcinoma. *Genome Med.* **2011**, *3*, 82. [CrossRef]
62. Ciarimboli, G.; Koepsell, H.; Iordanova, M.; Gorboulev, V.; Durner, B.; Lang, D.; Edemir, B.; Schroter, R.; Van Le, T.; Schlatter, E. Individual PKC-phosphorylation sites in organic cation transporter 1 determine substrate selectivity and transport regulation. *J. Am. Soc. Nephrol.* **2005**, *16*, 1562–1570. [CrossRef]
63. Keller, T.; Gorboulev, V.; Mueller, T.D.; Dotsch, V.; Bernhard, F.; Koepsell, H. Rat Organic Cation Transporter 1 Contains Three Binding Sites for Substrate 1-Methyl-4-phenylpyridinium per Monomer. *Mol. Pharmacol.* **2019**, *95*, 169–182. [CrossRef]
64. Shu, Y.; Sheardown, S.A.; Brown, C.; Owen, R.P.; Zhang, S.; Castro, R.A.; Ianculescu, A.G.; Yue, L.; Lo, J.C.; Burchard, E.G.; et al. Effect of genetic variation in the organic cation transporter 1 (OCT1) on metformin action. *J. Clin. Investig.* **2007**, *117*, 1422–1431. [CrossRef]
65. Manzetti, S.; Zhang, J.; van der Spoel, D. Thiamin function, metabolism, uptake, and transport. *Biochemistry* **2014**, *53*, 821–835. [CrossRef]
66. Chen, L.; Shu, Y.; Liang, X.; Chen, E.C.; Yee, S.W.; Zur, A.A.; Li, S.; Xu, L.; Keshari, K.R.; Lin, M.J.; et al. OCT1 is a high-capacity thiamine transporter that regulates hepatic steatosis and is a target of metformin. *Proc. Natl. Acad. Sci. USA* **2014**, *111*, 9983–9988. [CrossRef]

67. Nies, A.T.; Schwab, M. Organic cation transporter pharmacogenomics and drug-drug interaction. *Expert Rev. Clin. Pharmacol.* **2010**, *3*, 707–711. [CrossRef]
68. Tzvetkov, M.V.; Matthaei, J.; Pojar, S.; Faltraco, F.; Vogler, S.; Prukop, T.; Seitz, T.; Brockmoller, J. Increased Systemic Exposure and Stronger Cardiovascular and Metabolic Adverse Reactions to Fenoterol in Individuals with Heritable OCT1 Deficiency. *Clin. Pharmacol. Ther.* **2018**, *103*, 868–878. [CrossRef]
69. Sundelin, E.; Gormsen, L.C.; Jensen, J.B.; Vendelbo, M.H.; Jakobsen, S.; Munk, O.L.; Christensen, M.; Brosen, K.; Frokiaer, J.; Jessen, N. Genetic Polymorphisms in Organic Cation Transporter 1 Attenuates Hepatic Metformin Exposure in Humans. *Clin. Pharmacol. Ther.* **2017**, *102*, 841–848. [CrossRef]
70. Tzvetkov, M.V. OCT1 pharmacogenetics in pain management: Is a clinical application within reach? *Pharmacogenomics* **2017**, *18*, 1515–1523. [CrossRef]
71. Zolk, O. Disposition of metformin: Variability due to polymorphisms of organic cation transporters. *Ann. Med.* **2012**, *44*, 119–129. [CrossRef]
72. Lanvers-Kaminsky, C.; Sprowl, J.A.; Malath, I.; Deuster, D.; Eveslage, M.; Schlatter, E.; Mathijssen, R.H.; Boos, J.; Jurgens, H.; Am Zehnhoff-Dinnesen, A.G.; et al. Human OCT2 variant c.808G>T confers protection effect against cisplatin-induced ototoxicity. *Pharmacogenomics* **2015**, *16*, 323–332. [CrossRef]
73. Grundemann, D.; Schechinger, B.; Rappold, G.A.; Schomig, E. Molecular identification of the corticosterone-sensitive extraneuronal catecholamine transporter. *Nat. Neurosci.* **1998**, *1*, 349–351. [CrossRef]
74. Vollmar, J.; Kim, Y.O.; Marquardt, J.U.; Becker, D.; Galle, P.R.; Schuppan, D.; Zimmermann, T. Deletion of organic cation transporter Oct3 promotes hepatic fibrosis via upregulation of TGFbeta. *Am. J. Physiol. Gastrointest. Liver Physiol.* **2019**, *317*, G195–G202. [CrossRef]
75. Kunzmann, S.; Schmidt-Weber, C.; Zingg, J.M.; Azzi, A.; Kramer, B.W.; Blaser, K.; Akdis, C.A.; Speer, C.P. Connective tissue growth factor expression is regulated by histamine in lung fibroblasts: Potential role of histamine in airway remodeling. *J. Allergy Clin. Immunol.* **2007**, *119*, 1398–1407. [CrossRef]
76. Bonnefont-Rousselot, D.; Mahmoudi, A.; Mougenot, N.; Varoquaux, O.; Le Nahour, G.; Fouret, P.; Lechat, P. Catecholamine effects on cardiac remodelling, oxidative stress and fibrosis in experimental heart failure. *Redox Rep.* **2002**, *7*, 145–151. [CrossRef]
77. Vaz, F.M.; Wanders, R.J. Carnitine biosynthesis in mammals. *Biochem. J.* **2002**, *361 Pt 3*, 417–429. [CrossRef]
78. Almannai, M.; Alfadhel, M.; El-Hattab, A.W. Carnitine Inborn Errors of Metabolism. *Molecules* **2019**, *24*, 3251. [CrossRef]
79. Longo, N.; Frigeni, M.; Pasquali, M. Carnitine transport and fatty acid oxidation. *Biochim. et Biophys. Acta* **2016**, *1863*, 2422–2435. [CrossRef]
80. Yokogawa, K.; Higashi, Y.; Tamai, I.; Nomura, M.; Hashimoto, N.; Nikaido, H.; Hayakawa, J.; Miyamoto, K.; Tsuji, A. Decreased tissue distribution of L-carnitine in juvenile visceral steatosis mice. *J. Pharmacol. Exp. Ther.* **1999**, *289*, 224–230.
81. Nezu, J.; Tamai, I.; Oku, A.; Ohashi, R.; Yabuuchi, H.; Hashimoto, N.; Nikaido, H.; Sai, Y.; Koizumi, A.; Shoji, Y.; et al. Primary systemic carnitine deficiency is caused by mutations in a gene encoding sodium ion-dependent carnitine transporter. *Nat. Genet.* **1999**, *21*, 91–94. [CrossRef]
82. Ringseis, R.; Luci, S.; Spielmann, J.; Kluge, H.; Fischer, M.; Geissler, S.; Wen, G.; Hirche, F.; Eder, K. Clofibrate treatment up-regulates novel organic cation transporter (OCTN)-2 in tissues of pigs as a model of non-prolliferating species. *Eur. J. Pharmacol.* **2008**, *583*, 11–17. [CrossRef]
83. Ringseis, R.; Posel, S.; Hirche, F.; Eder, K. Treatment with pharmacological peroxisome proliferator-activated receptor alpha agonist clofibrate causes upregulation of organic cation transporter 2 in liver and small intestine of rats. *Pharmacol. Res. Off. J. Ital. Pharmacol. Soc.* **2007**, *56*, 175–183.
84. Maeda, T.; Wakasawa, T.; Funabashi, M.; Fukushi, A.; Fujita, M.; Motojima, K.; Tamai, I. Regulation of Octn2 transporter (SLC22A5) by peroxisome proliferator activated receptor alpha. *Biol. Pharm. Bull.* **2008**, *31*, 1230–1236. [CrossRef]
85. Hirai, T.; Fukui, Y.; Motojima, K. PPARalpha agonists positively and negatively regulate the expression of several nutrient/drug transporters in mouse small intestine. *Biol. Pharm. Bull.* **2007**, *30*, 2185–2190. [CrossRef] [PubMed]
86. Koch, A.; Konig, B.; Stangl, G.I.; Eder, K. PPAR alpha mediates transcriptional upregulation of novel organic cation transporters-2 and -3 and enzymes involved in hepatic carnitine synthesis. *Exp. Biol. Med. (Maywood)* **2008**, *233*, 356–365. [CrossRef]

87. van Vlies, N.; Ferdinandusse, S.; Turkenburg, M.; Wanders, R.J.; Vaz, F.M. PPAR alpha-activation results in enhanced carnitine biosynthesis and OCTN2-mediated hepatic carnitine accumulation. *Biochim. et Biophys. Acta* **2007**, *1767*, 1134–1142. [CrossRef]
88. Kiens, B. Skeletal muscle lipid metabolism in exercise and insulin resistance. *Physiol. Rev.* **2006**, *86*, 205–243. [CrossRef]
89. Stephens, F.B.; Constantin-Teodosiu, D.; Laithwaite, D.; Simpson, E.J.; Greenhaff, P.L. Insulin stimulates L-carnitine accumulation in human skeletal muscle. *Faseb. J. Off. Publ. Fed. Am. Soc. Exp. Biol.* **2006**, *20*, 377–379. [CrossRef]
90. Tang, Y.; Masuo, Y.; Sakai, Y.; Wakayama, T.; Sugiura, T.; Harada, R.; Futatsugi, A.; Komura, T.; Nakamichi, N.; Sekiguchi, H.; et al. Localization of Xenobiotic Transporter OCTN1/SLC22A4 in Hepatic Stellate Cells and Its Protective Role in Liver Fibrosis. *J. Pharm. Sci.* **2016**, *105*, 1779–1789. [CrossRef]
91. McBride, B.F.; Yang, T.; Liu, K.; Urban, T.J.; Giacomini, K.M.; Kim, R.B.; Roden, D.M. The organic cation transporter, OCTN1, expressed in the human heart, potentiates antagonism of the HERG potassium channel. *J. Cardiovasc. Pharmacol.* **2009**, *54*, 63–71. [CrossRef]
92. Tamai, I.; Yabuuchi, H.; Nezu, J.; Sai, Y.; Oku, A.; Shimane, M.; Tsuji, A. Cloning and characterization of a novel human pH-dependent organic cation transporter, OCTN1. *FEBS Lett.* **1997**, *419*, 107–111. [CrossRef]
93. Motohashi, H.; Nakao, Y.; Masuda, S.; Katsura, T.; Kamba, T.; Ogawa, O.; Inui, K. Precise comparison of protein localization among OCT, OAT, and MATE in human kidney. *J. Pharm. Sci.* **2013**, *102*, 3302–3308. [CrossRef] [PubMed]
94. Wu, X.; Huang, W.; Prasad, P.D.; Seth, P.; Rajan, D.P.; Leibach, F.H.; Chen, J.; Conway, S.J.; Ganapathy, V. Functional characteristics and tissue distribution pattern of organic cation transporter 2 (OCTN2), an organic cation/carnitine transporter. *J. Pharmacol. Exp. Ther.* **1999**, *290*, 1482–1492. [PubMed]
95. Jonker, J.W.; Wagenaar, E.; Van Eijl, S.; Schinkel, A.H. Deficiency in the organic cation transporters 1 and 2 (Oct1/Oct2 [Slc22a1/Slc22a2]) in mice abolishes renal secretion of organic cations. *Mol. Cell Biol.* **2003**, *23*, 7902–7908. [CrossRef] [PubMed]
96. Chu, X.; Bleasby, K.; Chan, G.H.; Nunes, I.; Evers, R. The Complexities of Interpreting Reversible Elevated Serum Creatinine Levels in Drug Development: Does a Correlation with Inhibition of Renal Transporters Exist? *Drug Metab. Dispos.* **2016**, *44*, 1498–1509. [CrossRef]
97. Levey, A.S.; Perrone, R.D.; Madias, N.E. Serum creatinine and renal function. *Annu. Rev. Med.* **1988**, *39*, 465–490. [CrossRef] [PubMed]
98. Lepist, E.I.; Zhang, X.; Hao, J.; Huang, J.; Kosaka, A.; Birkus, G.; Murray, B.P.; Bannister, R.; Cihlar, T.; Huang, Y.; et al. Contribution of the organic anion transporter OAT2 to the renal active tubular secretion of creatinine and mechanism for serum creatinine elevations caused by cobicistat. *Kidney Int.* **2014**, *86*, 350–357. [CrossRef]
99. Perrone, R.D.; Madias, N.E.; Levey, A.S. Serum creatinine as an index of renal function: New insights into old concepts. *Clin. Chem.* **1992**, *38*, 1933–1953. [CrossRef] [PubMed]
100. Urakami, Y.; Kimura, N.; Okuda, M.; Inui, K. Creatinine transport by basolateral organic cation transporter hOCT2 in the human kidney. *Pharm. Res.* **2004**, *21*, 976–981. [CrossRef]
101. Scotcher, D.; Arya, V.; Yang, X.; Zhao, P.; Zhang, L.; Huang, S.M.; Rostami-Hodjegan, A.; Galetin, A. Mechanistic Models as Framework for Understanding Biomarker Disposition: Prediction of Creatinine-Drug Interactions. *CPT Pharmacomet. Syst. Pharmacol.* **2020**, *9*, 282–293. [CrossRef]
102. Gutierrez, F.; Fulladosa, X.; Barril, G.; Domingo, P. Renal tubular transporter-mediated interactions of HIV drugs: Implications for patient management. *Aids. Rev.* **2014**, *16*, 199–212.
103. Nakada, T.; Kudo, T.; Kume, T.; Kusuhara, H.; Ito, K. Estimation of changes in serum creatinine and creatinine clearance caused by renal transporter inhibition in healthy subjects. *Drug Metab. Pharm.* **2019**, *34*, 233–238. [CrossRef]
104. EMA Guideline on the Investigation of Drug Interactions. Available online: http://www.ema.europa.eu/docs/en_GB/document_library/Scientific_guideline/2012/07/WC500129606.pdf (accessed on 19 August 2020).
105. FDA, U. In Vitro Metabolism- and Transporter- Mediated Drug-Drug Interaction Studies Guidance for Industry. 2019. Available online: http://www.fda.gov/Drugs/GuidanceComplianceRegulatoryInformation/Guidances/default.htm (accessed on 19 August 2020).
106. Somogyi, A.; Stockley, C.; Keal, J.; Rolan, P.; Bochner, F. Reduction of metformin renal tubular secretion by cimetidine in man. *Br. J. Clin. Pharm.* **1987**, *23*, 545–551. [CrossRef] [PubMed]

107. Chen, E.C.; Liang, X.; Yee, S.W.; Geier, E.G.; Stocker, S.L.; Chen, L.; Giacomini, K.M. Targeted disruption of organic cation transporter 3 attenuates the pharmacologic response to metformin. *Mol. Pharm.* **2015**, *88*, 75–83. [CrossRef] [PubMed]
108. Wang, Z.J.; Yin, O.Q.; Tomlinson, B.; Chow, M.S. OCT2 polymorphisms and in-vivo renal functional consequence: Studies with metformin and cimetidine. *Pharm. Genom.* **2008**, *18*, 637–645. [CrossRef] [PubMed]
109. Ito, S.; Kusuhara, H.; Yokochi, M.; Toyoshima, J.; Inoue, K.; Yuasa, H.; Sugiyama, Y. Competitive inhibition of the luminal efflux by multidrug and toxin extrusions, but not basolateral uptake by organic cation transporter 2, is the likely mechanism underlying the pharmacokinetic drug-drug interactions caused by cimetidine in the kidney. *J. Pharmacol. Exp. Ther.* **2012**, *340*, 393–403. [CrossRef] [PubMed]
110. Tsuda, M.; Terada, T.; Ueba, M.; Sato, T.; Masuda, S.; Katsura, T.; Inui, K. Involvement of human multidrug and toxin extrusion 1 in the drug interaction between cimetidine and metformin in renal epithelial cells. *J. Pharmacol. Exp. Ther.* **2009**, *329*, 185–191. [CrossRef]
111. Wright, S.H. Molecular and cellular physiology of organic cation transporter 2. *Am. J. Physiol. Ren. Physiol.* **2019**, *317*, F1669–F1679. [CrossRef]
112. Sandoval, P.J.; Morales, M.; Secomb, T.W.; Wright, S.H. Kinetic basis of metformin-MPP interactions with organic cation transporter OCT2. *Am. J. Physiol. Ren. Physiol.* **2019**, *317*, F720–F734. [CrossRef]
113. Yonezawa, A.; Inui, K. Organic cation transporter OCT/SLC22A and H(+)/organic cation antiporter MATE/SLC47A are key molecules for nephrotoxicity of platinum agents. *Biochem. Pharm.* **2011**, *81*, 563–568. [CrossRef]
114. Manohar, S.; Leung, N. Cisplatin nephrotoxicity: A review of the literature. *J. Nephrol.* **2018**, *31*, 15–25. [CrossRef]
115. Ciarimboli, G. Membrane transporters as mediators of cisplatin side-effects. *Anticancer Res.* **2014**, *34*, 547–550. [CrossRef] [PubMed]
116. Ciarimboli, G. Membrane transporters as mediators of Cisplatin effects and side effects. *Science (Cairo)* **2012**, *2012*, 473829. [CrossRef]
117. Ciarimboli, G.; Ludwig, T.; Lang, D.; Pavenstadt, H.; Koepsell, H.; Piechota, H.J.; Haier, J.; Jaehde, U.; Zisowsky, J.; Schlatter, E. Cisplatin nephrotoxicity is critically mediated via the human organic cation transporter 2. *Am. J. Pathol.* **2005**, *167*, 1477–1484. [CrossRef]
118. Filipski, K.K.; Mathijssen, R.H.; Mikkelsen, T.S.; Schinkel, A.H.; Sparreboom, A. Contribution of organic cation transporter 2 (OCT2) to cisplatin-induced nephrotoxicity. *Clin. Pharm. Ther.* **2009**, *86*, 396–402. [CrossRef]
119. Harrach, S.; Ciarimboli, G. Role of transporters in the distribution of platinum-based drugs. *Front. Pharmacol.* **2015**, *6*, 85. [CrossRef]
120. Sleijfer, D.T.; Offerman, J.J.; Mulder, N.H.; Verweij, M.; van der Hem, G.K.; Schraffordt Koops, H.S.; Meijer, S. The protective potential of the combination of verapamil and cimetidine on cisplatin-induced nephrotoxicity in man. *Cancer* **1987**, *60*, 2823–2828. [CrossRef]
121. Zhang, J.; Zhou, W. Ameliorative effects of SLC22A2 gene polymorphism 808 G/T and cimetidine on cisplatin-induced nephrotoxicity in Chinese cancer patients. *Food Chem. Toxicol.* **2012**, *50*, 2289–2293. [CrossRef]
122. Katsuda, H.; Yamashita, M.; Katsura, H.; Yu, J.; Waki, Y.; Nagata, N.; Sai, Y.; Miyamoto, K. Protecting cisplatin-induced nephrotoxicity with cimetidine does not affect antitumor activity. *Biol. Pharm. Bull.* **2010**, *33*, 1867–1871. [CrossRef]
123. Fox, E.; Levin, K.; Zhu, Y.; Segers, B.; Balamuth, N.; Womer, R.; Bagatell, R.; Balis, F. Pantoprazole, an Inhibitor of the Organic Cation Transporter 2, Does Not Ameliorate Cisplatin-Related Ototoxicity or Nephrotoxicity in Children and Adolescents with Newly Diagnosed Osteosarcoma Treated with Methotrexate, Doxorubicin, and Cisplatin. *Oncologist* **2018**, *23*, 762–e79. [CrossRef]
124. Shen, Q.; Wang, J.; Yuan, Z.; Jiang, Z.; Shu, T.; Xu, D.; He, J.; Zhang, L.; Huang, X. Key role of organic cation transporter 2 for the nephrotoxicity effect of triptolide in rheumatoid arthritis. *Int. Immunopharmacol.* **2019**, *77*, 105959. [CrossRef]
125. Qi, X.; Zhu, L.; Yang, B.; Luo, H.; Xu, W.; He, X.; Huang, K. Mitigation of cell apoptosis induced by ochratoxin A (OTA) is possibly through organic cation transport 2 (OCT2) knockout. *Food Chem. Toxicol.* **2018**, *121*, 15–23. [CrossRef] [PubMed]
126. Uwai, Y.; Ida, H.; Tsuji, Y.; Katsura, T.; Inui, K. Renal transport of adefovir, cidofovir, and tenofovir by SLC22A family members (hOAT1, hOAT3, and hOCT2). *Pharm. Res.* **2007**, *24*, 811–815. [CrossRef] [PubMed]

127. Ciarimboli, G.; Holle, S.K.; Vollenbrocker, B.; Hagos, Y.; Reuter, S.; Burckhardt, G.; Bierer, S.; Herrmann, E.; Pavenstadt, H.; Rossi, R.; et al. New clues for nephrotoxicity induced by ifosfamide: Preferential renal uptake via the human organic cation transporter 2. *Mol. Pharm.* **2011**, *8*, 270–279. [CrossRef] [PubMed]
128. Yoon, H.; Cho, H.Y.; Yoo, H.D.; Kim, S.M.; Lee, Y.B. Influences of organic cation transporter polymorphisms on the population pharmacokinetics of metformin in healthy subjects. *AAPS J.* **2013**, *15*, 571–580. [CrossRef] [PubMed]
129. Ferdinandusse, S.; Te Brinke, H.; Ruiter, J.P.N.; Haasjes, J.; Oostheim, W.; van Lenthe, H.; IJlst, L.; Ebberink, M.S.; Wanders, R.J.A.; Vaz, F.M.; et al. A mutation creating an upstream translation initiation codon in SLC22A5 5'UTR is a frequent cause of primary carnitine deficiency. *Hum. Mutat.* **2019**, *40*, 1899–1904. [CrossRef] [PubMed]
130. Frigeni, M.; Balakrishnan, B.; Yin, X.; Calderon, F.R.O.; Mao, R.; Pasquali, M.; Longo, N. Functional and molecular studies in primary carnitine deficiency. *Hum. Mutat.* **2017**, *38*, 1684–1699. [CrossRef]
131. Li, F.Y.; El-Hattab, A.W.; Bawle, E.V.; Boles, R.G.; Schmitt, E.S.; Scaglia, F.; Wong, L.J. Molecular spectrum of SLC22A5 (OCTN2) gene mutations detected in 143 subjects evaluated for systemic carnitine deficiency. *Hum. Mutat.* **2010**, *31*, E1632–E1651. [CrossRef]
132. Kishimoto, S.; Suda, K.; Yoshimoto, H.; Teramachi, Y.; Nishino, H.; Koteda, Y.; Itoh, S.; Kudo, Y.; Iemura, M.; Matsuishi, T. Thirty-year follow-up of carnitine supplementation in two siblings with hypertrophic cardiomyopathy caused by primary systemic carnitine deficiency. *Int. J. Cardiol.* **2012**, *159*, e14–e15. [CrossRef]
133. Spiekerkoetter, U.; Huener, G.; Baykal, T.; Demirkol, M.; Duran, M.; Wanders, R.; Nezu, J.; Mayatepek, E. Silent and symptomatic primary carnitine deficiency within the same family due to identical mutations in the organic cation/carnitine transporter OCTN2. *J. Inherit. Metab. Dis.* **2003**, *26*, 613–615. [CrossRef]
134. Rose, E.C.; di San Filippo, C.A.; Ndukwe Erlingsson, U.C.; Ardon, O.; Pasquali, M.; Longo, N. Genotype-phenotype correlation in primary carnitine deficiency. *Hum. Mutat.* **2012**, *33*, 118–123. [CrossRef]
135. Vasiljevski, E.R.; Summers, M.A.; Little, D.G.; Schindeler, A. Lipid storage myopathies: Current treatments and future directions. *Prog. Lipid Res.* **2018**, *72*, 1–17. [CrossRef] [PubMed]
136. Jeong, E.S.; Kim, G.; Moon, K.S.; Kim, Y.B.; Oh, J.H.; Kim, H.S.; Jeong, J.; Shin, J.G.; Kim, D.H. Characterization of urinary metabolites as biomarkers of colistin-induced nephrotoxicity in rats by a liquid chromatography/mass spectrometry-based metabolomics approach. *Toxicol. Lett.* **2016**, *248*, 52–60. [CrossRef] [PubMed]
137. Tune, B.M. Effects of L-carnitine on the renal tubular transport of cephaloridine. *Biochem. Pharmacol.* **1995**, *50*, 562–564. [CrossRef]
138. Tune, B.M.; Hsu, C.Y. Toxicity of cephaloridine to carnitine transport and fatty acid metabolism in rabbit renal cortical mitochondria: Structure-activity relationships. *J. Pharmacol. Exp. Ther.* **1994**, *270*, 873–880.
139. Gai, Z.; Samodelov, S.L.; Kullak-Ublick, G.A.; Visentin, M. Molecular Mechanisms of Colistin-Induced Nephrotoxicity. *Molecules* **2019**, *24*, 653. [CrossRef]
140. Ganapathy, M.E.; Huang, W.; Rajan, D.P.; Carter, A.L.; Sugawara, M.; Iseki, K.; Leibach, F.H.; Ganapathy, V. beta-lactam antibiotics as substrates for OCTN2, an organic cation/carnitine transporter. *J. Biol. Chem.* **2000**, *275*, 1699–1707. [CrossRef]
141. Peltekova, V.D.; Wintle, R.F.; Rubin, L.A.; Amos, C.I.; Huang, Q.; Gu, X.; Newman, B.; Van Oene, M.; Cescon, D.; Greenberg, G.; et al. Functional variants of OCTN cation transporter genes are associated with Crohn disease. *Nat. Genet.* **2004**, *36*, 471–475. [CrossRef]
142. Kekuda, R.; Prasad, P.D.; Wu, X.; Wang, H.; Fei, Y.J.; Leibach, F.H.; Ganapathy, V. Cloning and functional characterization of a potential-sensitive, polyspecific organic cation transporter (OCT3) most abundantly expressed in placenta. *J. Biol. Chem.* **1998**, *273*, 15971–15979. [CrossRef]
143. Grundemann, D.; Liebich, G.; Kiefer, N.; Koster, S.; Schomig, E. Selective substrates for non-neuronal monoamine transporters. *Mol. Pharmacol.* **1999**, *56*, 1–10. [CrossRef]
144. Sinclair, C.J.; Chi, K.D.; Subramanian, V.; Ward, K.L.; Green, R.M. Functional expression of a high affinity mammalian hepatic choline/organic cation transporter. *J. Lipid Res.* **2000**, *41*, 1841–1848.
145. Busch, A.E.; Quester, S.; Ulzheimer, J.C.; Waldegger, S.; Gorboulev, V.; Arndt, P.; Lang, F.; Koepsell, H. Electrogenic properties and substrate specificity of the polyspecific rat cation transporter rOCT1. *J. Biol. Chem.* **1996**, *271*, 32599–32604. [CrossRef] [PubMed]

146. Sugiura, T.; Kato, S.; Shimizu, T.; Wakayama, T.; Nakamichi, N.; Kubo, Y.; Iwata, D.; Suzuki, K.; Soga, T.; Asano, M.; et al. Functional expression of carnitine/organic cation transporter OCTN1/SLC22A4 in mouse small intestine and liver. *Drug Metab. Dispos.* **2010**, *38*, 1665–1672. [CrossRef]
147. Kato, Y.; Kubo, Y.; Iwata, D.; Kato, S.; Sudo, T.; Sugiura, T.; Kagaya, T.; Wakayama, T.; Hirayama, A.; Sugimoto, M.; et al. Gene knockout and metabolome analysis of carnitine/organic cation transporter OCTN1. *Pharm. Res.* **2010**, *27*, 832–840. [CrossRef] [PubMed]
148. Kawasaki, Y.; Kato, Y.; Sai, Y.; Tsuji, A. Functional characterization of human organic cation transporter OCTN1 single nucleotide polymorphisms in the Japanese population. *J. Pharm. Sci.* **2004**, *93*, 2920–2926. [CrossRef]
149. Newman, B.; Gu, X.J.; Wintle, R.; Cescon, D.; Yazdanpanah, M.; Liu, X.D.; Peltekova, V.; Van Oene, M.; Amos, C.I.; Siminovitch, K.A. A risk haplotype in the solute carrier family 22A4/22A5 gene cluster influences phenotypic expression of Crohn's disease. *Gastroenterology* **2005**, *128*, 260–269. [CrossRef] [PubMed]
150. Palmieri, O.; Latiano, A.; Valvano, R.; D'Inca, R.; Vecchi, M.; Sturniolo, G.C.; Saibeni, S.; Peyvandi, F.; Bossa, F.; Zagaria, C.; et al. Variants of OCTN1-2 cation transporter genes are associated with both Crohn's disease and ulcerative colitis. *Aliment. Pharmacol. Ther.* **2006**, *23*, 497–506. [CrossRef] [PubMed]
151. Babusukumar, U.; Wang, T.; McGuire, E.; Broeckel, U.; Kugathasan, S. Contribution of OCTN variants within the IBD5 locus to pediatric onset Crohn's disease. *Am. J. Gastroenterol.* **2006**, *101*, 1354–1361. [CrossRef]
152. Russell, R.K.; Drummond, H.E.; Nimmo, E.R.; Anderson, N.H.; Noble, C.L.; Wilson, D.C.; Gillett, P.M.; McGrogan, P.; Hassan, K.; Weaver, L.T.; et al. Analysis of the influence of OCTN1/2 variants within the IBD5 locus on disease susceptibility and growth indices in early onset inflammatory bowel disease. *Gut* **2006**, *55*, 1114–1123. [CrossRef] [PubMed]
153. Waller, S.; Tremelling, M.; Bredin, F.; Godfrey, L.; Howson, J.; Parkes, M. Evidence for association of OCTN genes and IBD5 with ulcerative colitis. *Gut* **2006**, *55*, 809–814. [CrossRef]
154. Silverberg, M.S.; Duerr, R.H.; Brant, S.R.; Bromfield, G.; Datta, L.W.; Jani, N.; Kane, S.V.; Rotter, J.I.; Philip Schumm, L.; Hillary Steinhart, A.; et al. Refined genomic localization and ethnic differences observed for the IBD5 association with Crohn's disease. *Eur. J. Hum. Genet.* **2007**, *15*, 328–335. [CrossRef]
155. Tarasova, L.; Kalnina, I.; Geldnere, K.; Bumbure, A.; Ritenberga, R.; Nikitina-Zake, L.; Fridmanis, D.; Vaivade, I.; Pirags, V.; Klovins, J. Association of genetic variation in the organic cation transporters OCT1, OCT2 and multidrug and toxin extrusion 1 transporter protein genes with the gastrointestinal side effects and lower BMI in metformin-treated type 2 diabetes patients. *Pharm. Genom.* **2012**, *22*, 659–666. [CrossRef] [PubMed]
156. Wang, D.S.; Jonker, J.W.; Kato, Y.; Kusuhara, H.; Schinkel, A.H.; Sugiyama, Y. Involvement of organic cation transporter 1 in hepatic and intestinal distribution of metformin. *J. Pharmacol. Exp. Ther.* **2002**, *302*, 510–515. [CrossRef]
157. Dawed, A.Y.; Zhou, K.; van Leeuwen, N.; Mahajan, A.; Robertson, N.; Koivula, R.; Elders, P.J.M.; Rauh, S.P.; Jones, A.G.; Holl, R.W.; et al. Variation in the Plasma Membrane Monoamine Transporter (PMAT) (Encoded by SLC29A4) and Organic Cation Transporter 1 (OCT1) (Encoded by SLC22A1) and Gastrointestinal Intolerance to Metformin in Type 2 Diabetes: An IMI DIRECT Study. *Diabetes Care* **2019**, *42*, 1027–1033. [CrossRef]
158. Nakamichi, N.; Shima, H.; Asano, S.; Ishimoto, T.; Sugiura, T.; Matsubara, K.; Kusuhara, H.; Sugiyama, Y.; Sai, Y.; Miyamoto, K.; et al. Involvement of carnitine/organic cation transporter OCTN1/SLC22A4 in gastrointestinal absorption of metformin. *J. Pharm. Sci.* **2013**, *102*, 3407–3417. [CrossRef]
159. Busch, A.E.; Karbach, U.; Miska, D.; Gorboulev, V.; Akhoundova, A.; Volk, C.; Arndt, P.; Ulzheimer, J.C.; Sonders, M.S.; Baumann, C.; et al. Human neurons express the polyspecific cation transporter hOCT2, which translocates monoamine neurotransmitters, amantadine, and memantine. *Mol. Pharmacol.* **1998**, *54*, 342–352. [CrossRef]
160. Haag, C.; Berkels, R.; Grundemann, D.; Lazar, A.; Taubert, D.; Schomig, E. The localisation of the extraneuronal monoamine transporter (EMT) in rat brain. *J. Neurochem.* **2004**, *88*, 291–297. [CrossRef]
161. Vialou, V.; Balasse, L.; Callebert, J.; Launay, J.M.; Giros, B.; Gautron, S. Altered aminergic neurotransmission in the brain of organic cation transporter 3-deficient mice. *J. Neurochem.* **2008**, *106*, 1471–1482. [CrossRef]
162. Gasser, P.J.; Lowry, C.A.; Orchinik, M. Corticosterone-sensitive monoamine transport in the rat dorsomedial hypothalamus: Potential role for organic cation transporter 3 in stress-induced modulation of monoaminergic neurotransmission. *J. Neurosci. Off. J. Soc. Neurosci.* **2006**, *26*, 8758–8766. [CrossRef]
163. Cui, M.; Aras, R.; Christian, W.V.; Rappold, P.M.; Hatwar, M.; Panza, J.; Jackson-Lewis, V.; Javitch, J.A.; Ballatori, N.; Przedborski, S.; et al. The organic cation transporter-3 is a pivotal modulator of

neurodegeneration in the nigrostriatal dopaminergic pathway. *Proc. Natl. Acad. Sci. USA* **2009**, *106*, 8043–8048. [CrossRef]
164. Bacq, A.; Balasse, L.; Biala, G.; Guiard, B.; Gardier, A.M.; Schinkel, A.; Louis, F.; Vialou, V.; Martres, M.P.; Chevarin, C.; et al. Organic cation transporter 2 controls brain norepinephrine and serotonin clearance and antidepressant response. *Mol. Psychiatry* **2012**, *17*, 926–939. [CrossRef]
165. Courousse, T.; Bacq, A.; Belzung, C.; Guiard, B.; Balasse, L.; Louis, F.; Le Guisquet, A.M.; Gardier, A.M.; Schinkel, A.H.; Giros, B.; et al. Brain organic cation transporter 2 controls response and vulnerability to stress and GSK3beta signaling. *Mol. Psychiatry* **2015**, *20*, 889–900. [CrossRef] [PubMed]
166. Sprowl, J.A.; Ciarimboli, G.; Lancaster, C.S.; Giovinazzo, H.; Gibson, A.A.; Du, G.; Janke, L.J.; Cavaletti, G.; Shields, A.F.; Sparreboom, A. Oxaliplatin-induced neurotoxicity is dependent on the organic cation transporter OCT2. *Proc. Natl. Acad. Sci. USA* **2013**, *110*, 11199–11204. [CrossRef] [PubMed]
167. Huang, K.M.; Leblanc, A.F.; Uddin, M.E.; Kim, J.Y.; Chen, M.; Eisenmann, E.D.; Gibson, A.A.; Li, Y.; Hong, K.W.; DiGiacomo, D.; et al. Neuronal uptake transporters contribute to oxaliplatin neurotoxicity in mice. *J. Clin. Investig.* **2020**. [CrossRef] [PubMed]
168. Chaves, C.; Campanelli, F.; Chapy, H.; Gomez-Zepeda, D.; Glacial, F.; Smirnova, M.; Taghi, M.; Pallud, J.; Perriere, N.; Decleves, X.; et al. An Interspecies Molecular and Functional Study of Organic Cation Transporters at the Blood-Brain Barrier: From Rodents to Humans. *Pharmaceutics* **2020**, *12*, 308. [CrossRef]
169. Laurell, G. Pharmacological intervention in the field of ototoxicity. *HNO* **2019**, *67*, 434–439. [CrossRef]
170. Hellberg, V.; Gahm, C.; Liu, W.; Ehrsson, H.; Rask-Andersen, H.; Laurell, G. Immunohistochemical localization of OCT2 in the cochlea of various species. *Laryngoscope* **2015**, *125*, E320–E325. [CrossRef]
171. Ben Said, M.; Grati, M.; Ishimoto, T.; Zou, B.; Chakchouk, I.; Ma, Q.; Yao, Q.; Hammami, B.; Yan, D.; Mittal, R.; et al. A mutation in SLC22A4 encoding an organic cation transporter expressed in the cochlea strial endothelium causes human recessive non-syndromic hearing loss DFNB60. *Hum. Genet.* **2016**, *135*, 513–524. [CrossRef]
172. Grundemann, D. The ergothioneine transporter controls and indicates ergothioneine activity—A review. *Prev. Med.* **2012**, *54*, S71–S74. [CrossRef]
173. Koeth, R.A.; Wang, Z.; Levison, B.S.; Buffa, J.A.; Org, E.; Sheehy, B.T.; Britt, E.B.; Fu, X.; Wu, Y.; Li, L.; et al. Intestinal microbiota metabolism of L-carnitine, a nutrient in red meat, promotes atherosclerosis. *Nat. Med.* **2013**, *19*, 576–585. [CrossRef]
174. Tang, W.H.; Wang, Z.; Levison, B.S.; Koeth, R.A.; Britt, E.B.; Fu, X.; Wu, Y.; Hazen, S.L. Intestinal microbial metabolism of phosphatidylcholine and cardiovascular risk. *N. Engl. J. Med.* **2013**, *368*, 1575–1584. [CrossRef] [PubMed]
175. Teft, W.A.; Morse, B.L.; Leake, B.F.; Wilson, A.; Mansell, S.E.; Hegele, R.A.; Ho, R.H.; Kim, R.B. Identification and Characterization of Trimethylamine-N-oxide Uptake and Efflux Transporters. *Mol. Pharm.* **2017**, *14*, 310–318. [CrossRef]
176. Miyake, T.; Mizuno, T.; Mochizuki, T.; Kimura, M.; Matsuki, S.; Irie, S.; Ieiri, I.; Maeda, K.; Kusuhara, H. Involvement of Organic Cation Transporters in the Kinetics of Trimethylamine N-oxide. *J. Pharm. Sci.* **2017**, *106*, 2542–2550. [CrossRef] [PubMed]
177. Pathak, P.; Helsley, R.N.; Brown, A.L.; Buffa, J.A.; Choucair, I.; Nemet, I.; Gogonea, C.B.; Gogonea, V.; Wang, Z.; Garcia-Garcia, J.C.; et al. Small molecule inhibition of gut microbial choline trimethylamine lyase activity alters host cholesterol and bile acid metabolism. *Am. J. Physiol. Heart Circ. Physiol.* **2020**, *318*, H1474–H1486. [CrossRef]
178. Miller, M.J.; Bostwick, B.L.; Kennedy, A.D.; Donti, T.R.; Sun, Q.; Sutton, V.R.; Elsea, S.H. Chronic Oral L-Carnitine Supplementation Drives Marked Plasma TMAO Elevations in Patients with Organic Acidemias Despite Dietary Meat Restrictions. *JIMD Rep.* **2016**, *30*, 39–44. [PubMed]
179. Vallance, H.D.; Koochin, A.; Branov, J.; Rosen-Heath, A.; Bosdet, T.; Wang, Z.; Hazen, S.L.; Horvath, G. Marked elevation in plasma trimethylamine-N-oxide (TMAO) in patients with mitochondrial disorders treated with oral l-carnitine. *Mol. Genet. Metab. Rep.* **2018**, *15*, 130–133. [CrossRef] [PubMed]
180. Samulak, J.J.; Sawicka, A.K.; Hartmane, D.; Grinberga, S.; Pugovics, O.; Lysiak-Szydlowska, W.; Olek, R.A. L-Carnitine Supplementation Increases Trimethylamine-N-Oxide but not Markers of Atherosclerosis in Healthy Aged Women. *Ann. Nutr. Metab.* **2019**, *74*, 11–17. [CrossRef] [PubMed]

181. Fukami, K.; Yamagishi, S.; Sakai, K.; Kaida, Y.; Yokoro, M.; Ueda, S.; Wada, Y.; Takeuchi, M.; Shimizu, M.; Yamazaki, H.; et al. Oral L-carnitine supplementation increases trimethylamine-N-oxide but reduces markers of vascular injury in hemodialysis patients. *J. Cardiovasc. Pharmacol.* **2015**, *65*, 289–295. [CrossRef]
182. Bordoni, L.; Sawicka, A.K.; Szarmach, A.; Winklewski, P.J.; Olek, R.A.; Gabbianelli, R. A Pilot Study on the Effects of l-Carnitine and Trimethylamine-N-Oxide on Platelet Mitochondrial DNA Methylation and CVD Biomarkers in Aged Women. *Int. J. Mol. Sci.* **2020**, *21*, 1047. [CrossRef]
183. Olek, R.A.; Samulak, J.J.; Sawicka, A.K.; Hartmane, D.; Grinberga, S.; Pugovics, O.; Lysiak-Szydlowska, W. Increased Trimethylamine N-Oxide Is Not Associated with Oxidative Stress Markers in Healthy Aged Women. *Oxid. Med. Cell Longev.* **2019**, *2019*, 6247169. [CrossRef]
184. Verhaar, B.J.H.; Prodan, A.; Nieuwdorp, M.; Muller, M. Gut Microbiota in Hypertension and Atherosclerosis: A Review. *Nutrients* **2020**, *12*, 2982. [CrossRef]
185. Heianza, Y.; Ma, W.; Manson, J.E.; Rexrode, K.M.; Qi, L. Gut Microbiota Metabolites and Risk of Major Adverse Cardiovascular Disease Events and Death: A Systematic Review and Meta-Analysis of Prospective Studies. *J. Am. Heart Assoc.* **2017**, *6*, e004947. [CrossRef]
186. Mueller, D.M.; Allenspach, M.; Othman, A.; Saely, C.H.; Muendlein, A.; Vonbank, A.; Drexel, H.; von Eckardstein, A. Plasma levels of trimethylamine-N-oxide are confounded by impaired kidney function and poor metabolic control. *Atherosclerosis* **2015**, *243*, 638–644. [CrossRef]
187. Jia, J.; Dou, P.; Gao, M.; Kong, X.; Li, C.; Liu, Z.; Huang, T. Assessment of Causal Direction Between Gut Microbiota-Dependent Metabolites and Cardiometabolic Health: A Bidirectional Mendelian Randomization Analysis. *Diabetes* **2019**, *68*, 1747–1755. [CrossRef] [PubMed]
188. Getz, G.S.; Reardon, C.A. Animal models of atherosclerosis. *Arterioscler. Thromb. Vasc. Biol.* **2012**, *32*, 1104–1115. [CrossRef]
189. Aldana-Hernandez, P.; Leonard, K.A.; Zhao, Y.Y.; Curtis, J.M.; Field, C.J.; Jacobs, R.L. Dietary Choline or Trimethylamine N-oxide Supplementation Does Not Influence Atherosclerosis Development in Ldlr-/- and Apoe-/- Male Mice. *J. Nutr.* **2020**, *150*, 249–255. [CrossRef] [PubMed]
190. Chen, L.; Pawlikowski, B.; Schlessinger, A.; More, S.S.; Stryke, D.; Johns, S.J.; Portman, M.A.; Chen, E.; Ferrin, T.E.; Sali, A.; et al. Role of organic cation transporter 3 (SLC22A3) and its missense variants in the pharmacologic action of metformin. *Pharm. Genom.* **2010**, *20*, 687–699. [CrossRef] [PubMed]
191. Pochini, L.; Scalise, M.; Galluccio, M.; Indiveri, C. OCTN cation transporters in health and disease: Role as drug targets and assay development. *J. Biomol. Screen* **2013**, *18*, 851–867. [CrossRef]
192. Pochini, L.; Galluccio, M.; Scalise, M.; Console, L.; Indiveri, C. OCTN: A Small Transporter Subfamily with Great Relevance to Human Pathophysiology, Drug Discovery, and Diagnostics. *Slas. Discov.* **2019**, *24*, 89–110. [CrossRef]

Publisher's Note: MDPI stays neutral with regard to jurisdictional claims in published maps and institutional affiliations.

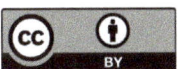

© 2020 by the authors. Licensee MDPI, Basel, Switzerland. This article is an open access article distributed under the terms and conditions of the Creative Commons Attribution (CC BY) license (http://creativecommons.org/licenses/by/4.0/).

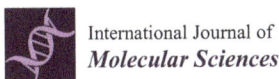

Review

The Impact of Genetic Polymorphisms in Organic Cation Transporters on Renal Drug Disposition

Zulfan Zazuli [1,2,*,†], Naut J. C. B. Duin [3,†], Katja Jansen [3], Susanne J. H. Vijverberg [1], Anke H. Maitland-van der Zee [1] and Rosalinde Masereeuw [3,*]

1. Department of Respiratory Medicine, Amsterdam UMC, University of Amsterdam, 1105 AZ Amsterdam, The Netherlands; s.j.vijverberg@amsterdamumc.nl (S.J.H.V.); a.h.maitland@amsterdamumc.nl (A.H.M.-v.d.Z.)
2. Department of Pharmacology-Clinical Pharmacy, School of Pharmacy, Bandung Institute of Technology, Jawa Barat 40132, Indonesia
3. Division of Pharmacology, Utrecht Institute for Pharmaceutical Sciences, Utrecht University, 3584 CG Utrecht, The Netherlands; n.j.c.b.duin@students.uu.nl (N.J.C.B.D.); k.jansen@uu.nl (K.J.)
* Correspondence: zulfan@fa.itb.ac.id (Z.Z.); r.masereeuw@uu.nl (R.M.)
† These authors contributed equally to this work.

Received: 20 August 2020; Accepted: 7 September 2020; Published: 10 September 2020

Abstract: A considerable number of drugs and/or their metabolites are excreted by the kidneys through glomerular filtration and active renal tubule secretion via transporter proteins. Uptake transporters in the proximal tubule are part of the solute carrier (SLC) superfamily, and include the organic cation transporters (OCTs). Several studies have shown that specific genetic polymorphisms in OCTs alter drug disposition and may lead to nephrotoxicity. Multiple single nucleotide polymorphisms (SNPs) have been reported for the OCT genes (*SLC22A1*, *SLC22A2* and *SLC22A3*), which can influence the proteins' structure and expression levels and affect their transport function. A gain-in-function mutation may lead to accumulation of drugs in renal proximal tubule cells, eventually leading to nephrotoxicity. This review illustrates the impact of genetic polymorphisms in OCTs on renal drug disposition and kidney injury, the clinical significances and how to personalize therapies to minimize the risk of drug toxicity.

Keywords: organic cation transporters; drug disposition; genetic polymorphisms; kidney; drug-induced kidney injury; nephrotoxicity

1. Introduction

The kidney is an important excretory organ for drugs and their metabolites in mammalian species, including humans. To facilitate this, in addition to filtration, the kidneys contain several transporters in their proximal tubule cells, including the solute carriers (SLCs) belonging to organic anion transporters (OATs), organic cation transporters (OCTs) and multidrug and toxic compound extrusion proteins (MATEs) and several other transporters of the ATP binding cassette (ABC) family, such as multidrug resistance proteins (MRPs) [1]. Most renally cleared drugs are excreted by multiple transporters that, in concerted action, take up molecules from the blood and efflux them into the lumen.

Positively charged (cationic) drugs and drug metabolites at a physiological pH are mainly handled by OCTs (Figure 1). The OCTs facilitate the movement of endogenous and exogenous organic cationic compounds into (and from) the cell [2]. Organic cations cover a myriad of molecular structures and dimensions, which make the OCTs polyspecific transporters [2]. Multiple studies have been published on the structure and function of OCTs and at least three different subtypes have been confirmed, OCT1-OCT3 [2–6]. The genes encoding for OCT1 (*SLC22A1*) and OCT2 (*SLC22A2*) are clustered on the same chromosome, 2q26, whereas the gene encoding OCT3 (*SLC22A3*) is located on chromosome

6q27 [7]. All subtypes are electrogenic, facilitative transporters, independent of sodium and chloride ions and function bidirectionally [3,8]. The OCTs are jointly dependent on the electrochemical gradient caused by the cationic substrate and the membrane potential to translocate substrates [9].

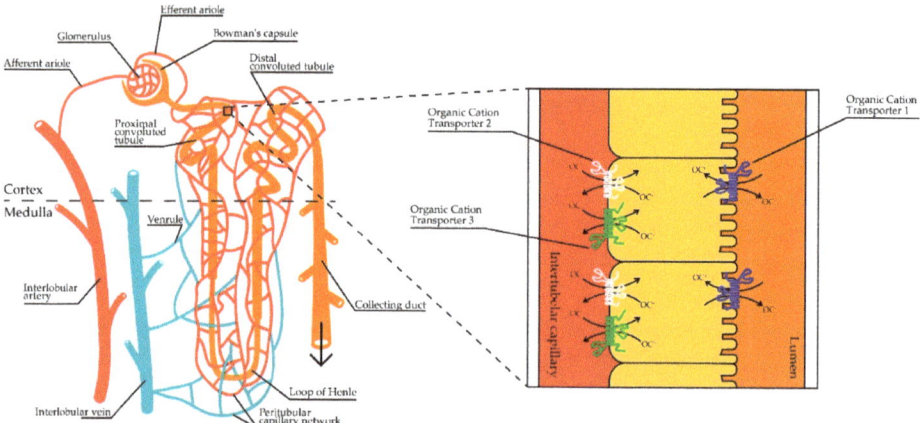

Figure 1. Schematic view of a nephron and a close-up of proximal tubule cells with organic cation transporters (OCTs) present in plasma membranes. In addition to glomerular filtration, organic cations (OCs) can be excreted in the proximal convoluted tubules, where OCT2 and OCT3 facilitate the uptake of compounds from the peritubular capillaries over the basolateral membrane into the intracellular space, and OCT1 mediates the uptake from the ultrafiltrate over the apical membrane.

Genetic variations in OCT-encoded genes might influence the functioning of OCTs and, in the end, contribute to interindividual differences in drug disposition. The advancement of genomic technologies has led to the completion of influential human genetic mapping, such as the Human Genome Project [10]. By utilizing abundance genetic information available from this project, researchers have been able to look into the genes, genetic variations and their prevalence in the population. This progress has also driven the development of the pharmacogenomics and pharmacogenetics field, resulting in the identification of genetic markers mostly in the form of single nucleotide polymorphisms (SNPs) that affect treatment efficacy and safety through their influence on drug pharmacokinetics and pharmacodynamics [11], including polymorphisms in genes that regulate transporter proteins like OCTs [12]. It is important to not only investigate the impact of genetic polymorphisms on drug effectiveness and toxicity separately, but also to understand how we can alleviate drug toxicity without compromising its effectiveness.

In this review, we will discuss the *SLC22A* family members 1–3 encoding the OCTs, their physiological roles and expressions, their known polymorphisms and how they can affect drug disposition and drug-induced kidney injury, their clinical significances and potential to personalize therapies to avoid the development of toxicity.

2. Role of the Organic Cation Transporters

The SLC22A transporter family members consist of 12 α-helical transmembrane domains with an extracellular glycosylated loop between domains 1 and 2. The large intracellular loop with the designated phosphorylation sites is found between the 6th and 7th domain [2–4] (Figure 2).

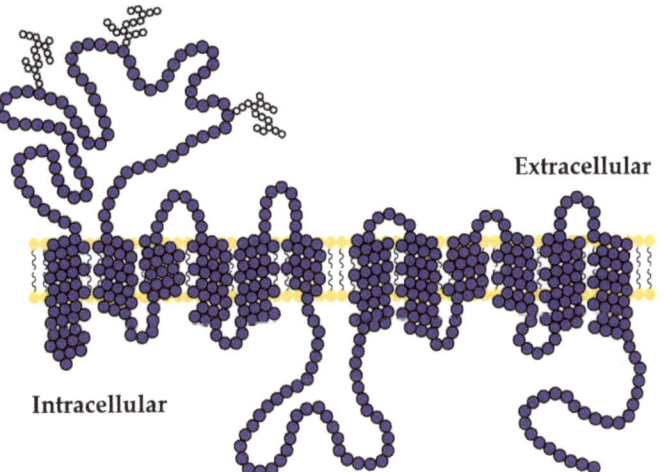

Figure 2. General topology of OCTs [3,13]. The proteins consist of twelve transmembranal α-helical domains. Between the first and the second loop, there is an extracellular loop that includes the N-glycolysation sites. The intracellular loop between the sixth and seventh domain includes phosphorylation sites.

2.1. Role of OCT1

OCT1 consists of 553 amino acids. It is predominantly expressed in the liver but is also found in other tissues, which indicates that OCT1 has a housekeeping role in the body [4,14–16]. OCT1 is involved in the release of acetylcholine in the lungs and the placenta [17,18] and is also capable of translocating several neurotransmitters, such as serotonin and norepinephrine [2,4,14,15,18]. In the liver, OCT1 is expressed at the sinusoidal (basolateral) membrane of the hepatocytes, where it mediates the hepatic uptake of organic cations [19]. OCT1 is also expressed at the apical membrane in trachea and bronchi, in neurons where it helps to maintain the electrochemical gradient [14,18,20], in the blood–brain barrier, immune cells and the kidney [20,21]. In the human kidney, one study showed apical expression of OCT1 mediating the reabsorption of cationic drugs [20]. In contrast, another study suggested that OCT1 is localized at the basolateral membrane [22], but significant functions in the kidney have thus far only been described for rodent Oct1. Since both rOCT1 and rOCT2 were localized to the basolateral membranes of proximal tubule cells, it is hypothesized that in rodents rOct1 and rOct2 fulfill the role of OCT2 in humans [23]. As human OCT1 shows very low expression in the kidney, it is hard to specify the localization and functional relevance of the protein [16]. Differences in OCT1 expression between humans and rodents may also explain this functional variation. Basit et al. reported that OCT1 was not detected in kidneys from humans and monkeys, but was abundantly expressed in rats and mice [24].

Detailed information on OCT1 substrates, both endogenous and pharmacological compounds, can be found in Table 1.

Table 1. Organic cation transporters and their endogenous and drug substrates.

Type of OCT	Endogenous Substrates	Drug Substrates			References
OCT1	monoamine neurotransmitters ** norepinephrine ** serotonin ** histamine ** dopamine **	Acyclovir albuterol * amiloride * amisulpride ** atenolol * atropine * barberine ** cimetidine * clidinium daunorubicin debrisoquine diltiazem evafirenz fenoterol *	furamidine ganciclovir ipratropium * irinotecan lamivudine ** lamotrigine metformin ** metoclopramide * oxaliplatin ** paclitacel pentamidine picoplatin * procainamide *	Ranitidine * salbutamol selegiline sumatriptan * terazosin * terbutaline * tiotropium * triamterene * trimethoprim * tropisetron varenicline * zalcitabine	[8,21,25,26]
OCT2	creatinine monoamine neurotransmitters ** norepinephrine ** serotonin ** histamine ** dopamine **	Albuterol * amantadine amiloride * amiodarone amisulpride ** atenolol * atropine * barberine ** cimetidine * cisplatin famotidine fenoterol *	ganciclovir ifosfamide ipratropium * lamivudine ** memantine metformin ** metoclopramide * oxaliplatin ** picoplatin * procainamide *	Ranitidine * Sumatriptan * Terazosin * Terbutaline * Tiotropium * Triamterene * Trimethoprim * Varenicline * zalcitabine zidovudine	[1,21,27]
OCT3	monoamine neurotransmitters ** dopamine ** norepinephrine ** serotonin ** histamine **	Amisulpride ** berberine ** cisplatin etilefrine	Lamuvidine ** lidocaine metformin **	pramipexole oxaliplatin ** quinidine	[8,21]

* Substrate of both OCT1 and OCT2. ** Substrate of OCT1, OCT2 and OCT3.

2.2. Role of OCT2

OCT2 consists of 555 amino acids. It is predominantly expressed at the basolateral side of the renal proximal tubules cells, but is also found in central nervous system (CNS) tissues, such as the brain and spinal cord [3,14,16,28]. In general, OCT2 plays a role in the uptake of cationic compounds from blood to the intracellular space. Like OCT1, the expressions of OCT2 differs between humans and other species, especially in rodents, a widely used model for drug-induced nephrotoxicity screening. Expressions of OCT2 are significantly higher in rats and mice than in the human kidney cortex [24]. Pharmacological substrates that have been reported as OCT2 substrates can be found in Table 1. Several OCT1 substrates overlap with those of OCT2. In addition, OCT2 displays a decisive role in the excretion of endogenous substrates, such as creatinine [29], which is widely accepted in clinical settings to estimate glomerular filtration. Consequently, creatinine excretion, potentially inhibited by OCT2 substrates, hinders its accuracy as a kidney function marker.

In the brain, a widespread array of OCT1 substrates can bind to OCT2, including monoamine neurotransmitters, norepinephrine, serotonin, histamine and dopamine [2,30]. Yet, it has a preference for smaller hydrophilic compounds, in contrast to OCT1 that interacts more with bigger hydrophobic compounds [31]. Furthermore, OCT2 mediates the transport of anti-Parkinson's drugs, such as amantadine and memantine through the brain–blood barrier [21]. Urakami et al. reported the existence of a splice variant of OCT2, namely OCT2A, consisting of 483 amino acids and nine transmembrane domains, which does not follow the predictable topology of the *SLC22A* family. OCT2A is suggested to have a narrower spectrum of substrates in comparison to OCT2, as it might not transport metformin [32], but it has a high affinity towards its substrates [33].

2.3. Role of OCT3

OCT3 consists of 556 amino acids and is widely expressed, but to a lesser extent than the other two subtypes. The transporter is predominantly found in skeletal muscles, the placenta and CNS; but is also present in the colon, the kidney, the heart and the liver [2,3,15,16,34–36]. OCT3 plays a role in the biliary excretion of cationic compounds in the liver and regulates the interstitial concentration of neurotransmitters in the CNS, ganglia and the heart [3,36]. The biliary excretion function is suggested to be crucial for substrates which are not transported by OCT1 or if OCT1 is inhibited by OCT1-specific substrates [21]. In the placenta, it helps the regulation of acetylcholine and the transport of organic cations [17]. OCT3 is also known as an extraneuronal monoamine transporter because of its role in the release and uptake of neurotransmitters. It plays a major role in the clearance of dopamine, norepinephrine, serotonin and histamine [36]. OCT3 is moderately expressed at the basolateral membrane of human kidney proximal tubule cells and has been regarded as less important than OCT2 [37,38], but is perceived to play a more significant role in the brain, heart and liver. In contrast with OCT1 and OCT2, the expression of OCT3 was detectable in human kidneys but not in monkeys, dogs or rodents [24]. OCT3 substrates can be found in Table 1.

3. Drug-Related Genetic Polymorphisms in the Organic Cation Transporter Genes

Several studies discovered polymorphisms in the OCT genes that affect the transporters' function. These effects range from loss of transporter function and misfolded protein to a gain in transporter function. Common SNPs (minor allele frequency (MAF) ≥ 1%) in OCT genes (*SLC22A1*, *SLC22A2* and *SLC22A3*) and investigated SNPs that affect the OCTs' function are presented in the Supplementary Materials (Supplementary Materials Figure S1) and Table 2, respectively. In addition, the following sections show that metformin, the first-line antidiabetic agent, and cisplatin, a widely used chemotherapeutic agent, are OCT substrates with the most important clinical read-outs.

Table 2. Studied OCT1-3 polymorphisms with minor allele frequency (MAF).

Gene	Polymorphism	AA *	Allele Change	Annotation (DNA Strand **)	Alleles		MAF per Ethnicity #							References
					Minor	Major	EU	Af	As	EA	SA	C	LA	Other	
SLC22A1 (OCT1)	rs12208357	R61C	181C>T	Coding (plus)	T	C	0.0723	0.0281	0	0	0.04	0.037	0.0216	0.0701	[12,20,39–43]
	rs55918055	C88R	262T>C	Coding (plus)	C	T	0.00303	0.006	0	0	0	0	0	0	[12,44,45]
	rs34130495	G401S	1201G>A	Coding (plus)	A	G	0.0261	0.005	0	0	0	0.02	0.0127	0.0197	[39,45,46]
	rs72552763	M420del	1260-1262delGAT	Coding (plus)	del	GAT	0.1148	0.053	0	0	0	0	0	0.0805	[12,20,39–41,43,44]
	rs34059508	G465R	1393G>A	Coding (plus)	A	G	0.02274	0.008	0	0	0	0	0	0.0194	[12,20,39,40,43,45,47]
	rs628031	M408V	1222A>G	Coding (plus)	A	G	0.402712	0.2663	0.3	0.308	0.3466	N/D	0.2058	0.3701	[20,40,43,48,49]
	rs683369	F160L	480G>C	Coding (plus)	G	C	0.1977	0.123	0.22	0.36	0.2	N/D ***	0	0.1712	[48,50–52]
	N/A ****	R206C	616C>T	Coding (plus)	T	C	N/D	N/D	0.008 [1]	N/D	N/D	N/D	N/D	N/D	[48]
	N/A	Q97K	289C>A	Coding (plus)	A	C	N/D	N/D	0.017 [1]	N/D	N/D	N/D	N/D	N/D	[48]
	rs200684404	P117L	350C>T	Coding (plus)	T	C	0.00008	0.001	0.012	0.018	0	N/D	0	0.0004	[20,40,53]
	rs34447885	S14F	41C>T	Coding (plus)	T	C	0.00033	0.012	0	0	0	N/D	0	0.0011	[44]
	rs36103319	G220V	659G>T	Coding (plus)	T	G	0.00013	0	0	0	0	N/D	N/D	0	[47,53,54]
	rs34104736	S189L	566C>T	Coding (plus)	T	C	0.00152	0	0	0	N/D	N/D	N/D	0.0014	[44]
	rs2282143	P341L	1022C>T	Coding (plus)	T	C	0.014788	0.0621	0.094	0.086	0.08	0.069	0.0384	0.0181	[47,49,53]
	rs622342	N/A	C>A	Intron 9	C	A	0.363843	0.1871	0.192	0.155	0.2764	N/D	0.3689	0.3048	[53,55]

218

Table 2. Cont.

Gene	Polymorphism	AA *	Allele Change	Annotation (DNA Strand **)	Alleles		MAF per Ethnicity #							References
					Minor	Major	EU	Af	As	EA	SA	C	LA	Other	
SLC22A2 (OCT2)	rs316019	A270S	808A>C	Coding (minus)	A	C	0.103508	0.1541	0.11	0.11	0.1156	N/D	0.0533	0.102206	[20,43,56–63]
	rs8177516	R400S	1198G>T	Coding (minus)	T	G	0.000205	0.0121	0	0	0.0002	0.026	N/D	0.0014	[44,47]
	rs8177517	K432Q	1294A>G	Coding (minus)	G	A	0.001096	0.0243	0	0	0.0022	0.003	N/D	0.0022	[44,47]
	rs8177507	M165I	495G>A	Coding (minus)	A	G	0.000009	0.0062	0	0	0	0	N/D	0.0002	[44,64]
	rs201919874	T199I	596C>T	Coding (minus)	T	C	0^2	0^2	0^2	0.0007^2	0^2	N/D	N/D	N/D	[63,65]
	rs596881	N/A	T>C	3'UTR (plus)	T	C	0.101541	0.2983	0.104	0.102	0.1294	0.136	0.0707	0.1224	[66,67]
	rs145450955	T201M	602C>T	Coding (minus)	T	C	0.00001	0	0.045	0	N/D	N/D	N/D	0.0001	[57,58,62,68]
	rs2292334	A411	1233G>A	Coding (plus)	A	G	0.364435	0.1458	0.448	0.403	0.2702	0.331	0.5086	0.3458	[69–71]
	rs8187715	T44M	131C>T	Coding (plus)	T	T	0.006^4	0.006^3	0.012^3	N/D	N/D	N/D	N/D	0.0009	[72]
	rs8187717	A116S	346G>T	Coding (plus)	T	G	0	0.0017^4	0	0	0	0	0	0	[72]
	rs8187725	T400I	1199C>T	Coding (plus)	T	C	0.00005	0	0	0	0	0	0	0	[72–74]
SLC22A3 (OCT3)	rs12212246	A439V	1316C>T	Coding (plus)	T	C	0.00001	0	0	0	0	0	0	0	[73,74]
	rs9365165	G475S	1423G>A	Coding (plus)	A	G	0.00013	0	0	0	0	0	0	0	[73,74]
	rs8187722	L346	1038A>G	Coding (plus)	G	A	0.001233	0.0338	0	0	0.0002	0	0	0.0079	[69,72]

219

Table 2. *Cont.*

Gene	Polymorphism	AA *	Allele Change	Annotation (DNA Strand **)	Alleles		MAF per Ethnicity #								References
					Minor	Major	EU	Af	As	EA	SA	C	LA	Other	
	N/A	V423F	1267G>T	Coding (plus)	T	G	0[4]	0[4]	N/D	0.068[4]	N/D	N/D	N/D	N/D	[72]
	rs3088442	N/A	564G>A	3'UTR (plus)	A	G	0.36755	0.08969	0.35	0.35	0.08	0.5	0.92	0.335	[70,71]
	rs555754	N/A	-29G>A	5'UTR (plus)	A	G	0.46766	0.5441	0.25	0.21	0.33	0.515	0.3764	0.477	[75,76]
	rs60515630	N/A	-81G>delAG	Upstream	G	del	0.0029	0.1	N/D	N/D	N/D	N/D	N/D	N/D	[75,76]
	rs376563	N/A	976-6046T>C	Intron 5 (plus)	T	C	0.47480	0.2523	0.35	0.386	0.47	0.444	0.3652	0.4119	[67]
	rs2076828	N/A	698C>G	3'UTR (plus)	G	C	0.4249	0.46	0.8	0.5377	0.8	N/D	N/D	0.4	[77]
	rs2481030	N/A	A>G	Intergenic	G	A	0.3404	0.177	0.17	0.17	0.81	N/D	0.2671	0.306	[78]

* AA: Amino acid. ** Plus and minus signs mean on which DNA strand the polymorphisms is found. *** N/D: No data. **** N/A: Not available. # Frequency database used is ALFA (Allele Frequency Aggregator) if not otherwise mentioned. EU is European population; Af is African population; As is Asian population; EA is East Asian population; SA is South Asian population; C is Caribbean and Native American Population; LA is Latin American and Hispanic population; Other is small non-designated populations. [1] Frequency found in Chen (2010a) [48]. [2] Frequency was found in Kang et al. (2007) [79]. [3] Frequencies from HapMap project. [4] Frequencies found in Chen (2010b) [72].

Metformin is a high-affinity substrate for all OCT isoforms. Therefore, it is commonly used as a substrate prototype to investigate OCT transport activity. Metformin does not bind to plasma proteins and is excreted unchanged into the urine, which makes it a suitable candidate for studying OCTs and their genetic variations with regard to drug disposition [80,81]. To investigate the effect of genetic variations on susceptibility to drug-induced nephrotoxicity, the anti-cancer agent cisplatin is widely used due to its well-studied dose-limiting nephrotoxic effects.

3.1. Genetic Polymorphisms in the OCT1 Gene (SLC22A1)

SLC22A1 is the most extensively studied OCT gene in pharmacogenetics studies. Using a candidate gene approach, several studies showed significant associations between genetic variants in SLC22A1 and drug pharmacokinetics, although results were not always consistent. However, the genome-wide association studies carried out to date could not detect a significant association between SLC22A1 variants and drug disposition [82,83].

Six common polymorphisms have been reported to affect the transporter function: rs34130495 (G401S), rs72552763 (M420del), rs628031 (M408V), rs6383369 (F160L), rs2282143 (P341L) and intronic rs622342. These polymorphisms are found mostly in the European and African population and are associated with reduced uptake activity of metformin [20,44,47,48,53,55,84]. Some of these polymorphisms (e.g., rs34130495, rs72552763, rs683369 and rs622342) are found, but R206C and Q97K are rare variants reported exclusively in the Asian population [48,53]. In an in vitro setting using HEK293 cells, Shu et al. showed that seven of the 12 polymorphisms of OCT1 lead to a reduced uptake of metformin, of which two polymorphisms (rs12208357 (R61C) and rs72552763 (M420del)) are common variants in Caucasians [84]. In contrast, a clinical study by Tzvetkov et al. (2009) in 103 healthy male Caucasians showed that rs12208357 (R61C), rs55918055 (C88R), rs34130495 (G401S) and rs72552763 (M420del) were associated with a significantly higher renal clearance of metformin [20]. To study these contradictory findings, Tzvetkov et al. (2009) performed a histochemical expression study and showed that OCT1 is mainly expressed at the apical membrane of renal proximal tubules and hypothesized that OCT1 plays a role in the reabsorption of metformin. This explained the higher renal clearance with reduced transport function [20]. A Danish study on 159 type 2 diabetes melitus (T2DM) patients concluded that SLC22A1 polymorphisms decrease the steady state of metformin and are associated with a reduction in the absolute decrease in Hb1Ac [39]. However, a study in 34 healthy volunteers indicated no impact of different SLC22A1 genotypes both on metformin steady-state pharmacokinetics and glucose utilization [85,86]. In addition, a large cohort study in 251 intolerant and 1915 fully metformin-tolerant T2DM patients in the UK showed that two reduced function OCT1 alleles were associated with metformin intolerance [87]. Furthermore, the intronic polymorphism rs622342 has been associated with reduced metformin uptake [53]. Naja et al. showed that the rs622342 variant produced higher fasting blood sugar levels and more glycosylated hemoglobin, which suggest a role in the glycemic response of metformin in type 2 diabetes [55], while Becker et al. reported a smaller glucose-lowering effect (based on HbA1c) of metformin in patients with diabetes mellitus [88]. This higher risk of reduced glycemic response was also found in rs6383369 (F160L) [50]. Although the previous study reported polymorphisms at SLC22A1 associated with reduced metformin uptake, several clinical studies [51,89] and a meta-analyses of 5434 patients with T2DM across eight cohorts of the Metformin Genetics Consortium (MetGen) showed no significant association between SLC22A1 polymorphisms (R61C, M420del, combined genotype for R61C and M420del–number of reduced function alleles and rs622342) and glycemic response to metformin monotherapy [89]. Therefore, while in vitro experimental studies, as well as most hypothesis-driven clinical studies (e.g., candidate gene association studies), demonstrated that SLC22A1 polymorphisms may alter metformin disposition both in the liver and kidney and metformin intolerance, pooled analysis, like meta-analysis, indicated that these altered metformin dispositions might not be substantial enough to affect metformin effectiveness clinically.

The loss-of-function haplotypes of OCT1 were not only associated with reduced metformin transport, but also with reduced clearance of morphine [40,45,46]. OCT1 is primarily expressed in hepatocytes and the hepatic excretion of drugs will be influenced by the lower functioning haplotypes. Qiu et al. and Singh et al. showed that rs6383369 (F160L) and rs628031 (M480V) reduced the clearance of imatinib [49,52]. In OCT1, the loss-of-function genetic variants showed lower uptake activity in all reported polymorphisms for metformin and imatinib, and also showed a decreased clearance of morphine. These effects are summarized in Table 3 and discussed further in Section 4.

3.2. Genetic Polymorphism in the OCT2 Gene (SLC22A2)

SLC22A2 has two common polymorphisms that affect the activity of the protein, as shown in Table 2. These polymorphisms are rs316019 (A270S) and rs596881 in the 3′ untranslated region (UTR). The variants rs316019 and rs596881 are frequently found in almost all ethnicities with MAF above 80% and 70%, respectively.

Through in silico analysis, Sajib et al. found that substrates fit better to the binding site of the A270 variant as it is more open and has a wider space than the S270 variant [56]. The polymorphism rs316019 (A270S) is associated with reduced or no changes in transport activity. Song et al. (2008) and Wang et al. (2008) both showed significantly lower activity in metformin transport with the S270 variant in healthy Korean and Chinese subjects, resulting in lower renal clearance of metformin [57,58]. A study on 1056 T2DM subjects with mostly African American ethnicity (63%) strengthens this evidence, as the minor allele rs316019 was associated with more favorable trajectories (lower disease progression) of HbA1c levels compared to the major allele carrier [90]. In contrast, a study in 23 healthy volunteers of Caucasian and African American ancestries showed that renal clearance and the net secretion of metformin were significantly higher in the variant genotype of rs316019 than in the wildtype reference genotype [91]. Finally, a meta-analysis of 5434 patients with T2DM across eight cohorts of the Metformin Genetics Consortium (MetGen) showed no statistically significant association between rs316019 polymorphisms and glycemic response to metformin monotherapy [89].

Table 3. Organic cation transporter function and substrates affected by polymorphisms.

Gene	SNP	Ref	Drugs and Chemicals	Effect
SLC22A1 (OCT1)	rs12208357	[20,39,41–43,87]	Metformin, morphine	Reduced uptake activity; decrease in steady-state concentration of metformin; associated with metformin intolerance
	rs55918055	[44,45]	Metformin	Reduced uptake activity
	rs34130495	[39,45,46,87]	Metformin, * MPP+	Reduced uptake activity; decrease in steady-state concentration of metformin; associated with metformin intolerance
	rs72552763	[20,39–43,87]	Metformin, morphine, MPP+	Reduced uptake activity and decreased morphine clearance; decrease in steady-state concentration of metformin; associated with metformin intolerance
	rs34059508	[20,39,43,45,47,87]	Metformin, MPP+	Reduced uptake activity; decrease in steady-state concentration of metformin; associated with metformin intolerance
	rs628031	[20,43,48,49]	Metformin, imatinib	Reduced imatinib clearance
	rs683369	[48,50–52]	Metformin, imatinib	Reduced function and reduced imatinib clearance
	R206C	[48]	Metformin	Reduced uptake activity, reduced function
	Q97K	[48]	Metformin	Reduced uptake activity
	rs200684404	[48]	Metformin	Reduced uptake activity
	rs34447885	[20,53]	Metformin	Reduced uptake activity
	rs36103319	[44]	Metformin	Reduced uptake activity
	rs34104736	[47,53,54]	Metformin	Reduced uptake activity
	rs2282143	[47,49,53]	MPP+	Reduced uptake activity
	rs622342	[39,53,55,88]	Metformin	Reduced uptake activity; decrease in steady-state concentration of metformin; smaller HbA1c lowering effect
SLC22A2 (OCT2)	rs316019	[20,43,56–63,66,90–96]	Metformin, cisplatin, creatinine, MPP+, lamivudine	Reduced uptake activity, lower renal clearance of metformin, higher renal clearance of metformin, lower HbA1c levels in metformin users, lower nephrotoxicity, higher nephrotoxicity, lower hematotoxicity, lower hepatotoxicity
	rs8177516	[44,47]	Metformin, MPP+, ** TBA	Reduced uptake activity

Table 3. Cont.

Gene	SNP	Ref	Drugs and Chemicals	Effect
	rs8177517	[44,47]	Metformin, MPP+, TBA	Reduced uptake activity
	rs8177507	[44,64]	Metformin	Reduced uptake activity
	rs201919874	[63,65]	Metformin, MPP+, lamivudine	Damaged protein, reduced activity
	rs596881	[66,67]	N/A	Renoprotective effect and maintenance of eGFR, hypertension
	rs145450955	[57,58,62,68]	Metformin, MPP+, lamivudine, insulin	Reduced activity, changed insulin resistance
	rs2292334	[69–71]	Metformin	Reduced activity
	rs8187715	[72]	Metformin, * MPP+, *** catecholamines	Enhanced uptake activity
	rs8187717	[72]	Catecholamines, metformin, MPP+, histamine	Reduced uptake activity
	rs8187725	[72,73]	Catecholamines, metformin, MPP+, histamine	Reduced uptake activity
SLCC22A3 (OCT3)	rs12212246	[73]	Catecholamines, metformin, MPP+, histamine	Reduced uptake activity
	rs9365165	[73]	Histamine	Reduced histamine uptake
	rs8187722	[69,72]	Metformin	Reduced uptake activity
	V423F	[72]	Catecholamines	Reduced uptake activity
	rs3088442	[70,71]	Metformin	Genetic risk marker for T2DM #, A allele has protective effect
	rs555754	[75]	N/A	Higher transcription rate, higher expression
	rs60515630	[75]	N/A	Higher transcription rate, higher expression
	rs376563	[67]	N/A	Effect on diabetic nephropathy and hypertension
	rs2076828	[77]	Metformin	Reduced response to metformin
	rs2481030	[78]	Metformin	Metformin inefficiency

* MPP+: 1-methyl-4-phenylpyridinium. ** TBA: tetrabutylammonium. *** Catecholamines: serotonin, norepinephrine, acetylcholine and dopamine. # T2DM: type 2 diabetes.

A recent in vitro study using a 3-[4,5-dimethylthiazol-2-yl]-2,5 diphenyl tetrazolium bromide (MTT) assay showed that decreased expression of hOCT2 A270S resulted in protection against cisplatin cellular toxicity compared to hOCT2 wildtype cells [59]. However, creatinine displayed a higher affinity for hOCT2 A270S, resulting in higher serum creatinine clearance in A270S compared to wildtype, which suggested an increased function [59]. In addition, the reported associations between rs316019 polymorphisms and cisplatin-induced nephrotoxicity are also conflicting among clinical studies using serum creatinine as a renal function parameter. This is possibly due to the influence of age, sex, ethnicity and the nature of creatinine itself as an OCT2 substrate [97]. Three studies (a study on 80 Dutch patients [60] and two Japanese studies consisting of 31 children [92] and 53 adults [93]) reported that individuals carrying a variant of rs316019 less frequently experienced creatinine-based cisplatin nephrotoxicity compared to individuals with the wildtype genotype. A study in 123 Chinese patients also displayed lower changes of cystatin C in patients with a mutant genotype [94]. However, a study in 95 Japanese esophageal cancer patients reported no association [98]. Moreover, a study in 206 patients (92% Caucasians) even showed that patients who carried a variant genotype had higher levels of KIM-1, a novel biomarker of kidney injury, compared to wildtype carriers [66]. These findings were also confirmed by a study in 159 Canadian subjects that reported a higher risk of creatinine-based cisplatin nephrotoxicity in patients bearing the variant allele compared to the wildtype allele [61]. A study on 403 Chinese non-small cell lung cancer (NSCLC) patients displayed that rs316019 was associated with lower risk of hepato- and hematotoxicity in platinum-based chemotherapy [95]. Furthermore, this polymorphism was also associated with a lower risk of ototoxicity both in adult and pediatric patients treated with cisplatin according to a German study [96].

The intronic rs596881 polymorphism was shown to have a renoprotective effect as the estimated glomerular filtration rate (eGFR, a combination of serum creatinine-, age- and sex-based renal function estimation) was preserved in the rs596881 haplotypes [66].

The less common polymorphisms, rs8177516 (R400S), rs8177517 (K432Q), rs8177507 (M165I), rs201919874 (T199I) and rs14540955 (T201M), all showed reduced transporter activity [44,47,57,62,63,65,79]. Moeez et al. (2019a) investigated the T199I variant in which threonine199 is changed to isoleucine199, which alters the protein structure by acquiring a catalytic residue, losing the loop and glycosylation site. Furthermore, it gains an α-helix structure and a molecular recognition feature. These changes affect the binding pocket of OCT2 and reduces the transporter's activity [65]. Leabman et al. (2002) showed that rs8177516 (R400C) and rs8177507 (M165I) had reduced dose–response curves of 1-methyl-4-phenylpyridinium (MPP$^+$) than the wildtype, by saturating OCT2 with this substrate. Of these three variants, the rs8177516 (R400C) variant had the lowest activity. The polymorphisms rs316019 (A270S) and rs8177517 (K432Q) had similar dose responses to a saturating amount of MPP$^+$ when compared to wildtype. They also studied the effect of inhibiting compounds on the transporter variants, rs8177516 (R400S), rs8177517 (K432Q), rs8177507 (M165I) and rs316019 (A270S), and suggested that tetrabutylammonium is the more potent inhibitor for the rs8177516 (R400S) and rs8177517 (K432Q) variants, whereas rs316019 (A270S) showed decreased inhibition by tetrabutylammonium [64]. Song et al. (2008) and Choi et al. (2012) showed that rs201919874 (T199I) and rs14540955 (T201M) variants have a lower renal clearance of metformin and consequentially a higher plasma concentration [58,63]. Choi et al. (2012) also showed a lower renal clearance for MPP$^+$ and lamivudine in rs201919874 (T199I), rs14540955 (T201M) and rs316019 (A270S) variants [63]. Furthermore, Choi et al. (2013) showed that only the homozygous rs14540955 (T201M) had a significantly lower lamivudine clearance [68]. Kashi et al. (2015) suggested that rs14540955 (T201M) changes resistance to insulin, as the study showed an increase in the Homeostatic Model Assessment for Insulin Resistance (HOMA-IR) in this variant. This is probably due to the reduced transport of metformin [62].

3.3. Genetic Polymorphisms in the OCT3 Gene (SLC22A3)

SLC22A3 has four common polymorphisms found in European, African, Asian, East Asian, South Asian, Caribbean and Native American, Latin American and Hispanic populations, as shown in Table 2. The polymorphisms include: rs2292334 (A411), rs3088442 in the 3′ UTR, rs555754 in the 5′ UTR and intronic rs376563. These polymorphisms account for more than 10% of the MAF in the ethnicities described above. Other non-synonymous polymorphisms have a MAF of ≤ 1%.

The rs8187717 (A116S), rs8187725 (T400I), rs1221246 (A439V) and rs8187722 (L346) variants are all associated with a reduced uptake of metformin [72–74] as well as catecholamines and histamine [69,73,74]. The latter substrates are also affected by the polymorphisms rs9365165 (G475S) and V423F. Chen et al. (2010) investigated several polymorphisms, of which only the rs8187715 (T44M) variant showed enhanced uptake activity of OCT3 [72]. Hakooz et al. (2017) investigated the synonymous polymorphisms rs2292334 (A411) and rs8187722 (L346) in which the heterozygous variant rs2292334 showed a higher plasma concentration and lower clearance for metformin compared to the wildtype. On the other hand, the rs8187722 (L346) polymorphism showed no significant reduction in metformin clearance [69]. Analysis of pharmacodynamic data in 57 healthy volunteers with mixed ethnicities (majority African American, $n = 33$; Asian, $n = 18$; Caucasian, $n = 6$) showed that the variant rs2076828 was associated with reduced response to metformin during an oral glucose tolerance test [77]. Furthermore, a study in 233 newly diagnosed Caucasian T2DM patients showed that minor alleles of rs2481030 located in the intergenic region between *SLC22A2* and *SLC22A3* are associated with metformin inefficiency [78]. However, another study in 103 healthy male Caucasians reported no significant effect of several *SLC22A3* variants in the disposition to metformin [20].

Besides polymorphisms affecting uptake activity, a polymorphism acting as genetic marker was found. Mahrooz et al. (2017) and Moeez et al. (2019b) investigated the polymorphism rs3088442 in the 3′ UTR of the *SLC22A3* gene. They hypothesized that this polymorphism could be a genetic marker for an increased risk of type 2 diabetes, but the study showed a protective effect on the susceptibility to type 2 diabetes. The minor A allele was shown to have a positive effect, in contrast to the major G allele showing a negative effect on the metformin response [70,71]. Furthermore, Chen et al. (2013) suggested that the polymorphisms rs555754 and rs60515630, both in the 5′ upstream region, are involved in the transcription rate of the *SLC22A3* gene. The rs555754 and rs60515630 variants showed a higher transcription rate of *SLC22A3* and a higher expression of OCT3 in the liver [75]. Furthermore, OCT3 has a low expression in prostate cancer lines and higher expression levels of OCT3 have been associated with cancer suppressive effects, possibly due to the enhanced transcription rate and higher expression caused by the rs555754 and rs60515630 polymorphisms [75]. It has been suggested that OCT3 could be a candidate genetic biomarker to predict therapy effectiveness in various diseases, especially cancer [4,36,75].

Previously, an epidemiological study highlighted the differences in metformin response between various self-reported ethnic origins, in which patients with an African American background appear to have a better glycemic response to metformin than European American patients [99]. One might hypothesize that differences in allele distributions of pharmacogenomic variants among various ethnicities could be associated with variations in metformin response. In general, individuals with an African background have lower MAF in metformin-related OCT variants than European individuals, as observed in rs628031 (Table 2). However, there is limited evidence that racial or ethnic variations account for differences in metformin response to date. Furthermore, most of the pharmacogenetic research in metformin has been focused on European and Asian individuals. Further research will be needed to characterize the response to metformin in pharmacogenomic variants across ethnicities, especially African.

4. Impact of Pharmacogenetic Variants in OCTs in Precision Medicine

Overall, the antidiabetic drug metformin and antineoplastic drug cisplatin are the most extensively studied drugs related to pharmacogenetic variants in OCTs. Based on in vitro, in vivo and clinical pharmacogenetic studies in *SLC22A1-3* genes, metformin is the most comprehensively studied drug, covering pharmacokinetics and drug response outcomes due to its high affinity to all three OCT subtypes. Pharmacogenetic variants in OCTs related to cisplatin are also widely studied, especially variants in *SLC22A2* since cellular cisplatin uptake is mainly regulated by OCT2. Published studies have covered both the efficacy and adverse drug reaction aspects of cisplatin. The impacts of *SLC22A3* pharmacogenetic variants are still insufficiently unraveled, especially in clinical settings. More information on how OCT polymorphisms affect OCT substrates is presented in Table 3.

Metformin is considered to be the first-line antidiabetic drug to treat T2DM and has been used for more than 60 years. Metformin itself is perceived as the safest antidiabetic agent in chronic kidney disease. In addition, independent of its hypoglycemic effect, it reduces the risk of myocardial infarction, stroke and mortality in patients with T2DM and chronic kidney disease (CKD) [100]. However, its use has been limited in severe renal impairment patients because of a higher risk of lactic acidosis [100,101]. Apart from that, the clinical utility of *SLC22A1* and *SLC22A2* variants to assist the precision medicine of metformin is questionable, as a meta-analysis of 5434 patients with T2DM across eight cohorts of the Metformin Genetics Consortium (MetGen) showed no significant association between *SLC22A1* (R61C, M420del, combined genotype for R61C and M420del–number of reduced function alleles and rs622342) and *SLC22A2* polymorphisms (rs316019) and glycemic response to metformin monotherapy [89], and no organic cation transporter variants were found to be associated with metformin disposition through genome-wide studies. Through a three-stage genome-wide association study (GWAS) in 10,577 subjects of European ancestry, the MetGen Consortium reported that rs8192675 in the intron of *SLC2A2*, which encodes the facilitated glucose transporter GLUT2, was associated with a greater reduction in HbA1c [82]. A GWAS on 1312 white and black participants in the ACCORD trial showed that common and rare variants in *PRPF31*, *CPA6* and *STAT3* were associated with metformin response [83]. In addition, a recent systematic review suggested that the role of *SLC22A1* variants in individual responses to metformin is population-specific due to high heterogeneity among studied populations [102]. However, the combined effect of the *SLC22A1* genotype is valuable to predict metformin intolerance [87,103].

Cisplatin is arguably one of the most studied nephrotoxic drugs. It is a highly potent chemotherapeutic agent, but its therapeutic use is limited due to the development of nephrotoxicity and ototoxicity. Cytotoxic events include oxidative stress, cytoplasmic organelle dysfunction (endoplasmic reticulum stress and mitochondrial dysfunction), DNA damage and activation of apoptotic pathways (death receptor and caspase-dependent pathway) [104]. This leads to cell necrosis. OCTs have been proven to play an important role in cisplatin nephrotoxicity. When cisplatin is taken up by a basolateral transporter, predominantly OCT2, but also the copper transport protein (copper transporter receptor 1, CTR1), but not excreted as fast or at all by apical transporters, such as the multidrug and toxic compound extrusion proteins (MATEs), it will accumulate inside the cell and affect multiple cell functions, eventually resulting in cell death [104]. As mentioned before, rs316019 (A270S) is shown to modify the nephrotoxicity of cisplatin, although the result was not consistent [43,60]. Instead of OCT variants, a GWAS on 1010 testicular cancer survivors reported that rs1377817 of *MYH14* was associated with the serum platinum residuals [105]. Besides nephrotoxicity, ototoxicity is another unwanted effect of cisplatin that is extensively studied. However, none of the OCT genetic variants was proven to be associated with cisplatin-induced ototoxicity. Through candidate gene studies, rs9332377 *COMT* [106–108] and rs12201199 *TPMT* [106,109,110] were associated with ototoxicity, although the direction of association is not consistent among studies. Meanwhile, the rs4788863 *SLC16A5* variant demonstrated an otoprotective effect [111,112]. Two GWASs reported SNPs that are associated with an increased risk of ototoxicity: rs1872328 in *ACYP2* [113] and rs62283056 in *WFS1* [114]. The clinical evidence for those SNPs was also supported with functional validation studies [115].

The development of genomic technologies has allowed the unbiased investigation of genetic variation across the genome, like GWASs. GWASs on metformin are a good example on how such an approach may reveal new and relevant variants through observed outcomes. In cisplatin nephrotoxicity, however, differences in outcome definition were proven to contribute to inconsistent associations between the genetic variant and the outcome [61]. Thus, such an effort should be accompanied by more robust kidney injury biomarkers than serum creatinine for a better phenotyping, such as kidney injury molecule-1 (KIM-1), β2-microglobulin (B2M), cystatin C, clusterin and trefoil factor-3 (TFF-3), to define nephrotoxicity [116]. The selection of more sensitive and specific drug-induced kidney injury biomarkers will be a feasible solution for the creatinine limitations we mentioned earlier. However, it should be noted that the large sample size of specific ethnicity populations and similar clinical characteristics of the population required to detect a significant genome-wide association might be a major challenge, as demonstrated by the metformin GWAS. Alternatively, functional validations in in vitro settings using gene-editing techniques such as CRISPR-Cas9 and pharmacokinetic validation of current associated SNPs may lead to robust evidence on the mechanistic role of the associated SNPs on cisplatin disposition. Moreover, multilayer omics profiling, such as genomics, epigenomics, transcriptomics, metabolomics and proteomics, observed in the same subject would generate valuable knowledge to reveal the whole mechanism of action, how drugs affect the body's physiological processes and demonstrate their efficacy and toxicity, especially for metformin and cisplatin. Such comprehensive information would be a significant step to precision therapy of metformin and cisplatin to reduce their toxicity and optimize their effectiveness at an individual level. Finally, a clinical study on genotype-guided prescribing would also offer an answer on how utilizing individual genetic information is clinically significant in metformin and cisplatin therapy.

5. Conclusions

The current evidence and literature show several promising genetic biomarkers in the prediction of OCT drug substrate disposition, especially metformin and cisplatin. Meanwhile, the evidence on OCT genetic variants' influence on renal drug disposition remains inconsistent, especially for *SLC22A2* in cisplatin. Therefore, in addition to current findings, data from larger cohorts with multiomics approaches whenever possible, along with the necessary functional validation, would be significantly beneficial to explain comprehensively interindividual variability in the pharmacokinetic, pharmacodynamic, effectiveness and toxicity profiles of drugs, including nephrotoxicity. Finally, these data could drive the precision therapy of drugs: avoiding and minimizing unwanted effects and enhancing drug effectiveness simultaneously.

Supplementary Materials: The following are available online at http://www.mdpi.com/1422-0067/21/18/6627/s1, Figure S1: Common SNPs (MAF≥1%) in *SLC22A1*, *SLC22A2* and *SLC22A3* (Extracted from UCSC Genome Browser on Human).

Author Contributions: Conceptualization, Z.Z., N.J.C.B.D. and R.M.; writing—original draft preparation, N.J.C.B.D., Z.Z., K.J.; writing—review and editing, all authors; visualization, N.J.C.B.D. and Z.Z.; supervision, S.J.H.V., A.H.M.-v.d.Z. and R.M. All authors contributed to the overall writing and reviewing of the manuscript. All authors have read and agreed to the published version of the manuscript.

Funding: This work was supported by the Indonesia Endowment Fund for Education (LPDP), Ministry of Finance, the Republic of Indonesia (as a part of Z.Z.'s Ph.D. project, grant no. 20161022049506, 2016). The funder had no role in the design of the study; in the collection, analyses or interpretation of data; in the writing of the manuscript or in the decision to publish the results.

Conflicts of Interest: The authors declare no conflict of interest.

Abbreviations

SLC	Solute carrier
OAT	Organic anion transporters
OCT	Organic cation transporter
SNP	Single nucleotide polymorphism
MATE	Multidrug and toxic compound extrusion
CTR	Copper transporter

ABC	ATP-binding cassette
MRP	Multidrug resistance protein
OC	Organic cation
CNS	Central nervous system
MAF	Minor allele frequency
HEK293	Human embryonic kidney 293 cells
T2DM	Type 2 diabetes mellitus
eGFR	Estimated glomerular filtration rate
MPP+	1-methyl-4-phenylpyridinium
TBA	Tetrabutylammonium
HOMA-IR	Homeostatic model assessment for insulin resistance
3'UTR	Three prime untranslated region
MTT	3-[4,5-dimethylthiazol-2-yl]-2,5 diphenyl tetrazolium bromide
KIM-1	Kidney injury molecule-1
B2M	β2-microglobulin
TFF-3	Trefoil factor-3
NSCLC	Non-small cell lung cancer
CKD	Chronic kidney disease
GWAS	Genome-wide association studies
CRISPR-Cas9	Clustered Regularly Interspaced Short Palindromic Repeats and Cas genes

References

1. Ivanyuk, A.; Livio, F.; Biollaz, J.; Buclin, T. Renal Drug Transporters and Drug Interactions. *Clin. Pharmacokinet.* **2017**, *56*, 825–892. [CrossRef] [PubMed]
2. Ciarimboli, G. Organic Cation Transporters. *Xenobiotica* **2008**, *38*, 936–971. [CrossRef] [PubMed]
3. Koepsell, H.; Endou, H. The SLC22 drug transporter family. *Pflug. Arch. Eur. J. Physiol.* **2004**, *447*, 666–676. [CrossRef]
4. Koepsell, H.; Lips, K.; Volk, C. Polyspecific organic cation transporters: Structure, function, physiological roles, and biopharmaceutical implications. *Pharm. Res.* **2007**, *24*, 1227–1251. [CrossRef] [PubMed]
5. Koepsell, H.; Schmitt, B.M.; Gorboulev, V. Organic cation transporters. *Rev. Physiol. Biochem. Pharmacol.* **2003**, *150*, 36–90. [CrossRef] [PubMed]
6. Van Montfoort, J.; Hagenbuch, B.; Groothuis, G.; Koepsell, H.; Meier, P.; Meijer, D. Drug Uptake Systems in Liver and Kidney. *Curr. Drug Metab.* **2005**, *4*, 185–211. [CrossRef]
7. Zhang, L.; Gorset, W.; Dresser, M.J.; Giacomini, K.M. The Interaction of n-Tetraalkylammonium Compounds with a Human Organic Cation Transporter, hOCT1. *J. Pharmacol. Exp. Ther.* **1999**, *288*, 1192–1198.
8. Wagner, D.J.; Hu, T.; Wang, J. Polyspecific organic cation transporters and their impact on drug intracellular levels and pharmacodynamics. *Pharmacol. Res.* **2016**, *111*, 237–246. [CrossRef]
9. Koepsell, H. Polyspecific organic cation transporters: Their functions and interactions with drugs. *Trends Pharmacol. Sci.* **2004**, *25*, 375–381. [CrossRef]
10. Moraes, F.; Góes, A. A decade of human genome project conclusion: Scientific diffusion about our genome knowledge. *Biochem. Mol. Biol. Educ.* **2016**, *44*, 215–223. [CrossRef]
11. Roden, D.M.; McLeod, H.L.; Relling, M.V.; Williams, M.S.; Mensah, G.A.; Peterson, J.F.; Van Driest, S.L. Pharmacogenomics. *Lancet* **2019**, *394*, 521–532. [CrossRef]
12. Yee, S.W.; Brackman, D.J.; Ennis, E.A.; Sugiyama, Y.; Kamdem, L.K.; Blanchard, R.; Galetin, A.; Zhang, L.; Giacomini, K.M. Influence of Transporter Polymorphisms on Drug Disposition and Response: A Perspective From the International Transporter Consortium. *Clin. Pharmacol. Ther.* **2018**, *104*, 803–817. [CrossRef] [PubMed]
13. Pelis, R.M.; Zhang, X.; Dangprapai, Y.; Wright, S.H. Cysteine accessibility in the hydrophilic cleft of human organic cation transporter 2. *J. Biol. Chem.* **2006**, *281*, 35272–35280. [CrossRef] [PubMed]

14. Gorboulev, V.; Ulzheimer, J.C.; Akhoundova, A.; Ulzheimer-Teuber, I.; Karbach, U.; Quester, S.; Baumann, C.; Lang, F.; Koepsell, H. Cloning and characterization of two human polyspecific organic cation transporters. *DNA Cell Biol.* **1997**, *16*, 871–881. [CrossRef] [PubMed]
15. Nies, A.T.; Koepsell, H.; Winter, S.; Burk, O.; Klein, K.; Kerb, R.; Zanger, U.M.; Keppler, D.; Schwab, M.; Schaeffeler, E. Expression of organic cation transporters OCT1 (SLC22A1) and OCT3 (SLC22A3) is affected by genetic factors and cholestasis in human liver. *Hepatology* **2009**, *50*, 1227–1240. [CrossRef]
16. Nishimura, M.; Naito, S. Tissue-specific mRNA Expression Profiles of Human ATP-binding Cassette and Solute Carrier Transporter Superfamilies. *Drug Metab. Pharmacokinet.* **2005**, *20*, 452–477. [CrossRef]
17. Wessler, I.; Roth, E.; Deutsch, C.; Brockerhoff, P.; Bittinger, F.; Kirkpatrick, C.J.; Kilbinger, H. Release of non-neuronal acetylcholine from the isolated human placenta is mediated by organic cation transporters. *Br. J. Pharmacol.* **2001**, *134*, 951–956. [CrossRef]
18. Lips, K.S.; Volk, C.; Schmitt, B.M.; Pfeil, U.; Arndt, P.; Miska, D.; Ermert, L.; Kummer, W.; Koepsell, H. Polyspecific cation transporters mediate luminal release of acetylcholine from bronchial epithelium. *Am. J. Respir. Cell Mol. Biol.* **2005**, *33*, 79–88. [CrossRef]
19. Nies, A.T.; Koepsell, H.; Damme, K.; Schwab, M. Organic Cation Transporters (OCTs, MATEs), In Vitro and In Vivo Evidence for the Importance in Drug Therapy. In *Handbook of Experimental Pharmacology*; Springer: Berlin, Germany, 2011; Volume 201, pp. 105–167. ISBN 9783642145407.
20. Tzvetkov, M.V.; Vormfelde, S.J.H.V.; Balen, D.; Meineke, I.; Schmidt, T.; Sehrt, D.; Sabolić, I.; Koepsell, H.; Brockmöller, J. The effects of genetic polymorphisms in the organic cation transporters OCT1, OCT2, and OCT3 on the renal clearance of metformin. *Clin. Pharmacol. Ther.* **2009**, *86*, 299–306. [CrossRef]
21. Koepsell, H. The SLC22 family with transporters of organic cations, anions and zwitterions. *Mol. Asp. Med.* **2013**, *34*, 413–435. [CrossRef]
22. Motohashi, H.; Inui, K.I. Organic cation transporter OCTs (SLC22) and MATEs (SLC47) in the human kidney. *AAPS J.* **2013**, *15*, 581–588. [CrossRef]
23. Sugawara-Yokoo, M.; Urakami, Y.; Koyama, H.; Fujikura, K.; Masuda, S.; Saito, H.; Naruse, T.; Inui, K.I.; Takata, K. Differential localization of organic cation transporters rOCT1 and rOCT2 in the basolateral membrane of rat kidney proximal tubules. *Histochem. Cell Biol.* **2000**, *114*, 175–180. [CrossRef] [PubMed]
24. Prasad, B. Kidney cortical transporter expression across species using quantitative proteomics. *Drug Metab. Dispos.* **2019**, *47*, 802–808. [CrossRef]
25. Andreev, E.; Brosseau, N.; Carmona, E.; Mes-Masson, A.M.; Ramotar, D. The human organic cation transporter OCT1 mediates high affinity uptake of the anticancer drug daunorubicin. *Sci. Rep.* **2016**, *6*. [CrossRef] [PubMed]
26. Koepsell, H. Role of organic cation transporters in drug-drug interaction. *Expert Opin. Drug Metab. Toxicol.* **2015**, *11*, 1619–1633. [CrossRef]
27. Hendrickx, R.; Johansson, J.G.; Lohmann, C.; Jenvert, R.M.; Blomgren, A.; Börjesson, L.; Gustavsson, L. Identification of novel substrates and structure-activity relationship of cellular uptake mediated by human organic cation transporters 1 and 2. *J. Med. Chem.* **2013**, *56*, 7232–7242. [CrossRef]
28. Tojo, A.; Sekine, T.; Nakajima, N.; Hosoyamada, M.; Kanai, Y.; Kimura, K.; Endou, H. Immunohistochemical localization of multispecific renal organic anion transporter 1 in rat kidney. *J. Am. Soc. Nephrol.* **1999**, *10*, 464–471.
29. Ciarimboli, G.; Lancaster, C.S.; Schlatter, E.; Franke, R.M.; Sprowl, J.A.; Pavenstädt, H.; Massmann, V.; Guckel, D.; Mathijssen, R.H.J.; Yang, W.; et al. Proximal tubular secretion of creatinine by organic cation transporter OCT2 in cancer patients. *Clin. Cancer Res.* **2012**, *18*, 1101–1108. [CrossRef]
30. Busch, A.E.; Karbach, U.; Miska, D.; Gorboulev, V.; Akhoundova, A.; Volk, C.; Arndt, P.; Ulzheimer, J.C.; Sonders, M.S.; Baumann, C.; et al. Human neurons express the polyspecific cation transporter hOCT2, which translocates monoamine neurotransmitters, amantadine, and memantine. *Mol. Pharmacol.* **1998**, *54*, 342–352. [CrossRef]
31. Dresser, M.J.; Xiao, G.; Leabman, M.K.; Gray, A.T.; Giacomini, K.M. Interactions of n-tetraalkylammonium compounds and biguanides with a human renal organic cation transporter (hOCT2). *Pharm. Res.* **2002**, *19*, 1244–1247. [CrossRef]
32. Kimura, N.; Masuda, S.; Tanihara, Y.; Ueo, H.; Okuda, M.; Katsura, T.; Inui, K.I. Metformin is a superior substrate for renal organic cation transporter OCT2 rather than hepatic OCT1. *Drug Metab. Pharmacokinet.* **2005**, *20*, 379–386. [CrossRef] [PubMed]

33. Urakami, Y.; Akazawa, M.; Saito, H.; Okuda, M.; Inui, K.I. cDNA cloning, functional characterization, and tissue distribution of an alternatively spliced variant of organic cation transporter hOCT2 predominantly expressed in the human kidney. *J. Am. Soc. Nephrol.* **2002**, *13*, 1703–1710. [CrossRef] [PubMed]
34. Sata, R.; Ohtani, H.; Tsujimoto, M.; Murakami, H.; Koyabu, N.; Nakamura, T.; Uchiumi, T.; Kuwano, M.; Nagata, H.; Tsukimori, K.; et al. Functional analysis of organic cation transporter 3 expressed in human placenta. *J. Pharmacol. Exp. Ther.* **2005**, *315*, 888–895. [CrossRef] [PubMed]
35. Kekuda, R.; Prasad, P.D.; Wu, X.; Wang, H.; Fei, Y.-J.; Leibach, F.H.; Ganapathy, V. Cloning and Functional Characterization of a Potential-sensitive, Polyspecific Organic Cation Transporter (OCT3) Most Abundantly Expressed in Placenta. *J. Biol. Chem.* **1998**, *273*, 15971–15979. [CrossRef] [PubMed]
36. Gasser, P.J.; Lowry, C.A. Organic cation transporter 3: A cellular mechanism underlying rapid, non-genomic glucocorticoid regulation of monoaminergic neurotransmission, physiology, and behavior. *Horm. Behav.* **2018**, *104*, 173–182. [CrossRef] [PubMed]
37. Wu, X.; Wei, H.; Ganapathy, M.E.; Wang, H.; Kekuda, R.; Conway, S.J.; Leibach, F.H.; Ganapathy, V. Structure, function, and regional distribution of the organic cation transporter OCT3 in the kidney. *Am. J. Physiol.-Ren. Physiol.* **2000**, *279*. [CrossRef]
38. Dresser, M.J.; Leabman, M.K.; Giacomini, K.M. Transporters involved in the elimination of drugs in the kidney: Organic anion transporters and organic cation transporters. *J. Pharm. Sci.* **2001**, *90*. [CrossRef]
39. Christensen, M.M.H.; Brasch-Andersen, C.; Green, H.; Nielsen, F.; Damkier, P.; Beck-Nielsen, H.; Brosen, K. The pharmacogenetics of metformin and its impact on plasma metformin steady-state levels and glycosylated hemoglobin A1c. *Pharmacogenet. Genom.* **2011**, *21*, 837–850. [CrossRef]
40. Tzvetkov, M.V.; Dos Santos Pereira, J.N.; Meineke, I.; Saadatmand, A.R.; Stingl, J.C.; Brockmöller, J. Morphine is a substrate of the organic cation transporter OCT1 and polymorphisms in OCT1 gene affect morphine pharmacokinetics after codeine administration. *Biochem. Pharmacol.* **2013**, *86*, 666–678. [CrossRef]
41. Pedersen, A.J.T.; Stage, T.B.; Glintborg, D.; Andersen, M.; Christensen, M.M.H. The Pharmacogenetics of Metformin in Women with Polycystic Ovary Syndrome: A Randomized Trial. *Basic Clin. Pharmacol. Toxicol.* **2018**, *122*, 239–244. [CrossRef]
42. Santoro, A.B.; Botton, M.R.; Struchiner, C.J.; Suarez-Kurtz, G. Influence of pharmacogenetic polymorphisms and demographic variables on metformin pharmacokinetics in an admixed Brazilian cohort. *Br. J. Clin. Pharmacol.* **2018**, *84*, 987–996. [CrossRef] [PubMed]
43. Tarasova, L.; Kalnina, I.; Geldnere, K.; Bumbure, A.; Ritenberga, R.; Nikitina-Zake, L.; Fridmanis, D.; Vaivade, I.; Pirags, V.; Klovins, J. Association of genetic variation in the organic cation transporters OCT1, OCT2 and multidrug and toxin extrusion 1 transporter protein genes with the gastrointestinal side effects and lower BMI in metformin-treated type 2 diabetes patients. *Pharmacogenet. Genom.* **2012**, *22*, 659–666. [CrossRef] [PubMed]
44. Cheong, H.S.; Kim, H.D.; Na, H.S.; Kim, J.O.; Kim, L.H.; Kim, S.H.; Bae, J.S.; Chung, M.W.; Shin, H.D. Screening of genetic variations of SLC15A2, SLC22A1, SLC22A2 and SLC22A6 genes. *J. Hum. Genet.* **2011**, *56*, 666–670. [CrossRef] [PubMed]
45. Venkatasubramanian, R.; Fukuda, T.; Niu, J.; Mizuno, T.; Chidambaran, V.; Vinks, A.A.; Sadhasivam, S. ABCC3 and OCT1 genotypes influence pharmacokinetics of morphine in children. *Pharmacogenomics* **2014**, *15*, 1297–1309. [CrossRef]
46. Balyan, R.; Zhang, X.; Chidambaran, V.; Martin, L.J.; Mizuno, T.; Fukuda, T.; Vinks, A.A.; Sadhasivam, S. OCT1 genetic variants are associated with postoperative morphine-related adverse effects in children. *Pharmacogenomics* **2017**, *18*, 621–629. [CrossRef]
47. Kroetz, D.L.; Yee, S.W.; Giacomini, K.M. The Pharmacogenomics of Membrane Transporters Project: Research at the Interface of Genomics and Transporter Pharmacology. *Clin. Pharmacol. Ther.* **2010**, *87*, 109–116. [CrossRef]
48. Chen, L.; Takizawa, M.; Chen, E.; Schlessinger, A.; Segenthelar, J.; Choi, J.H.; Sali, A.; Kubo, M.; Nakamura, S.; Iwamoto, Y.; et al. Genetic Polymorphisms in Organic Cation Transporter 1 (OCT1) in Chinese and Japanese Populations Exhibit Altered Function. *J. Pharmacol. Exp. Ther.* **2010**, *335*, 42–50. [CrossRef]
49. Singh, O.; Chan, J.Y.; Lin, K.; Heng, C.C.T.; Chowbay, B. SLC22A1-ABCB1 Haplotype Profiles Predict Imatinib Pharmacokinetics in Asian Patients with Chronic Myeloid Leukemia. *PLoS ONE* **2012**, *7*, e51771. [CrossRef]

50. Altall, R.M.; Qusti, S.Y.; Filimban, N.; Alhozali, A.M.; Alotaibi, N.A.; Dallol, A.; Chaudhary, A.G.; Bakhashab, S. SLC22A1 And ATM Genes Polymorphisms Are Associated With The Risk Of Type 2 Diabetes Mellitus In Western Saudi Arabia: A Case-Control Study. *Appl. Clin. Genet.* **2019**, *12*, 213–219. [CrossRef]
51. Jablonski, K.A.; McAteer, J.B.; de Bakker, P.I.W.; Franks, P.W.; Pollin, T.I.; Hanson, R.L.; Saxena, R.; Fowler, S.; Shuldiner, A.R.; Knowler, W.C.; et al. Common Variants in 40 Genes Assessed for Diabetes Incidence and Response to Metformin and Lifestyle Intervention in the Diabetes Prevention Program. *Diabetes* **2010**, *59*, 2672–2681. [CrossRef] [PubMed]
52. Qiu, H.-B.; Zhuang, W.; Wu, T.; Xin, S.; Lin, C.-Z.; Ruan, H.-L.; Zhu, X.; Huang, M.; Li, J.-L.; Hou, X.-Y.; et al. Imatinib-induced ophthalmological side-effects in GIST patients are associated with the variations of EGFR, SLC22A1, SLC22A5 and ABCB1. *Pharm. J.* **2018**, *18*, 460–466. [CrossRef] [PubMed]
53. Arimany-Nardi, C.; Koepsell, H.; Pastor-Anglada, M. Role of SLC22A1 polymorphic variants in drug disposition, therapeutic responses, and drug-drug interactions. *Pharmacogenom. J.* **2015**, *15*, 473–487. [CrossRef] [PubMed]
54. Jacobs, C.; Pearce, B.; Du Plessis, M.; Hoosain, N.; Benjeddou, M. Genetic polymorphisms and haplotypes of the organic cation transporter 1 gene (SLC22A1) in the Xhosa population of South Africa. *Genet. Mol. Biol.* **2014**, *37*, 350–359. [CrossRef] [PubMed]
55. Naja, K.; El Shamieh, S.; Fakhoury, R. rs622342A>C in SLC22A1 is associated with metformin pharmacokinetics and glycemic response. *Drug Metab. Pharmacokinet.* **2020**, *35*, 160–164. [CrossRef] [PubMed]
56. Sajib, A.A.; Islam, T.; Paul, N.; Yeasmin, S. Interaction of rs316019 variants of SLC22A2 with metformin and other drugs- an in silico analysis. *J. Genet. Eng. Biotechnol.* **2018**, *16*, 769–775. [CrossRef]
57. Wang, Z.J.; Yin, O.Q.P.; Tomlinson, B.; Chow, M.S.S. OCT2 polymorphisms and in-vivo renal functional consequence: Studies with metformin and cimetidine. *Pharmacogenet. Genom.* **2008**, *18*, 637–645. [CrossRef]
58. Song, I.; Shin, H.; Shim, E.; Jung, I.; Kim, W.; Shon, J.; Shin, J. Genetic Variants of the Organic Cation Transporter 2 Influence the Disposition of Metformin. *Clin. Pharmacol. Ther.* **2008**, *84*, 559–562. [CrossRef] [PubMed]
59. Frenzel, D.; Köppen, C.; Bolle Bauer, O.; Karst, U.; Schröter, R.; Tzvetkov, M.V.; Ciarimboli, G. Effects of Single Nucleotide Polymorphism Ala270Ser (rs316019) on the Function and Regulation of hOCT2. *Biomolecules* **2019**, *9*, 578. [CrossRef]
60. Filipski, K.K.; Mathijssen, R.H.; Mikkelsen, T.S.; Schinkel, A.H.; Sparreboom, A. Contribution of organic cation transporter 2 (OCT2) to cisplatin-induced nephrotoxicity. *Clin. Pharmacol. Ther.* **2009**, *86*, 396–402. [CrossRef]
61. Zazuli, Z.; Otten, L.S.; Drögemöller, B.I.; Medeiros, M.; Monzon, J.G.; Wright, G.E.; Kollmannsberger, C.K.; Bedard, P.L.; Chen, Z.; Gelmon, K.A.; et al. Outcome Definition Influences the Relationship between Genetic Polymorphisms of ERCC1, ERCC2, SLC22A2 and Cisplatin Nephrotoxicity in Adult Testicular Cancer Patients. *Genes (Basel)* **2019**, *10*, 364. [CrossRef]
62. Kashi, Z.; Masoumi, P.; Mahrooz, A.; Hashemi-Soteh, M.B.; Bahar, A.; Alizadeh, A. The variant organic cation transporter 2 (OCT2)–T201M contribute to changes in insulin resistance in patients with type 2 diabetes treated with metformin. *Diabetes Res. Clin. Pract.* **2015**, *108*, 78–83. [CrossRef] [PubMed]
63. Choi, M.-K.; Song, I.-S. Genetic variants of organic cation transporter 1 (OCT1) and OCT2 significantly reduce lamivudine uptake. *Biopharm. Drug Dispos.* **2012**, *33*, 170–178. [CrossRef]
64. Leabman, M.K.; Huang, C.C.; Kawamoto, M.; Johns, S.J.; Stryke, D.; Ferrin, T.E.; DeYoung, J.; Taylor, T.; Clark, A.G.; Herskowitz, I.; et al. Polymorphisms in a human kidney xenobiotic transporter, OCT2, exhibit altered function. *Pharmacogenetics* **2002**, *12*, 395–405. [CrossRef] [PubMed]
65. Moeez, S.; Khalid, Z.; Jalil, F.; Irfan, M.; Ismail, M.; Arif, M.A.; Niazi, R.; Khalid, S. Effects of SLC22A2 (rs201919874) and SLC47A2 (rs138244461) genetic variants on Metformin Pharmacokinetics in Pakistani T2DM patients. *J. Pak. Med. Assoc.* **2019**, *69*, 155–163. [PubMed]
66. Chang, C.; Hu, Y.; Hogan, S.L.; Mercke, N.; Gomez, M.; O'Bryant, C.; Bowles, D.W.; George, B.; Wen, X.; Aleksunes, L.M.; et al. Pharmacogenomic variants may influence the urinary excretion of novel kidney injury biomarkers in patients receiving cisplatin. *Int. J. Mol. Sci.* **2017**, *18*, 1333. [CrossRef]
67. Sallinen, R.; Kaunisto, M.A.; Forsblom, C.; Thomas, M.; Fagerudd, J.; Pettersson-Fernholm, K.; Groop, P.H.; Wessman, M. Association of the SLC22A1, SLC22A2, and SLC22A3 genes encoding organic cation transporters with diabetic nephropathy and hypertension. *Ann. Med.* **2010**, *42*, 296–304. [CrossRef]

68. Choi, C.-I.; Bae, J.-W.; Keum, S.-K.; Lee, Y.-J.; Lee, H.-I.; Jang, C.-G.; Lee, S.-Y. Effects of OCT2 c.602C > T genetic variant on the pharmacokinetics of lamivudine. *Xenobiotica* **2013**, *43*, 636–640. [CrossRef]
69. Hakooz, N.; Jarrar, Y.B.; Zihlif, M.; Imraish, A.; Hamed, S.; Arafat, T. Effects of the genetic variants of organic cation transporters 1 and 3 on the pharmacokinetics of metformin in Jordanians. *Drug Metab. Pers. Ther.* **2017**, *32*, 157–162. [CrossRef]
70. Mahrooz, A.; Alizadeh, A.; Hashemi-Soteh, M.B.; Ghaffari-Cherati, M.; Hosseyni-Talei, S.R. The Polymorphic Variants rs3088442 and rs2292334 in the Organic Cation Transporter 3 (OCT3) Gene and Susceptibility Against Type 2 Diabetes: Role of their Interaction. *Arch. Med. Res.* **2017**, *48*, 162–168. [CrossRef]
71. Moeez, S.; Riaz, S.; Masood, N.; Kanwal, N.; Arif, M.A.; Niazi, R.; Khalid, S. Evaluation of the rs3088442 G>A SLC22A3 Gene Polymorphism and the Role of microRNA 147 in Groups of Adult Pakistani Populations With Type 2 Diabetes in Response to Metformin. *Can. J. Diabetes* **2019**, *43*, 128–135.e3. [CrossRef] [PubMed]
72. Chen, L.; Pawlikowski, B.; Schlessinger, A.; More, S.S.; Stryke, D.; Johns, S.J.; Portman, M.A.; Chen, E.; Ferrin, T.E.; Sali, A.; et al. Role of organic cation transporter 3 (SLC22A3) and its missense variants in the pharmacologic action of metformin. *Pharmacogenet. Genom.* **2010**, *20*, 687–699. [CrossRef] [PubMed]
73. Sakata, T.; Anzai, N.; Kimura, T.; Miura, D.; Fukutomi, T.; Takeda, M.; Sakurai, H.; Endou, H. Functional Analysis of Human Organic Cation Transporter OCT3 (SLC22A3) Polymorphisms. *J. Pharmacol. Sci.* **2010**, *113*, 263–266. [CrossRef] [PubMed]
74. Lozano, E.; Briz, O.; Macias, R.; Serrano, M.; Marin, J.; Herraez, E. Genetic Heterogeneity of SLC22 Family of Transporters in Drug Disposition. *J. Pers. Med.* **2018**, *8*, 14. [CrossRef] [PubMed]
75. Chen, L.; Hong, C.; Chen, E.C.; Yee, S.W.; Xu, L.; Almof, E.U.; Wen, C.; Fujii, K.; Johns, S.J.; Stryke, D.; et al. Genetic and epigenetic regulation of the organic cation transporter 3, SLC22A3. *Pharmacogenom. J.* **2013**, *13*, 110–120. [CrossRef] [PubMed]
76. Cacabelos, R.; Torrellas, C. Epigenetics of Aging and Alzheimer's Disease: Implications for Pharmacogenomics and Drug Response. *Int. J. Mol. Sci.* **2015**, *16*, 30483–30543. [CrossRef]
77. Chen, E.C.; Liang, X.; Yee, S.W.; Geier, E.G.; Stocker, S.L.; Chen, L.; Giacomini, K.M. Targeted disruption of organic cation transporter 3 attenuates the pharmacologic response to metformin. *Mol. Pharmacol.* **2015**, *88*, 75–83. [CrossRef]
78. Zaharenko, L.; Kalnina, I.; Geldnere, K.; Konrade, I.; Grinberga, S.; Žīdzik, J.; Javorský, M.; Lejnieks, A.; Nikitina-Zake, L.; Fridmanis, D.; et al. Single nucleotide polymorphisms in the intergenic region between metformin transporter OCT2 and OCT3 coding genes are associated with short-Term response to metformin monotherapy in type 2 diabetes mellitus patients. *Eur. J. Endocrinol.* **2016**, *175*, 531–540. [CrossRef]
79. Kang, H.J.; Song, I.S.; Ho, J.S.; Kim, W.Y.; Lee, C.H.; Shim, J.C.; Zhou, H.H.; Sang, S.L.; Shin, J.G. Identification and functional characterization of genetic variants of human organic cation transporters in a Korean population. *Drug Metab. Dispos.* **2007**, *35*, 667–675. [CrossRef]
80. Graham, G.G.; Punt, J.; Arora, M.; Day, R.O.; Doogue, M.P.; Duong, J.K.; Furlong, T.J.; Greenfield, J.R.; Greenup, L.C.; Kirkpatrick, C.M.; et al. Clinical pharmacokinetics of metformin. *Clin. Pharmacokinet.* **2011**, *50*, 81–98. [CrossRef]
81. Scheen, A.J. Clinical pharmacokinetics of metformin. *Clin. Pharmacokinet.* **1996**, *30*, 359–371. [CrossRef]
82. Zhou, K.; Yee, S.W.; Seiser, E.L.; Van Leeuwen, N.; Tavendale, R.; Bennett, A.J.; Groves, C.J.; Coleman, R.L.; Van Der Heijden, A.A.; Beulens, J.W.; et al. Variation in the glucose transporter gene SLC2A2 is associated with glycemic response to metformin. *Nat. Genet.* **2016**, *48*, 1055–1059. [CrossRef] [PubMed]
83. Rotroff, D.M.; Yee, S.W.; Zhou, K.; Marvel, S.W.; Shah, H.S.; Jack, J.R.; Havener, T.M.; Hedderson, M.M.; Kubo, M.; Herman, M.A.; et al. Genetic variants in CPA6 and PRPF31 are associated with variation in response to metformin in individuals with type 2 diabetes. *Diabetes* **2018**, *67*, 1428–1440. [CrossRef] [PubMed]
84. Shu, Y.; Sheardown, S.A.; Brown, C.; Owen, R.P.; Zhang, S.; Castro, R.A.; Ianculescu, A.G.; Yue, L.; Lo, J.C.; Burchard, E.G.; et al. Effect of genetic variation in the organic cation transporter 1 (OCT1) on metformin action. *J. Clin. Investig.* **2007**, *117*, 1422–1431. [CrossRef] [PubMed]
85. Christensen, M.M.H.; Højlund, K.; Hother-Nielsen, O.; Stage, T.B.; Damkier, P.; Beck-Nielsen, H.; Brøsen, K. Steady-state pharmacokinetics of metformin is independent of the OCT1 genotype in healthy volunteers. *Eur. J. Clin. Pharmacol.* **2015**, *71*, 691–697. [CrossRef] [PubMed]
86. Christensen, M.M.H.; Højlund, K.; Hother-Nielsen, O.; Stage, T.B.; Damkier, P.; Beck-Nielsen, H.; Brøsen, K. Endogenous glucose production increases in response to metformin treatment in the glycogen-depleted state in humans: A randomised trial. *Diabetologia* **2015**, *58*, 2494–2502. [CrossRef]

87. Dujic, T.; Zhou, K.; Donnelly, L.A.; Tavendale, R.; Palmer, C.N.A.; Pearson, E.R. Association of organic cation transporter 1 with intolerance to metformin in type 2 diabetes: A GoDARTS study. *Diabetes* **2015**, *64*, 1786–17931. [CrossRef]
88. Becker, M.L.; Visser, L.E.; van Schaik, R.H.N.; Hofman, A.; Uitterlinden, A.G.; Stricker, B.H.C. Genetic variation in the organic cation transporter 1 is associated with metformin response in patients with diabetes mellitus. *Pharmacogenom. J.* **2009**, *9*, 242–247. [CrossRef]
89. Dujic, T.; Zhou, K.; Yee, S.W.; van Leeuwen, N.; de Keyser, C.E.; Javorský, M.; Goswami, S.; Zaharenko, L.; Hougaard Christensen, M.M.; Out, M.; et al. Variants in Pharmacokinetic Transporters and Glycemic Response to Metformin: A Metgen Meta-Analysis. *Clin. Pharmacol. Ther.* **2017**, *101*, 763–772. [CrossRef]
90. Goswami, S.; Yee, S.W.; Xu, F.; Sridhar, S.B.; Mosley, J.D.; Takahashi, A.; Kubo, M.; Maeda, S.; Davis, R.L.; Roden, D.M.; et al. A Longitudinal HbA1c Model Elucidates Genes Linked to Disease Progression on Metformin. *Clin. Pharmacol. Ther.* **2016**, *100*, 537–547. [CrossRef]
91. Chen, Y.; Li, S.; Brown, C.; Cheatham, S.; Castro, R.A.; Leabman, M.K.; Urban, T.J.; Chen, L.; Yee, S.W.; Choi, J.H.; et al. Effect of genetic variation in the organic cation transporter 2 on the renal elimination of metformin. *Pharmacogenet. Genom.* **2009**, *19*, 497–504. [CrossRef]
92. Yanagisawa, R.; Kubota, N.; Hidaka, E.; Sakashita, K.; Tanaka, M.; Nakazawa, Y.; Nakamura, T. Cisplatin-induced nephrotoxicity in patients with advanced neuroblastoma. *Pediatr. Blood Cancer* **2018**, *65*, 1–2. [CrossRef]
93. Iwata, K.; Aizawa, K.; Kamitsu, S.; Jingami, S.; Fukunaga, E.; Yoshida, M.; Yoshimura, M.; Hamada, A.; Saito, H. Effects of genetic variants in SLC22A2 organic cation transporter 2 and SLC47A1 multidrug and toxin extrusion 1 transporter on cisplatin-induced adverse events. *Clin. Exp. Nephrol.* **2012**, *16*, 843–851. [CrossRef] [PubMed]
94. Zhang, J.; Zhou, W. Ameliorative effects of SLC22A2 gene polymorphism 808 G/T and cimetidine on cisplatin-induced nephrotoxicity in Chinese cancer patients. *Food Chem. Toxicol.* **2012**, *50*, 2289–2293. [CrossRef] [PubMed]
95. Qian, C.-Y.; Zheng, Y.; Wang, Y.; Chen, J.; Liu, J.-Y.; Zhou, H.-H.; Yin, J.-Y.; Liu, Z.-Q. Associations of genetic polymorphisms of the transporters organic cation transporter 2 (OCT2), multidrug and toxin extrusion 1 (MATE1), and ATP-binding cassette subfamily C member 2 (ABCC2) with platinum-based chemotherapy response and toxicity in non-sma. *Chin. J. Cancer* **2016**, *35*, 85. [CrossRef]
96. Ciarimboli, G.; Deuster, D.; Knief, A.; Sperling, M.; Holtkamp, M.; Edemir, B.; Pavenstädt, H.; Lanvers-Kaminsky, C.; Zehnhoff-Dinnesen, A.A.; Schinkel, A.H.; et al. Organic cation transporter 2 mediates cisplatin-induced oto- and nephrotoxicity and is a target for protective interventions. *Am. J. Pathol.* **2010**, *176*, 1169–1180. [CrossRef]
97. Zazuli, Z.; Vijverberg, S.; Slob, E.; Liu, G.; Carleton, B.; Veltman, J.; Baas, P.; Masereeuw, R.; Maitland-Van Der Zee, A.H. Genetic variations and cisplatin nephrotoxicity: A systematic review. *Front. Pharmacol.* **2018**, *9*, 1111. [CrossRef]
98. Hinai, Y.; Motoyama, S.; Niioka, T.; Miura, M. Absence of effect of SLC22A2 genotype on cisplatin-induced nephrotoxicity in oesophageal cancer patients receiving cisplatin and 5-fluorouracil: Report of results discordant with those of earlier studies. *J. Clin. Pharm. Ther.* **2013**, *38*, 498–503. [CrossRef]
99. Williams, L.K.; Padhukasahasram, B.; Ahmedani, B.K.; Peterson, E.L.; Wells, K.E.; Burchard, E.G.; Lanfear, D.E. Differing effects of metformin on glycemic control by race-ethnicity. *J. Clin. Endocrinol. Metab.* **2014**, *99*, 3160–3168. [CrossRef]
100. Tanner, C.; Wang, G.; Liu, N.; Andrikopoulos, S.; Zajac, J.D.; Ekinci, E.I. Metformin: Time to review its role and safety in chronic kidney disease. *Med. J. Aust.* **2019**, *211*, 37–42. [CrossRef]
101. Rocha, A.; Almeida, M.; Santos, J.; Carvalho, A. Metformin in patients with chronic kidney disease: Strengths and weaknesses. *J. Nephrol.* **2013**, *26*, 55–60. [CrossRef]
102. Mato, E.P.M.; Guewo-Fokeng, M.; Essop, M.F.; Owira, P.M.O. Genetic polymorphisms of organic cation transporter 1 (OCT1) and responses to metformin therapy in individuals with type 2 diabetes. *Medicine* **2018**, *97*. [CrossRef]
103. Pearson, E.R. Diabetes: Is There a Future for Pharmacogenomics Guided Treatment? *Clin. Pharmacol. Ther.* **2019**, *106*, 329–337. [CrossRef]
104. Manohar, S.; Leung, N. Cisplatin nephrotoxicity: A review of the literature. *J. Nephrol.* **2018**, *31*, 15–25. [CrossRef]

105. Trendowski, M.R.; El-Charif, O.; Ratain, M.J.; Monahan, P.; Mu, Z.; Wheeler, H.E.; Dinh, P.C.; Feldman, D.R.; Ardeshir-Rouhani-Fard, S.; Hamilton, R.J.; et al. Clinical and genome-wide analysis of serum platinum levels after cisplatin-based chemotherapy. *Clin. Cancer Res.* **2019**, *25*, 5913–5924. [CrossRef]
106. Thiesen, S.; Yin, P.; Jorgensen, A.L.; Zhang, J.E.; Manzo, V.; McEvoy, L.; Barton, C.; Picton, S.; Bailey, S.; Brock, P.; et al. TPMT, COMT and ACYP2 genetic variants in paediatric cancer patients with cisplatin-induced ototoxicity. *Pharmacogenet. Genom.* **2017**, *27*, 213–222. [CrossRef]
107. Teft, W.A.; Winquist, E.; Nichols, A.C.; Kuruvilla, S.; Richter, S.; Parker, C.; Francis, P.; Trinnear, M.; Lukovic, J.; Bukhari, N.; et al. Predictors of cisplatin-induced ototoxicity and survival in chemoradiation treated head and neck cancer patients. *Oral Oncol.* **2019**, *89*, 72–78. [CrossRef] [PubMed]
108. Ross, C.J.D.; Katzov-Eckert, H.; Dubé, M.P.; Brooks, B.; Rassekh, S.R.; Barhdadi, A.; Feroz-Zada, Y.; Visscher, H.; Brown, A.M.K.; Rieder, M.J.; et al. Genetic variants in TPMT and COMT are associated with hearing loss in children receiving cisplatin chemotherapy. *Nat. Genet.* **2009**, *41*, 1345–1349. [CrossRef]
109. Yang, J.J.; Lim, J.Y.S.; Huang, J.; Bass, J.; Wu, J.; Wang, C.; Fang, J.; Stewart, E.; Harstead EH, E.S.; Robinson, G.W.; et al. The role of inherited TPMT and COMT genetic variation in cisplatin-induced ototoxicity in children with cancer. *Clin. Pharmacol. Ther.* **2013**, *94*, 252–259. [CrossRef]
110. Hagleitner, M.M.; Coenen, M.J.H.; Patino-Garcia, A.; De Bont, E.S.J.M.; Gonzalez-Neira, A.; Vos, H.I.; Van Leeuwen, F.N.; Gelderblom, H.; Hoogerbrugge, P.M.; Guchelaar, H.J.; et al. Influence of genetic variants in TPMT and COMT associated with cisplatin induced hearing loss in patients with cancer: Two new cohorts and a meta-analysis reveal significant heterogeneity between cohorts. *PLoS ONE* **2014**, *9*. [CrossRef]
111. Drögemöller, B.I.; Monzon, J.G.; Bhavsar, A.P.; Borrie, A.E.; Brooks, B.; Wright, G.E.B.; Liu, G.; Renouf, D.J.; Kollmannsberger, C.K.; Bedard, P.L.; et al. Association between slc16a5 genetic variation and cisplatin-induced ototoxic effects in adult patients with testicular cancer. *JAMA Oncol.* **2017**, *3*, 1558–1562. [CrossRef]
112. Lui, G.; Bouazza, N.; Denoyelle, F.; Moine, M.; Brugières, L.; Chastagner, P.; Corradini, N.; Entz-Werle, N.; Vérité, C.; Landmanparker, J.; et al. Association between genetic polymorphisms and platinuminduced ototoxicity in children. *Oncotarget* **2018**, *9*, 30883–30893. [CrossRef] [PubMed]
113. Xu, H.; Robinson, G.W.; Huang, J.; Lim, J.Y.S.; Zhang, H.; Bass, J.K.; Broniscer, A.; Chintagumpala, M.; Bartels, U.; Gururangan, S.; et al. Common variants in ACYP2 influence susceptibility to cisplatin-induced hearing loss. *Nat. Genet.* **2015**, *47*, 263–266. [CrossRef] [PubMed]
114. Wheeler, H.E.; Gamazon, E.R.; Frisina, R.D.; Perez-Cervantes, C.; El Charif, O.; Mapes, B.; Fossa, S.D.; Feldman, D.R.; Hamilton, R.J.; Vaughn, D.J.; et al. Variants in WFS1 and other mendelian deafness genes are associated with cisplatin-associated ototoxicity. *Clin. Cancer Res.* **2017**, *23*, 3325–3333. [CrossRef]
115. Drögemöller, B.I.; Wright, G.E.B.; Lo, C.; Le, T.; Brooks, B.; Bhavsar, A.P.; Rassekh, S.R.; Ross, C.J.D.; Carleton, B.C. Pharmacogenomics of Cisplatin-Induced Ototoxicity: Successes, Shortcomings, and Future Avenues of Research. *Clin. Pharmacol. Ther.* **2019**, *106*, 350–359. [CrossRef] [PubMed]
116. Griffin, B.R.; Faubel, S.; Edelstein, C.L. Biomarkers of drug-induced kidney toxicity. *Ther. Drug Monit.* **2019**, *41*, 213–226. [CrossRef]

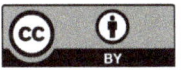

© 2020 by the authors. Licensee MDPI, Basel, Switzerland. This article is an open access article distributed under the terms and conditions of the Creative Commons Attribution (CC BY) license (http://creativecommons.org/licenses/by/4.0/).

MDPI
St. Alban-Anlage 66
4052 Basel
Switzerland
Tel. +41 61 683 77 34
Fax +41 61 302 89 18
www.mdpi.com

International Journal of Molecular Sciences Editorial Office
E-mail: ijms@mdpi.com
www.mdpi.com/journal/ijms

www.ingramcontent.com/pod-product-compliance
Lightning Source LLC
LaVergne TN
LVHW070439100526
838202LV00014B/1630